Emerging Technology Applications to Promote Physical Activity and Health

Emerging Technology Applications to Promote Physical Activity and Health

Special Issue Editors

Zan Gao
Jung Eun Lee

MDPI • Basel • Beijing • Wuhan • Barcelona • Belgrade

MDPI

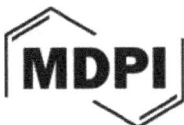

Special Issue Editors

Zan Gao
The University of Minnesota
USA

Jung Eun Lee
The University of Minnesota
USA

Editorial Office
MDPI
St. Alban-Anlage 66
4052 Basel, Switzerland

This is a reprint of articles from the Special Issue published online in the open access journal *Journal of Clinical Medicine* (ISSN 2077-0383) in 2018 (available at: https://www.mdpi.com/journal/jcm/special_issues/eta_physicalactivity_health).

For citation purposes, cite each article independently as indicated on the article page online and as indicated below:

LastName, A.A.; LastName, B.B.; LastName, C.C. Article Title. *Journal Name* **Year**, *Article Number, Page Range*.

ISBN 978-3-03897-708-7 (Pbk)
ISBN 978-3-03897-709-4 (PDF)

© 2019 by the authors. Articles in this book are Open Access and distributed under the Creative Commons Attribution (CC BY) license, which allows users to download, copy and build upon published articles, as long as the author and publisher are properly credited, which ensures maximum dissemination and a wider impact of our publications.

The book as a whole is distributed by MDPI under the terms and conditions of the Creative Commons license CC BY-NC-ND.

Contents

About the Special Issue Editors

Zan Gao, Prof., is a faculty member at University of Minnesota-Twin Cities. His research has primarily focused on promoting health and preventing diseases through field-based physical activity interventions with emerging technologies such as active video games, health wearables, and virtual reality. He has published 27 book chapters and 100 research articles in peer-reviewed journals such as *Obesity Review and American Journal of Preventive Medicine*. Dr. Gao has been the principal investigator of two National Institute of Health research grants and a Robert Wood Johnson Foundation Grant. He has received 4 Young Scholar Awards from various international and national organizations. Dr. Gao also serves as an Editorial Board Member for the *International Journal of Behavioral Nutrition and Physical Activity*, *Games for Health Journal*, *Journal of Sport and Health Science*, and *Journal of Clinical Medicine*, and has served as the Editor-in-Chief for *Journal of Research, Teaching, and Media in Kinesiology*. He is currently a Fellow of the American College of Sports Medicine, and a Fellow of the SHAPE America Research Council.

Jung Eun (June) Lee, Dr., is an Assistant Professor in the Department of Applied Human Sciences at the University of Minnesota at Duluth (UMD), USA. She completed her Ph.D. in the School of Kinesiology at the University of Minnesota, Twin Cities. Her research interests are psychosocial correlates of physical activity, technology-based physical activity promotion, and motor skill enhancement among children, the sedentary population, and individuals with depressive symptoms. She enjoys teaching Motor Learning and Development, and Exercise Adherence at UMD, and she is a member of the American College of Sport Medicine (ACSM), Society of Behavioral Medicine (SBM), Society of Health and Physical Educators (SHAPE), and International Society of Behavioral Nutrition and Physical Activity (ISBNPA). In her leisure time, she enjoys traveling, reading, hiking, and dancing.

Preface to "Emerging Technology Applications to Promote Physical Activity and Health"

Sedentary behavior has been identified as one of the major causes of many chronic diseases such as cardiovascular disease, stroke, cancer, type 2 diabetes, and obesity. Emerging technology plays a complex role in sedentary behavior, very much like a double-edged sword. On the one hand, some emerging technologies (e.g., sedentary video games and computer games) have contributed to the epidemic of sedentary behavior and physical inactivity. On the other hand, other innovative technologies have been increasingly utilized to promote physical activity and health. For example, newly emerging technologies such as mobile device applications, health wearable devices, and active video games have been adopted to promote health. As technology becomes an ever-more prevalent part of everyday life and population-based health programs seek new ways to increase life-long engagement with physical activity, the two have become increasingly linked.

This Special Issue offers a thorough, critical examination of emerging technologies in physical activity and health promotion, considering technological interventions in different contexts (communities, clinics, schools, homes, etc.) among various populations, exploring the challenges of integrating technology into physical activity promotion and offering solutions for its implementation. This Special Issue further aims to take a broadly positive stance toward interactive technology initiatives and, while discussing some negative implications of an increased use of technology, offers practical recommendations for promoting physical activity through various emerging technologies, including but not limited: active video games (exergaming); social media; mobile device apps; health wearables; mobile games, augmented reality games, global positioning and geographic information systems; and virtual reality.

As is well-known, technology is continuously evolving over time and constantly changing our lives. On the horizon are novel and exciting cutting-edge technologies that have great potential for physical activity and health promotion. Offering a logical and clear critique of emerging technologies in physical activity and health promotion, this Special Issue provides useful suggestions and practical implications for researchers, practitioners, and educators in the fields of public health, kinesiology, physical activity and health, and healthcare.

Zan Gao, Jung Eun Lee
Special Issue Editors

Journal of
Clinical Medicine

MDPI

Article

Examining Young Children's Physical Activity and Sedentary Behaviors in an Exergaming Program Using Accelerometry

Minghui Quan [1,*], Zachary Pope [2] and Zan Gao [1,3,*]

1   School of Kinesiology, Shanghai University of Sport, Shanghai 200438, China
2   School of Public Health, University of Minnesota-Twin Cities, Minneapolis, MN 55455, USA;
    popex157@umn.edu
3   School of Kinesiology, University of Minnesota-Twin Cities, Minneapolis, MN 55455, USA
*   Correspondence: quanminghui@163.com (M.Q.); gaoz@umn.edu (Z.G.); Tel.: 86-21-65507363 (M.Q.);
    +86-(612)-626-4639 (Z.G.); Fax: +86-(612)-626-7700 (Z.G.)

Received: 17 July 2018; Accepted: 23 September 2018; Published: 25 September 2018

Abstract: Exergaming has been observed to be a viable supplemental approach in promoting physical activity (PA) among children. However, whether sex differences in PA and sedentary behaviors exist during exergaming is inconsistent. Thus, this study aimed to quantify, via accelerometry, young children's PA and sedentary behaviors during exergaming as well as examine sex differences in these PA and sedentary behaviors during gameplay. In total, 121 first- and second-grade children (mean age = 6.89 ± 0.9 years; 73 girls) were included in the analysis. Children were a part of a large 18-week parent study. Children wore ActiGraph GT1M accelerometers during exergaming play, with four measurements purposely selected from the 28 total exergaming sessions to capture children's PA and sedentary behaviors during exergaming play. Outcome variables included mean percentages of time spent in moderate-to-vigorous PA (MVPA), light PA (LPA), and sedentary behavior during each exergaming session. One-way ANOVA was performed to determine whether there were differences in the percentage of time engaged in MVPA, LPA, and sedentary behavior during exergaming by sex. Accelerometry data indicated that children's mean percentage of exergaming time spent in MVPA, LPA, and sedentary behavior were 19.9%, 32.9%, and 47.2%, respectively. However, no sex differences were present. Observations in this study indicated that boys and girls have similar PA levels during exergaming and suggests that features inherent to exergaming may assist in PA promotion among both sexes.

Keywords: active video game; light physical activity; moderate-to-vigorous physical activity; sedentary behavior; sex difference

1. Introduction

Increased physical activity (PA) and reduced sedentary behavior among children and adolescents have been positively associated with improvements in physiological and cognitive outcomes, such as body composition, cardiorespiratory fitness, bone health, cognition, and academic achievement [1]. Consequently, it is recommended that children and adolescents accumulate at least 60 minutes (min) of moderate-to-vigorous PA (MVPA) per day [2]. However, a recent study's observations among 6128 children aged 9–11 years from 12 countries suggested that only 44.1% of participants met the MVPA recommendation [3]. Indeed, physical inactivity, along with dietary behaviors, has been highlighted as an important determinant of overweightness and obesity among children worldwide [4]. Furthermore, evidence has suggested that physical inactivity and overweightness/obesity during childhood may track into later life [5,6], leading to higher risks of many chronic diseases including stroke, type 2 diabetes, and heart disease [7]. Thus, researchers have been investigating effective and novel methods of promoting PA among children.

Exergaming, a new generation of video games, requires players to physically interact with video games during gameplay through various arm, leg, or whole-body movements such as dancing, jogging, and kicking [8]. Given the fact that children spend a large proportion of their time engaging in screen-based sedentary behavior [9,10], exergaming's physically active screen-based nature has been considered a promising way to promote PA levels in children and a feasible manner to facilitate population-level attenuation of the increasing obesity prevalence among children and adolescents [8,11].

Over the past decade, the beneficial health effects of exergaming have been extensively examined by researchers. Previous studies have suggested that exergaming may improve children's PA levels and attitudes [11–14], energy expenditure [15,16], and perceived motor skills [17], and reduce sedentary screen time [18,19] and waist circumference [20] and improve body composition [21,22]. However, whether exergaming is an effective approach to promote PA levels and help children meet the PA recommendations (i.e., 60 min of MVPA per day) is still unclear. One study indicated that children had marginally higher energy expenditure during exergaming gameplay than sedentary computer games, but that such gameplay was not enough to meet the PA recommendations for children [23]. This observation was supported by subsequent reviews, which suggested that many exergames could not engage children in moderate-intensity PA [24], with most exergames only eliciting light PA [25,26]. Nevertheless, we cannot ignore exergaming's potential role in facilitating PA and health promotion—particularly as increasing evidence has indicated that light PA (LPA) can confer health benefits [27]. Undoubtedly, it is easier for previously inactive children to accumulate more daily PA time during LPA before progressing toward greater MVPA participation. Hence, exergaming studies must also quantify children's LPA during exergaming instead of concentrating exclusively on MVPA.

As exergaming has also been posited as a potential approach to promote PA levels among both sexes, observations of exergaming's effectiveness at promoting PA between boys and girls are relevant, but have been mixed thus far. Some studies have reported that girls were less physically active than boys during exergaming play [23,28], while other studies did not observe a difference [29,30]. Considering the inconsistency of the observations, the relatively small sample sizes of previous studies [23,28–30], and the fact that girls are considered a high-priority group for PA promotion [31], more investigation of exergaming's ability to promote PA among both sexes is needed within larger and more diverse samples.

Therefore, the current study aims to: (1) quantify young children's PA and sedentary behaviors during exergaming using accelerometry; and (2) examine the sex differences in PA and sedentary behaviors during exergaming play. Study observations may provide a rationale for using exergaming as a supplement for more traditional PA promotion (e.g., physical education) in community-based contexts (e.g., school-based exergaming programs), particularly among girls.

2. Methods

2.1. Participants and Research Setting

A convenience sample of 158 (91 girls) first- and second-grade children, aged 6–8 years, were recruited from one Title-I Texas elementary school in the U.S. All children's parents were fully informed of the study's protocol, which was included on an informational sheet in children's take-home backpacks. Parents interested in having their child participate subsequently signed an informed consent document. Furthermore, children provided assent to participate as well. No data collection occurred on any child before parental consent and child assent were obtained. Notably, all study procedures were approved by the University's Institutional Review Board (IRB) and the school district prior to data collection commencing. Moreover, all procedures performed with the children were in accordance with the ethical standards of the institution and/or national research committee and with the 1964 Helsinki declaration and its later amendments or comparable ethical standards [32].

2.2. Measurements

PA levels and sedentary behaviors were assessed using ActiGraph GT1M accelerometers (ActiGraph, Pensacola, FL, USA), which have been proven to be valid and reliable in assessing PA and sedentary behaviors among children [33]. A 1-s epoch and cutoff points developed by Evenson and colleagues for children's PA were used in the present study [34]. Sedentary behavior was corresponded to 0–100 counts per minute, with LPA and MVPA corresponding to 101–2295 counts and ≥2296 counts per minute, respectively. Outcome variables were mean percentages of time spent in MVPA, LPA, and sedentary behavior during exergaming play during each exergaming session. To elaborate, approximately 20–22 min of PA data was collected during each 30-min exergaming session, with research assistants documenting the exact gameplay start and stop times. Following data collection, PA data were cut within ActiLife software to reflect the start and stop times of exergaming gameplay, meaning the percentages of time in MVPA, LPA, and sedentary behavior reflect the 20–22-min gameplay periods.

2.3. Procedures

Children in this cross-sectional study were part of a large 18-week exergaming intervention [35]. Throughout the intervention, an alternating two-week schedule was used. The first week included three days of a 30-min physical education session and two days of a 30-min exergaming session, whereas the second week was comprised of three and two days of exergaming and physical education sessions (30 min per session), respectively. Due to holidays and other unexpected class cancellations/activities, children actually participated in a total of 28 exergaming sessions and attended the exergaming sessions as a class (17–22 students per class). The accelerometers were placed on each children's right hip at the level of the superior iliac crest using an elastic waistband during each exergaming session by trained research assistants.

Twelve exergaming stations were set up in a large classroom, allowing up to 24 children to play the games simultaneously (i.e., each station accommodated up to two children). Each station included eight different Wii games, such as Wii Fit, Just Dance, and Wii Sports, which required children to perform a series of body movements to interact with onscreen characters and navigate through/successfully complete each game. Prior to testing, children were instructed how to play each game and were allowed to familiarize themselves with the games for 8 weeks prior to testing. During each exergaming session, a trained teacher or research assistant supervised the children during gameplay, with children transitioning between exergaming stations every 8–10 min. These transitions usually took less than two minutes, with these transitions allowing children to play all Wii games provided over the course of the school year, as the children were not allowed to pick the exergames played during these sessions. Notably, the teacher or research assistant supervising the children did not allow children to choose with whom they played exergaming, randomly assigning children to play with one another. This is important as it ensured that highly active friends did not bias exergaming PA measurements upward and, conversely, that highly sedentary friends did not bias exergaming PA measurements downward. Following this 18-week intervention, four days of accelerometer measurements were purposively selected from the 28 exergaming sessions to represent children's regular PA and sedentary behaviors well when participating in this PA modality. It is important to note that several sessions lasted longer or shorter than originally scheduled due to school events or class activities, beyond the different time spent engaging in line-up/warm-up and cool-down activities in each session. Furthermore, it should be noted that there were two different seasons (winter and spring) during the data collection period. As such, the researchers believed it best to select two sessions from each season for each child. This ensured that any seasonality effect possibly present could be controlled for. Therefore, it was more accurate for the researchers to purposively select the representative four sessions.

2.4. Data Analyses

Assuming the coefficient of variation (CV) of MVPA (CV = 0.39) based on the previous study [36], confidence level as 95%, and 8% level of precision, the required sample size was at least 90 in this study. Kolmogorov–Smirnov tests assessed normality, with variables described as the mean ± SD for normally distributed variables. Next, one-way ANOVA and Bonferroni post-hoc tests were used to determine whether sex differences existed in MVPA, LPA, and sedentary behavior time percentages. All analyses were conducted using SPSS version 22.0 (SPSS Inc.; Chicago, IL, USA), with a two-sided *p* value of ≤0.05 considered as statistically significant.

3. Results

Thirty-seven children were removed from the final analysis due to missing data on one or more of the purposively selected four exergaming sessions. The final sample was comprised of 37 six-year-old children (13 boys; 24 girls), 61 seven-year-old children (24 boys; 37 girls), and 23 eight-year-old children (11 boys; 12 girls). Table 1 presents descriptive statistics for children's mean percentages of time spent in MVPA, LPA, and sedentary behavior. Accelerometer data indicated that children's mean percentages of time spent in MVPA, LPA, and sedentary behavior were 19.86%, 32.94%, and 47.20%, respectively. Table 1 also shows the mean percentages of time that children were engaged in MVPA, LPA, and sedentary behavior during exergaming play by sex. No statistically significant sex differences were identified for MVPA, LPA, and sedentary behavior. Of note, children of any gender spent more than 50% of their time in MVPA and LPA.

Table 1. Percentage of time spent in physical activity and sedentary behavior during exergaming.

	MVPA		LPA		Sedentary	
	Mean	SD	Mean	SD	Mean	SD
Total (*n* = 121)	19.86	7.16	32.94	6.29	47.20	10.68
Gender						
Boys (*n* = 48)	19.31	7.15	33.09	5.67	47.60	9.91
Girls (*n* = 73)	20.22	7.19	32.84	6.70	46.94	11.21

Note: LPA = light physical activity; MVPA = moderate-to-vigorous physical activity; SD = standard deviation.

4. Discussion

As exergaming may be a viable supplemental approach to promote children's PA participation, it is important to objectively quantify children's PA and sedentary behavior during exergaming gameplay. These observations indicated that regardless of sex, children spent more than 50% of exergaming session time participating in PA (MVPA and LPA).

Study observations suggest that exergaming may be able to supplement other PA promotion strategies among children (e.g., physical education, in-class activity breaks, etc.), particularly for programs with the objective to increase LPA among previously inactive children. Thus, despite the current study's observation that the LPA percentage was greater than the MVPA percentage, reasons are present as to why exergaming may still be considered a potentially effective supplemental PA promotion strategy. First, the combined mean percentages for MVPA and LPA participation still accounted for more than 50% of each exergaming session. Although current recommendations stress that more than 50% of any PA session should be comprised of MVPA [37], the potential health benefits derived from engaging in LPA are emerging. Indeed, there is increasing evidence suggesting that LPA is independently and positively associated with improved health outcomes in children and adolescents, including reduced total body fat mass [38], some cardiometabolic risk factors [39], and improved body bone health [40], in addition to cognitive function improvements among boys [41]. Indeed, evidence has suggested the effectiveness of regular PA for health benefits—benefits partially explained by the increased energy expenditure that any intensity of PA confers versus sedentary behavior [42], but also because regular PA participation at any intensity (even LPA) results in improved cardiorespiratory health (e.g., increased arterial elasticity which lowers blood pressure, enhanced ability to deliver oxygen and other nutrients to muscles, etc.) [43]. Finally, LPA plays an important role in contributing to the children's daily total energy expenditure (LPA vs. MVPA: around to 26.6% vs. 25.1%) [44]. Therefore, LPA promotion may still be considered an alternative strategy in improving health-related outcomes, particularly as children replace sedentary behavior with exergaming or similar technology-based programs. In fact, considering the potential effect of LPA on health-related outcomes, the updated youth PA guidelines for youth not only emphasize the importance of MVPA, but also highlight that several hours of LPA should be performed each day [2].

Exergaming is also not constrained by seasonal weather conditions, meaning this PA modality could be used to supplement daily segments such as recess or physical education when adverse weather conditions prohibit outdoor PA engagement. Finally, exergaming may act as an alternative supplement to physical education and recess as studies have indicated exergaming to increase children's PA-related intrinsic motivation [45]—a psychosocial construct considered to be a crucial determinant in children's long-term PA engagement [46,47]. Thus, exergaming might be employed as a "stepping stone" to promote increased PA outside of exergaming sessions, as shown in previous literature [12,48].

The current study also observed no sex differences in PA levels during exergaming gameplay. Recent studies on sex-related differences in daily PA levels noted that boys had higher PA and sedentary behaviors than girls—observations consistent across different countries such as the U.S. [49] and China [9,50]. However, exergaming gameplay did not appear to exhibit these trends. Our observations are consistent with the previous studies, indicating that there was no difference between boys and girls for total PA time [51] or average metabolic equivalent (METs) during exergaming [52]. These observations are promising as it indicates that health professionals may be able use exergaming as an appropriate PA promotion strategy for all children, regardless of sex. However, more investigations in larger samples akin to the sample in the present study are needed, as past investigations have reported sex differences for exergaming-related intrinsic motivation and enjoyment [52,53]—constructs which were significantly related to PA levels [46]. Nonetheless, the fact that exergaming developers strive to develop games which are appealing to both sexes may partially explain the current study's observations.

A few study limitations need to be noted for future direction. First, all participants were part of a convenience sample recruited from a single school in Texas, which limits the generalizability of the study's observations to other populations from other geographic locations. Second, it is realized that the implementation of an exergaming program (or similar programs) is contingent upon school resources, as the setup of the exergaming classroom within the study school cost approximately US$3600. Notably, as the exergaming program was able to be implemented by one teacher coordinating up to 24 children playing on 12 different exergaming stations, this type of exergaming program does appear feasible to promote both LPA and MVPA among children. Fortunately, this configuration has been implemented in more than 750 public schools in the State of West Virginia for PA promotion [54]. Third, while this study does highlight the feasibility of implementing an exergaming program for PA promotion, other technologies may also be used in future studies (e.g., mobile devices), given the everchanging nature of youths' current technology interests. Finally, the current study did not include an analysis of children's anthropometric, physiological, or psychosocial outcomes—important components of overall health and wellness, which should be investigated thoroughly and in a longitudinal manner during future school-based exergaming or technology-based programs.

5. Conclusions

In conclusion, the current study's observations indicated that exergaming could facilitate LPA and MVPA in young children, with no difference in PA participation observed between sexes. Given exergaming's cost-effectiveness and resistance to weather conditions, exergaming may be a supplemental apparatus in promoting PA among young children [55,56]. Future large studies akin to the current investigation are needed to determine exergaming effectiveness among different age groups (e.g., older children and adolescents) and settings (e.g., school-based vs. home-based) to further evaluate the effectiveness of this PA modality for promoting children's PA.

Author Contributions: M.Q. performed the literature search, analyzed the data, and drafted the manuscript. Z.P. advised on analysis and interpretation of the data and critically revised the manuscript. Z.G. conceived and designed the study, collected the data, and helped to draft the manuscript.

Funding: This research was funded by National Natural Science Foundation of China (81703252).

Acknowledgments: The authors would like to thank the research assistants who helped with data collection and students who cooperated with the data collection.

Conflicts of Interest: The author has no financial disclosures and declare no conflicts of interest.

References

1. Poitras, V.J.; Gray, C.E.; Borghese, M.M.; Carson, V.; Chaput, J.P.; Janssen, I.; Katzmarzyk, P.T.; Pate, R.R.; Connor Gorber, S.; Kho, M.E.; et al. Systematic review of the relationships between objectively measured physical activity and health indicators in school-aged children and youth. *Appl. Physiol. Nutr. Metab.* **2016**, *41*, S197–S239. [CrossRef] [PubMed]
2. Tremblay, M.S.; Carson, V.; Chaput, J.P.; Connor Gorber, S.; Dinh, T.; Duggan, M.; Faulkner, G.; Gray, C.E.; Gruber, R.; Janson, K.; et al. Canadian 24-hour movement guidelines for children and youth: An integration of physical activity, sedentary behaviour, and sleep. *Appl. Physiol. Nutr. Metab.* **2016**, *41*, S311–S327. [CrossRef] [PubMed]
3. Romanviñas, B.; Chaput, J.P.; Katzmarzyk, P.T.; Fogelholm, M.; Lambert, E.V.; Maher, C.; Maia, J.; Olds, T.; Onywera, V.; Sarmiento, O.L. Proportion of children meeting recommendations for 24-hour movement guidelines and associations with adiposity in a 12-country study. *Int. J. Behav. Nutr. Phys. Act.* **2016**, *13*, 123. [CrossRef] [PubMed]
4. Abarca-Gómez, L.; Abdeen, Z.A.; Hamid, Z.A.; Dika, Z.; Ivkovic, V.; Jelakovic, A.; Jelakovic, B.; Kos, J.; Jureša, V.; Majer, M. Worldwide trends in body-mass index, underweight, overweight, and obesity from 1975 to 2016: A pooled analysis of 2416 population-based measurement studies in 128.9 million children, adolescents, and adults. *Lancet* **2017**, *390*, 2627–2642. [CrossRef]
5. Jones, R.A.; Hinkley, T.; Okely, A.D.; Salmon, J. Tracking physical activity and sedentary behavior in childhood: A systematic review. *Am. J. Prev. Med.* **2013**, *44*, 651–658. [CrossRef] [PubMed]
6. Evensen, E.; Wilsgaard, T.; Furberg, A.S.; Skeie, G. Tracking of overweight and obesity from early childhood to adolescence in a population-based cohort—The tromso study, fit futures. *BMC Pediatr.* **2016**, *16*, 64. [CrossRef] [PubMed]
7. Kyu, H.H.; Bachman, V.F.; Alexander, L.T.; Mumford, J.E.; Afshin, A.; Estep, K.; Veerman, J.L.; Delwiche, K.; Iannarone, M.L.; Moyer, M.L.; et al. Physical activity and risk of breast cancer, colon cancer, diabetes, ischemic heart disease, and ischemic stroke events: Systematic review and dose-response meta-analysis for the global burden of disease study 2013. *BMJ* **2016**, *354*, i3857. [CrossRef] [PubMed]
8. Zeng, N.; Gao, Z. Exergaming and obesity in youth: Current perspectives. *Int. J. Gen. Med.* **2016**, *9*, 275–284. [PubMed]
9. Cai, Y.; Zhu, X.; Wu, X. Overweight, obesity, and screen-time viewing among Chinese school-aged children: National prevalence estimates from the 2016 physical activity and fitness in China—The youth study. *J. Sport Health Sci.* **2017**, *6*, 404–409. [CrossRef]

10. Sisson, S.B.; Church, T.S.; Martin, C.K.; Tudorlocke, C.; Smith, S.R.; Bouchard, C.; Earnest, C.P.; Rankinen, T.; Newton, R.L., Jr.; Katzmarzyk, P.T. Profiles of sedentary behavior in children and adolescents: The US national health and nutrition examination survey, 2001–2006. *Pediatr. Obes.* **2011**, *4*, 353–359. [CrossRef] [PubMed]

11. Gao, Z.; Pope, Z.; Lee, J.E.; Stodden, D.; Roncesvalles, N.; Pasco, D.; Huang, C.; Feng, D. Impact of exergaming on young children's school day energy expenditure and moderate-to-vigorous physical activity levels. *J. Sport Health Sci.* **2017**, *6*, 11–16. [CrossRef]

12. Gao, Z.; Xiang, P. Effects of exergaming based exercise on urban children's physical activity participation and body composition. *J. Phys. Act. Health* **2014**, *11*, 992–998. [CrossRef] [PubMed]

13. Gao, Z.; Zhang, T.; Stodden, D. Children's physical activity levels and psychological correlates in interactive dance versus aerobic dance. *J. Sport Health Sci.* **2013**, *2*, 146–151. [CrossRef]

14. Denis, P.; Cédric, R.; Gilles, K.; Pope, Z.; Gao, Z. The effects of a bike active video game on players' physical activity and motivation. *J. Sport Health Sci.* **2017**, *6*, 25–32.

15. Leatherdale, S.T.; Woodruff, S.J.; Manske, S.R. Energy expenditure while playing active and inactive video games. *Am. J. Health Behav.* **2010**, *34*, 31–35. [CrossRef] [PubMed]

16. Miyachi, M.; Yamamoto, K.; Ohkawara, K.; Tanaka, S. METs in adults while playing active video games: A metabolic chamber study. *Med. Sci. Sports Exerc.* **2010**, *42*, 1149–1153. [CrossRef] [PubMed]

17. Edwards, J.; Jeffrey, S.; May, T.; Rinehart, N.J.; Barnett, L.M. Does playing a sports active video game improve object control skills of children with autism spectrum disorder? *J. Sport Health Sci.* **2017**, *6*, 17–24. [CrossRef]

18. Maloney, A.E.; Bethea, T.C.; Kelsey, K.S.; Marks, J.T.; Paez, S.; Rosenberg, A.M.; Catellier, D.J.; Hamer, R.M.; Sikich, L. A pilot of a video game (DDR) to promote physical activity and decrease sedentary screen time. *Obesity* **2008**, *16*, 2074–2080. [CrossRef] [PubMed]

19. Staiano, A.E.; Beyl, R.A.; Hsia, D.S.; Katzmarzyk, P.T.; Newton, R.L., Jr. Twelve weeks of dance exergaming in overweight and obese adolescent girls: Transfer effects on physical activity, screen time, and self-efficacy. *J. Sport Health Sci.* **2017**, *6*, 4–10. [CrossRef] [PubMed]

20. Mhurchu, C.N.; Maddison, R.; Jiang, Y.; Jull, A.; Prapavessis, H.; Rodgers, A. Couch potatoes to jumping beans: A pilot study of the effect of active video games on physical activity in children. *Int. J. Behav. Nutr. Phys. Act.* **2008**, *5*, 1–5. [CrossRef] [PubMed]

21. Maddison, R.; Foley, L.; Ni Mhurchu, C.; Jiang, Y.; Jull, A.; Prapavessis, H.; Hohepa, M.; Rodgers, A. Effects of active video games on body composition: A randomized controlled trial. *Am. J. Clin. Nutr.* **2011**, *94*, 156–163. [CrossRef] [PubMed]

22. Maddison, R.; Mhurchu, C.N.; Jull, A.; Prapavessis, H.; Foley, L.S.; Jiang, Y. Active video games: The mediating effect of aerobic fitness on body composition. *Int. J. Behav. Nutr. Phys. Act.* **2012**, *9*, 54. [CrossRef] [PubMed]

23. Graves, L.; Stratton, G.; Ridgers, N.D.; Cable, N.T. Energy expenditure in adolescents playing new generation computer games. *Br. J. Sports Med.* **2007**, *335*, 1282–1284.

24. Daley, A.J. Can exergaming contribute to improving physical activity levels and health outcomes in children? *Pediatrics* **2009**, *124*, 763–771. [CrossRef] [PubMed]

25. Foley, L.; Maddison, R. Use of active video games to increase physical activity in children: A (virtual) reality? *Pediatr. Exerc. Sci.* **2010**, *22*, 7–20. [CrossRef] [PubMed]

26. Gao, Z.; Chen, S. Are field-based exergames useful in preventing childhood obesity? A systematic review. *Obes. Rev.* **2014**, *15*, 676–691. [CrossRef] [PubMed]

27. Fuzeki, E.; Engeroff, T.; Banzer, W. Health benefits of light-intensity physical activity: A systematic review of accelerometer data of the national health and nutrition examination survey (NHANES). *Sports Med.* **2017**, *47*, 1769–1793. [CrossRef] [PubMed]

28. Sit, C.H.; Lam, J.W.; Mckenzie, T.L. Direct observation of children's preferences and activity levels during interactive and online electronic games. *J. Phys. Act. Health* **2010**, *7*, 484–489. [CrossRef]

29. Maddison, R.; Mhurchu, C.N.; Jull, A.; Jiang, Y.; Prapavessis, H.; Rodgers, A. Energy expended playing video console games: An opportunity to increase children's physical activity? *Pediatr. Exerc. Sci.* **2007**, *19*, 334–343. [CrossRef] [PubMed]

30. Lanningham-Foster, L.; Jensen, T.B.; Foster, R.C.; Redmond, A.B.; Walker, B.A.; Heinz, D.; Levine, J.A. Energy expenditure of sedentary screen time compared with active screen time for children. *Pediatrics* **2006**, *118*, 1831–1835. [CrossRef] [PubMed]

31. Centers for Disease Control and Prevention. *Youth Risk Behavior Sourveillance-United States, 2009*; Surveillance Summaries, MMWR: Atlanta, GA, USA, 2010.
32. General Assembly of the World Medical Association. World medical association declaration of Helsinki: Ethical principles for medical research involving human subjects. *J. Am. Coll. Dent.* **2014**, *81*, 14–18.
33. De Vries, S.I.; Bakker, I.; Hopman-Rock, M.; Hirasing, R.A.; van Mechelen, W. Clinimetric review of motion sensors in children and adolescents. *J. Clin. Epidemiol.* **2006**, *59*, 670–680. [CrossRef] [PubMed]
34. Evenson, K.R.; Catellier, D.J.; Gill, K.; Ondrak, K.S.; Mcmurray, R.G. Calibration of two objective measures of physical activity for children. *J. Sports Sci.* **2008**, *24*, 1557–1565. [CrossRef] [PubMed]
35. Zeng, N.; Gao, X.; Liu, Y.; Lee, J.E.; Gao, Z. Reliability of using motion sensors to measure children's physical activity levels in exergaming. *J. Clin. Med.* **2018**, *7*. [CrossRef] [PubMed]
36. Pope, Z.; Chen, S.; Pasco, D.; Gao, Z. Effects of body mass index on children's physical activity levels in school-based "dance dance revolution". *Games Health J.* **2016**, *5*, 183–188. [CrossRef] [PubMed]
37. U.S. Department of Health and Human Services. Strategies to Improve the Quality of Physical Education. 2010. Available online: www.cdc.gov/Healthyyouth/physicalactivity/pdf/quality_pe.pdf (accessed on 29 September 2014).
38. Kwon, S.; Janz, K.F.; Burns, T.L.; Levy, S.M. Association between light-intensity physical activity and adiposity in childhood. *Pediatr. Exerc. Sci.* **2011**, *23*, 218–229. [CrossRef] [PubMed]
39. Carson, V.; Ridgers, N.D.; Howard, B.J.; Winkler, E.A.; Healy, G.N.; Owen, N.; Dunstan, D.W.; Salmon, J. Light-intensity physical activity and cardiometabolic biomarkers in US adolescents. *PLoS ONE* **2013**, *8*, e71417. [CrossRef] [PubMed]
40. Tobias, J.H.; Steer, C.D.; Mattocks, C.G.; Riddoch, C.; Ness, A.R. Habitual levels of physical activity influence bone mass in 11-year-old children from the United Kingdom: Findings from a large population-based cohort. *J. Bone Miner. Res.* **2007**, *22*, 101–109. [CrossRef] [PubMed]
41. Quan, M.; Zhang, H.; Zhang, J.; Zhou, T.; Zhang, J.; Zhao, G.; Fang, H.; Sun, S.; Wang, R.; Chen, P. Preschoolers' technology-assessed physical activity and cognitive function: A cross-sectional study. *J. Clin. Med.* **2018**, *7*. [CrossRef] [PubMed]
42. Warburton, D.E.; Nicol, C.W.; Bredin, S.S. Health benefits of physical activity: The evidence. *CMAJ* **2006**, *174*, 801–809. [CrossRef] [PubMed]
43. Physical Activity Guidelines Advisory Committee. *2018 Physical Activity Guidelines Advisory Committee Scientific Report*; Physical Activity Guidelines Advisory Committee: Washington, DC, USA, 2018.
44. Owen, C.G.; Nightingale, C.M.; Rudnicka, A.R.; Cook, D.G.; Ekelund, U.; Whincup, P.H. Ethnic and gender differences in physical activity levels among 9–10-year-old children of white European, South Asian and African-Caribbean origin: The child heart health study in England (CHASE study). *Int. J. Epidemiol.* **2009**, *38*, 1082–1093. [CrossRef] [PubMed]
45. Gao, Z.; Podlog, L.; Huang, C. Associations among children's situational motivation, physical activity participation, and enjoyment in an active dance video game. *J. Sport Health Sci.* **2013**, *2*, 122–128. [CrossRef]
46. Dishman, R.K.; McIver, K.L.; Dowda, M.; Saunders, R.P.; Pate, R.R. Motivation and behavioral regulation of physical activity in middle school students. *Med. Sci. Sports Exerc.* **2015**, *47*, 1913–1921. [CrossRef] [PubMed]
47. Gao, Z.; Chen, S.; Pasco, D.; Pope, Z. Effects of active video games on physiological and psychological outcomes among children and adolescents: A meta-analysis. *Obes. Rev.* **2015**, *16*, 783–794. [CrossRef] [PubMed]
48. Gao, Z.; Huang, C.; Liu, T.; Xiong, W. Impact of interactive dance games on urban children's physical activity correlates and behavior. *J. Exerc. Sci. Fit.* **2012**, *10*, 107–112. [CrossRef]
49. Belcher, B.R.; Berrigan, D. Physical activity in us youth: Effect of race/ethnicity, age, gender, and weight status. *Med. Sci. Sports Exerc.* **2010**, *42*, 2211–2221. [CrossRef] [PubMed]
50. Fan, X.; Cao, Z.B. Physical activity among Chinese school-aged children: National prevalence estimates from the 2016 physical activity and fitness in China—The youth study. *J. Sport Health Sci.* **2017**, *6*, 388–394. [CrossRef]
51. Lam, J.W.K.; Sit, C.H.P.; Mcmanus, A.M. Play pattern of seated video game and active "exergame" alternatives. *J. Exerc. Sci. Fit.* **2011**, *9*, 24–30. [CrossRef]

52. Sun, H. Impact of exergames on physical activity and motivation in elementary school students: A follow-up study. *J. Sport Health Sci.* **2013**, *2*, 138–145. [CrossRef]
53. Gao, Z.; Zhang, P.; Podlog, L.W. Examining elementary school children's level of enjoyment of traditional tag games vs. Interactive dance games. *Psychol. Health Med.* **2014**, *19*, 605–613. [CrossRef] [PubMed]
54. CAMESPOT. Dance Dance Revolution Breaks Out in WV Schools. Available online: https://www.gamespot.com/articles/dance-dance-revolution-breaks-out-in-wv-schools/1100-6143007 (accessed on 25 January 2006).
55. Baranowski, T. Exergaming: Hope for future physical activity? Or blight on mankind? *J. Sport Health Sci.* **2017**, *6*, 44–46. [CrossRef]
56. Gao, Z. Fight fire with fire? Promoting physical activity and health through active video games. *J. Sport Health Sci.* **2017**, *6*, 1–3. [CrossRef]

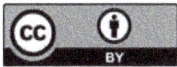

Journal of
Clinical Medicine

MDPI

Article

The Effect of Gamification through a Virtual Reality on Preoperative Anxiety in Pediatric Patients Undergoing General Anesthesia: A Prospective, Randomized, and Controlled Trial

Jung-Hee Ryu [1,2,†], Jin-Woo Park [1,2,†] , Francis Sahngun Nahm [1,2] , Young-Tae Jeon [1,2],
Ah-Young Oh [1,2] , Hak Jong Lee [3], Jin Hee Kim [1,2,*,‡] and Sung-Hee Han [1,2,*,‡]

[1]   Department of Anaesthesiology and Pain Medicine, Medical Virtual Reality Research Group, Seoul National
      University College of Medicine, Seoul 03080, Korea; jinaryu74@gmail.com (J.-H.R.);
      jinul8282@gmail.com (J.-W.P.); hiitsme@hanmail.net (F.S.N.); ytjeon@snubh.org (Y.-T.J.);
      ohahyoung@hanmail.net (A.-Y.O.)
[2]   Department of Anaesthesiology and Pain Medicine, Seoul National University Bundang Hospital,
      Seongnam 13620, Korea
[3]   Department of Radiology, Medical Device Research and Development Center, Seoul National University
      Bundang Hospital, Seongnam 13620, Korea; hakjlee@gmail.com
*   Correspondence: anesing1@snu.ac.kr (J.-H.K.); anesthesiology@snubh.org (S.-H.H.); Tel.: +82-31-787-7499
      (J.-H.K. & S.-H.H.)
†   The authors contributed equally to this project as co-first authors.
‡   The authors contributed equally to this project as co-corresponding authors.

Received: 8 August 2018; Accepted: 14 September 2018; Published: 17 September 2018

Abstract: The use of gamification in healthcare has been gaining popularity. This prospective, randomized, clinical trial was designed to evaluate whether gamification of the preoperative process—via virtual reality (VR) gaming that provides a vivid, immersive and realistic experience—could reduce preoperative anxiety in children. Seventy children scheduled for elective surgery under general anesthesia were randomly divided into either the control or gamification group. Children in the control group received conventional education regarding the preoperative process, whereas those in the gamification group played a 5 min VR game experiencing the preoperative experience. Preoperative anxiety, induction compliance checklist (ICC), and procedural behavior rating scale (PBRS) were measured. Sixty-nine children were included in the final analysis (control group = 35, gamification = 34). Preoperative anxiety (28.3 [23.3–36.7] vs. 46.7 [31.7–51.7]; $p < 0.001$) and intraoperative compliance measured using ICC ($p = 0.038$) were lower in the gamification group than in the control group. However, PBRS ($p = 0.092$) and parent/guardian satisfaction ($p = 0.268$) were comparable between the two groups. VR experience of the preoperative process could reduce preoperative anxiety and improve compliance during anesthetic induction in children undergoing elective surgery and general anesthesia.

Keywords: preoperative anxiety; virtual reality game; preoperative experience

---

1. Introduction

Gamification, defined as 'the use of game design elements in non-game contexts', has been gaining popularity in healthcare, incorporating elements like points and external rewards to encourage learning [1]. There are many examples of successful implementation of gamification to complement learning in medical education, given the integration of game-like features, including competition, narrative, leaderboards, graphics, and other game design elements, that may induce greater motivation and engagement [2,3]. In addition to medical education, gamification has been reported to be effective in patient education with various clinical conditions, such as psychological therapy and physical therapy [4].

With the recent advancement in technology, highly immersive, vivid virtual reality (VR) systems have been introduced into patient education [5,6]. The main characteristics offered by VR technology is the high immersion and real-time interaction [7]. A sense of presence in the VR is considered the major mechanism that enables anxiety to be felt. Meta-analysis demonstrated a positive relationship between the sense of presence and anxiety during VR exposure therapy to manage anxiety disorders [8]. Another study also examined the influence of real or virtual social stimuli on stress reactivity with a 5 min public speaking task, and the result showed comparable increases in salivary cortisol and cardiovascular reactivity in both the real and the virtual public speaking group [9]. These results show a promising future for the application of VR in various therapies. In a previous investigation, a 360 degree VR tour of the operating room was shown to be useful in providing a consistent, vivid, and immersive experience of the preoperative process, significantly reducing preoperative anxiety without physical and financial limitations [6].

Distress during the preoperative period usually leads to preoperative anxiety, with incidences of 40–60% [10]. Preoperative is also associated with adverse consequences, such as emergence delirium, higher postoperative pain, and postoperative maladaptive behavioral changes [11–13]. The authors hypothesized that the integration effect of gamification (motivation and engagement) and VR technology (immersion and reality) may provide a novel platform to increase active participation and motivation in pediatric patients. Therefore, this prospective, randomized, controlled study was performed to identify whether gamification of the preoperative process—via VR gaming—would induce a reduction in preoperative anxiety and an improvement in the compliance of pediatric patients undergoing general anesthesia and elective surgery.

2. Methods

2.1. Study

The protocol of this prospective, randomized, and controlled trial was approved by the institutional review board (IRB) of Seoul National University Bundang Hospital (IRB number: B-1801-445-302) and registered at University hospital Medical Information Network (UMIN) Clinical Trials Registry (registration number: UMIN000031252). Written informed consent was obtained from all parents/guardians of pediatric patients, and children aged 7 years or older signed additional agreements directly after receiving detailed instructions with their parents/guardians. This study was conducted at the Seoul National University Bundang Hospital between February and April of 2018.

2.2. Patients

A total of 70 American Society of Anesthesiologist (ASA) physical status I or II children, aged 4–10 years, undergoing elective day surgery and general anesthesia were enrolled in this study. The exclusion criteria were as follows: children requiring major surgery or postoperative intensive care; those with history of prematurity or congenital disease; those with hearing impairment; those with cognitive deficits or cognitive and intellectual developmental disabilities; those with prior experience of anesthesia; those taking psychoactive medications; and those with a history of epilepsy or seizure. Using a computer-generated randomization code (Random Allocation Software version 1.0; University of Medical Sciences, Isfahan, Iran), the enrolled patients were randomly allocated to one of two groups—the control or gamification group. Randomization was performed by an independent anesthesiologist who was only responsible for patient assignment 2 h before the arrival of patients in the reception area of the operating room.

2.3. VR Game

A 5 min VR game was produced in collaboration with a VR game producing company (JSC GAMES, Seoul, Korea). In the VR game, pediatric patients experienced the preoperative process and general anesthesia induction in a 360 degree, three-dimensional virtual environment, through first-person perspective (Figure 1a). Game elements, including virtual world, progression, exploration, challenge, and rewards, were incorporated. The player is first asked to change into a surgical gown after the confirmation of patient ID. Upon confirmation, the player is transported to the operating room (OR). The player is given the opportunity to explore and interact with the OR environment, including monitoring devices—i.e., ECG, saturation monitor, and non-invasive blood pressure (Figure 1b). When the player selects a device, a detailed description of its function is presented. In addition, the player is given the opportunity to learn how to properly breathe with the facial oxygen mask. The player is given the opportunity to choose a mask, based on the preferred fragrance, which included orange, cherry, or bubble gum. Following the instructions prompted in the game, the player is faced with challenges to defeat the germ monster. Each time the player advances to the following preoperative step, they are rewarded 'health points'. During the game, Chatan and Ace, famous animation characters of an animated film 'Hello Carbot' (ChoiRock Contents Factory, Seoul, Korea), explains the process in detail, encouraging players to cooperate appropriately. Permission to use these animation characters had been obtained (licensing agreement with ChoiRock Contents Factory). A head-mounted VR display, Oculus rift (Oculus VR, Menlo Park, CA, USA), and a hand and finger motion controller, Leap Motion Controller (Leap Motion, San Francisco, CA, USA) were used to play the VR game (Figure 1c).

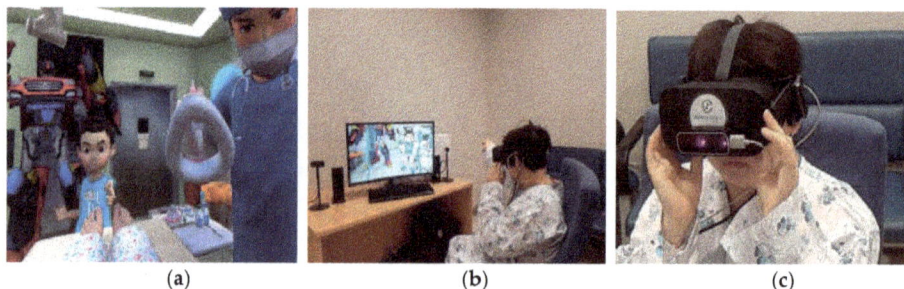

| (a) | (b) | (c) |

Figure 1. Virtual reality video game. (a) Players experience general anesthesia induction in a 360 degree, three-dimensional virtual environment, through first-person viewpoint; (b) can interact with virtual devices; (c) with a head-mounted VR display and a hand and finger motion controller.

2.4. Intervention

Baseline modified Yale Preoperative Anxiety Scale (m-YPAS) was performed by a blinded single evaluator at the time of admission. After measurement of the baseline m-YPAS, randomization was performed by an independent anesthesiologist, not otherwise involved in the trial using a computer-generated randomization code (Random Allocation Software version 1.0; University of Medical Sciences, Isfahan, Iran) with an allocation ratio of 1:1. An opaque envelope containing sequential numbers was transferred to a researcher, and the intervention was performed in an empty room 1 h prior to entering the operating room. For pediatric patients and parents/guardians in the control group, the conventional mode of education about the preoperative process was provided. Children in the gamification group played a 5 min VR game to experience the preoperative process. After the intervention, children and parents/guardians were encouraged to ask questions about the preoperative procedure and anesthesia to the researcher.

2.5. Anesthesia

Without premedication, children were transported to the operating room with their parent/guardian. Monitoring devices, including ECG, non-invasive blood pressure, and oxygen saturation, were applied. Induction of general anesthesia was performed by an anesthesiologist with at least 4 years of experience using intravenous (thiopental sodium, 5 mg/kg) or inhalation agent (sevoflurane) with a facial mask in oxygen. After confirming the loss of consciousness and disappearance of eyelid reflex, the concentration of sevoflurane was increased and intravenous muscle relaxant (rocuronium, 0.3–0.6 mg/kg) was administered. Then, parent/guardian was guided to the waiting room. Endotracheal intubation was performed following sufficient muscle relaxation. During the operation, anesthetic depth was maintained with 1–1.5 MAC sevoflurane. Reversal agents of muscle relaxant (glycopyrrolate and neostigmine) were administered after the surgery. Extubation was done, and patients were transferred to the post-anesthesia care unit (PACU).

2.6. Study Outcomes

All outcomes were assessed by a blinded single evaluator to exclude any possible interrater bias. The primary outcome was preoperative anxiety, which was measured using the validated Korean version of the modified Yale Preoperative Anxiety Scale (m-YPAS; Supplementary Table S1) [14]. The m-YPAS was evaluated twice: once at the time of admission prior to the intervention (baseline) and once just before the transportation from the reception area to the operating room for anesthetic induction (pre-anesthetic). Secondary outcomes included induction compliance checklist (ICC; Supplementary Table S2) [15], procedural behavior rating scale (PBRS; Supplementary Table S3) [16], and parent/guardian's satisfaction scores. ICC represents compliance of patients during induction of anesthesia, and PBRS describes the behavior in a stressful medical procedure. High scores of m-YPAS, ICC, and PBRS represented high anxiety, poor compliance, and increased stress, respectively. Parents/guardians were guided to the waiting room right after the induction of anesthesia, and they were asked to rate the satisfaction about the overall preoperative process of general anesthesia using a numerical rating scale (101 NRS; 0, very dissatisfied; 100, very satisfied).

2.7. Statistical Analysis

Power analysis was performed using G*Power 3.1.2 (Heinrich-Heine University, Düsseldorf, Germany). A previous study reported that the mean (SD) of m-YPAS score was 30.1 (8.4) in the control group undergoing elective surgery [17]. For clinical significance of the effect of the VR game, a reduction of 20% of the m-YPAS score was necessary. A sample size of 35 children per group was calculated with power of 0.8, significance level of 0.05, and 10% dropout rate. SPSS version 21.0 (SPSS Inc., IBM, Chicago, IL, USA) was utilized for all statistical analyses. The test of normal distribution was assessed using Shapiro-Wilk test. Continuous data (age, height, weight, BMI, induction time, anesthesia time, operation time, m-YPAS, PBRS score, and satisfaction scores) are presented as the median (interquartile range [IQR]), and categorical variables (gender, ASA physical class, induction agent, type of surgery, ICC score) are shown as numbers (%). Mann–Whitney U test was used for the analysis of continuous variables, and χ^2 test or Fisher's exact test was used for categorical variables. A full analysis set was used for data analysis. All of the reported p-values are two-sided. A p value of less than 0.050 was considered to indicate statistical significance.

3. Results

Of the 73 screened pediatric patients, 3 were excluded (2 declined to participate, and 1 met the exclusion criteria for cognitive deficit); the remaining 70 patients were randomly allocated to one of two groups: the control or gamification group (35 patients in each group). One child in the gamification group was excluded after randomization because the operation was cancelled. Thus, 69 children completed the study (Figure 2). There were no significant differences in the characteristics of patients, anesthesia, and surgery between the two groups (Table 1).

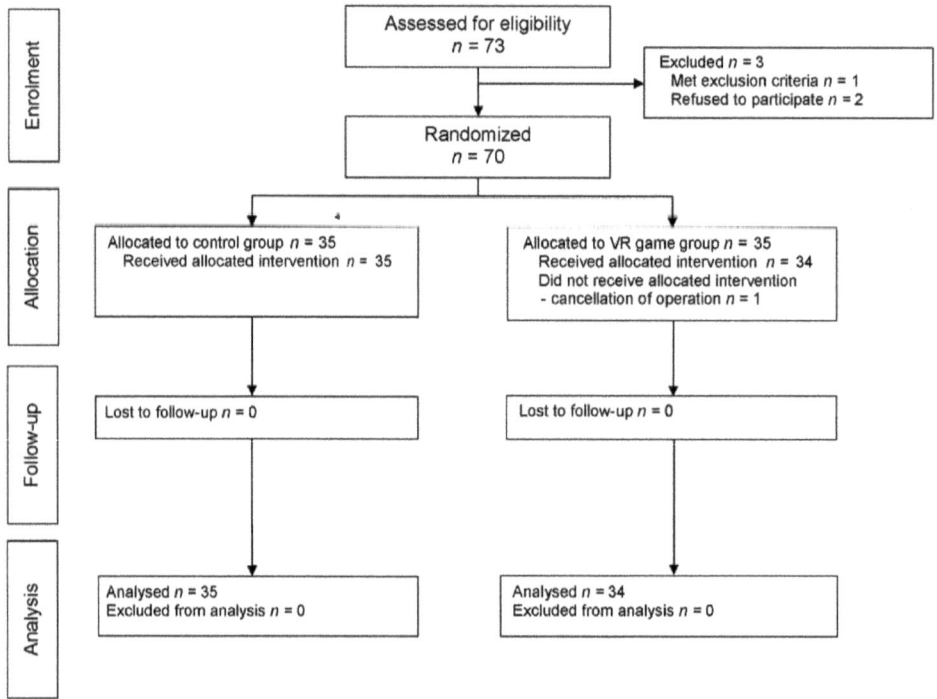

Figure 2. Consort diagram.

Table 1. Patients, anesthesia and surgery characteristics.

	Control Group (n = 35)	Gamification Group (n = 34)	p Value
Age (year)	6 (5–8)	5 (5–7)	0.170
Height (cm)	116.7 (109.8–127.3)	114.7 (108.7–125.7)	0.618
Weight (kg)	21.3 (18.9–28.6)	20.9 (18.4–28.9)	0.529
BMI (kg/m^2)	16.8 (15.7–17.6)	16.3 (15.2–17.3)	0.400
Gender (M/F)	22 (63)/13 (37)	18 (53)/16 (47)	0.469
ASA physical class (I/II)	34 (97)/1 (3)	33 (97)/1 (3)	>0.999
Induction time (min)	6 (4.5–8)	6 (5–7.8)	0.789
Anesthesia time (min)	40 (35–50)	42.5 (35–50)	0.479
Operation time (min)	20 (17.5–25)	20 (15–30)	0.997
Type of surgery			0.569
Otolaryngeal	12 (34)	17 (50)	
Ophthalmic	14 (40)	12 (35)	
Dental	4 (11)	2 (6)	
Others	5 (15)	3 (9)	

VR: virtual reality; ASA: American Society of Anesthesiologist; Induction time: time from the entrance into the operating room to intubation. Data are expressed as median (interquatile range [IQR]) or numbers (%).

There was no substantial difference between the two groups with respect to the baseline anxiety before the intervention. However, the pre-anesthetic m-YPAS scores of the gamification group were significantly lower than those of the control group after the intervention (28.3 [23.3–36.7] vs. 46.7 [31.7–51.7]; $p < 0.001$, Table 2). Moreover, the changes of m-YPAS scores before and after the intervention were also significantly different between the two groups (−22.5 [−29.6–14.2] vs. 0 [−20–4.2]; p = 0.002, Table 2).

Compliance during induction of anesthesia was measured with ICC; a greater number of pediatric patients in the gamification group showed better compliance than in the control group (p = 0.038, Table 2). However, stressful behaviors during anesthetic induction that were evaluated with PBRS were comparable between the two groups (p = 0.092, Table 2). Parent/guardian satisfaction about the overall preoperative process of general anesthesia was similar in both groups (p = 0.268, Table 2). This section may be divided by subheadings. It should provide a concise and precise description of the experimental results, their interpretation as well as the experimental conclusions that can be drawn.

Table 2. Preoperative anxiety, induction compliance, and stressful behaviors of children and parental satisfaction.

		Control Group (*n* = 35)	Gamification Group (*n* = 34)	*p* Value
m-YPAS	baseline	50.0 (43.3–65)	51.7 (46.7–67.5)	0.389
	preanesthetic	46.7 (31.7–51.7)	28.3 (23.3–36.7)	<0.001
	difference	0 (−20–4.2)	−22.5 (−29.6–−14.2)	0.002
ICC score	perfect (0)	19 (54)	27 (79)	0.038
	moderate (1–3)	13 (37)	7 (21)	
	poor (>4)	3 (9)	0 (0)	
PBRS score		1 (0–2)	0 (0–1)	0.092
Satisfaction Score (101 NRS)		100 (90–100)	100 (90–100)	0.268

m-YPAS: modified Yale Preoperative Anxiety; ICC: induction compliance checklist; PBRS: procedural behavior rating scale; NRS: numerical rating scale (0, very dissatisfied; 100, very satisfied). Data are expressed as median (IQR) or numbers (%).

4. Discussion

To the best of our knowledge, this is the first clinical study showing the outcome of using gamification—via VR technology—to educate pediatric patients in preparation for general anesthesia. The result of the current study showed that VR game reduced preoperative anxiety and improved compliance during anesthetic induction in children undergoing elective surgery and general anesthesia.

Gamification—as a means to educate patients to improve health outcomes—has previously been introduced and investigated, especially in the field of psychological and physical therapy [4]. Preoperative anxiety is a major concern in pediatric anesthesia because it may induce severe distress and various negative effects in children [10]. With the advancement of VR technology, a recent trial incorporated VR technology and found that preoperative anxiety was reduced by 30% in the VR group compared with the conventional education group [6]. During cognitive behavioral therapy for anxiety disorder, patients were exposed to anxiety-provoking situations, both in real life or via VR experience. They showed that the sense of presence is positively correlated with the level of anxiety [8]. Additionally, a comparable increases in stress response, such as salivary cortisol and cardiovascular reactivity, were observed in both the real and VR groups, suggesting the usefulness of VR applications in anxiety therapy [9]. Therefore, VR exposure can be considered as a practical alternative to traditional exposure, since it offers more control over the anxiety level of the stimulus. The current study evaluated the effects of gamification—via VR gaming—on preoperative anxiety. The result showed that experiencing the preoperative process via VR game may effectively reduce anxiety in pediatric patients (about 40%). The result of the current study may be explained by the combined effect of gamification (motivation and engagement) and VR experience (immersion and reality).

High ICC scores indicate less behavioral compliance [15], and the ICC scores of the present study were stratified into three categories (perfect, moderate, and poor) for the purpose of analysis. Children with VR game experience were more compliant during the induction of anesthesia than those with conventional education. Pediatric patients who played the VR game may be more familiar with the operating room environment and the preoperative process than those who received the conventional education, leading to higher compliance during the induction of anesthesia.

The PBRS score was measured during the induction of anesthesia to assess the degree of distress in children. However, there was no difference in PBRS between the two groups. This phenomenon may be because PBRS was more useful for assessing the distress and pain during painful procedures and postoperative period [16].

This study has some limitations. First, this study used the conventional preoperative education method in the control group. This is because our institution had been using this method to mitigate preoperative anxiety in children. The use of the same interactive VR intervention without the gamification component in the control group could reveal the true effect of gamification on preoperative anxiety. Second, there was no data available regarding the use of VR intervention or users' experiences, such as a measurement of the sense of presence. The current study was performed not to measure the effectiveness of VR intervention, but to identify whether gamification of the preoperative process, using VR, would reduce preoperative anxiety. Additionally, the sense of presence is measured with presence questionnaires [18], which is not clinically suitable for children undergoing anesthesia and surgery. Third, repeated measures analysis of variance (RM ANOVA) is the standard method for randomized controlled trials; however, it was not used for the analysis of the data in this study since the residual of the data did not follow a normal distribution. Therefore, the changes in preoperative anxiety (before and after treatment) were analyzed, and we found significant differences between the groups. Fourth, there is the possibility that the baseline m-YPAS may have been affected by randomization since children may figure out or explicitly ask the staff about their allocation at the time of collecting the pre-measurements. However, the baseline m-YPAS was collected before randomization, and the assessor was blinded to patient allocation.

5. Conclusions

Gamification—via the use of VR game—on the experience of the perioperative process appears to reduce preoperative anxiety and improve compliance during anesthetic induction in children undergoing elective surgery and general anesthesia. However, further study with the same interactive VR intervention without the gamification component as the control group may be necessary to investigate the true effect of gamification on preoperative anxiety. Gamification of the preoperative process may be a necessary component of pediatric patient education in reducing preoperative anxiety. It is a low-cost and easy-to-use tool with potential benefits. Nonetheless, a further investigation is needed to measure the effectiveness of users' experiences with gamification.

Supplementary Materials: The following are available online at http://www.mdpi.com/2077-0383/7/9/284/s1, Supplementary Table S1: modified Yale Preoperative Anxiety Scale, Supplementary Table S2: induction compliance checklist, Supplementary Table S3: procedural behavior rating scale.

Author Contributions: J.-H.R., J.-W.P., J.-H.K., and S.-H.H. conceptualized and designed the study; J.-W.P., A.-Y.O., Y.-T.J., and J.-H.K. collected the original data; J.-H.R., H.J.L., and S.-H.H. analyzed the data; F.S.N., A.-Y.O., Y.-T.J., and H.J.L. interpreted the analysis and helped with quality control; J.-H.R. and J.-W.P. prepared the original draft; J.-H.K., and S.-H.H. reviewed and edited the draft; J.-H.R., J.-W.P., F.S.N., J.-H.K., and S.-H.H. revised the manuscript.

Funding: This project was partially supported by Korea Creative Content Agency (No 1-17-F405-001).

Conflicts of Interest: The authors declare no conflict of interest.

References

1. King, D.; Greaves, F.; Exeter, C.; Darzi, A. 'Gamification': Influencing health behaviours with games. *J. R. Soc. Med.* **2013**, *106*, 76–78. [CrossRef] [PubMed]
2. McCoy, L.; Lewis, J.H.; Dalton, D. Gamification and multimedia for medical education: A landscape review. *J. Am. Osteopath. Assoc.* **2016**, *116*, 22–34. [CrossRef] [PubMed]

3. Theng, Y.L.; Lee, J.W.; Patinadan, P.V.; Foo, S.S. The use of videogames, gamification, and virtual environments in the self-management of diabetes: A systematic review of evidence. *Games Health J.* **2015**, *4*, 352–361. [CrossRef] [PubMed]

4. Primack, B.A.; Carroll, M.V.; McNamara, M.; Klem, M.L.; King, B.; Rich, M.; Chan, C.W.; Nayak, S. Role of video games in improving health-related outcomes: A systematic review. *Am. J. Prev. Med.* **2012**, *42*, 630–638. [CrossRef] [PubMed]

5. Bekelis, K.; Calnan, D.; Simmons, N.; MacKenzie, T.A.; Kakoulides, G. Effect of an immersive preoperative virtual reality experience on patient reported outcomes: A randomized controlled trial. *Ann. Surg.* **2017**, *265*, 1068–1073. [CrossRef] [PubMed]

6. Ryu, J.H.; Park, S.J.; Park, J.W.; Kim, J.W.; Yoo, H.J.; Kim, T.W.; Hong, J.S.; Han, S.H. Randomized clinical trial of immersive virtual reality tour of the operating theatre in children before anaesthesia. *Br. J. Surg.* **2017**, *104*, 1628–1633. [CrossRef] [PubMed]

7. Willaert, W.I.; Aggarwal, R.; Van Herzeele, I.; Cheshire, N.J.; Vermassen, F.E. Recent advancements in medical simulation: Patient-specific virtual reality simulation. *World J. Surg.* **2012**, *36*, 1703–1712. [CrossRef] [PubMed]

8. Ling, Y.; Nefs, H.T.; Morina, N.; Heynderickx, I.; Brinkman, W.P. A meta-analysis on the relationship between self-reported presence and anxiety in virtual reality exposure therapy for anxiety disorders. *PLoS ONE* **2014**, *9*, e96144. [CrossRef] [PubMed]

9. Kothgassner, O.D.; Felnhofer, A.; Hlavacs, H.; Beutl, L.; Palme, R.; Kryspin-Exner, I.; Glenk, L.M. Salivary cortisol and cardiovascular reactivity to a public speaking task in a virtual and real-life environment. *Comput. Hum. Behav.* **2016**, *62*, 124–135. [CrossRef]

10. Banchs, R.J.; Lerman, J. Preoperative anxiety management, emergence delirium, and postoperative behavior. *Anesthesiol. Clin.* **2014**, *32*, 1–23. [CrossRef] [PubMed]

11. Aouad, M.T.; Nasr, V.G. Emergence agitation in children: An update. *Curr. Opin. Anaesthesiol.* **2005**, *18*, 614–619. [CrossRef] [PubMed]

12. Kain, Z.N.; Mayes, L.C.; Caldwell-Andrews, A.A.; Karas, D.E.; McClain, B.C. Preoperative anxiety, postoperative pain, and behavioral recovery in young children undergoing surgery. *Pediatrics* **2006**, *118*, 651–658. [CrossRef] [PubMed]

13. Litke, J.; Pikulska, A.; Wegner, T. Management of perioperative stress in children and parents. Part 1–The preoperative period. *Anaesthesiol. Intensive Ther.* **2012**, *44*, 165–169. [PubMed]

14. Jung, K.; Im, M.H.; Hwang, J.M.; Oh, A.Y.; Park, M.S.; Jeong, W.J.; Kim, S.C.; Jung, S.W.; Sohn, H.; Yoon, M.O.; et al. Reliability and validity of korean version of modified: Yale preoperative anxiety scale. *Ann. Surg. Treat. Res.* **2016**, *90*, 43–48. [CrossRef] [PubMed]

15. Kain, Z.N.; Mayes, L.C.; Wang, S.M.; Caramico, L.A.; Hofstadter, M.B. Parental presence during induction of anesthesia versus sedative premedication: Which intervention is more effective? *Anesthesiology* **1998**, *89*, 1147–1156. [CrossRef] [PubMed]

16. Blount, R.L.; Loiselle, K.A. Behavioural assessment of pediatric pain. *Pain Res. Manag.* **2009**, *14*, 47–52. [CrossRef] [PubMed]

17. Moura, L.A.; Dias, I.M.; Pereira, L.V. Prevalence and factors associated with preoperative anxiety in children aged 5–12 years. *Rev. Lat. Am. Enfermagem.* **2016**, *24*. [CrossRef] [PubMed]

18. De Leo, G.; Diggs, L.A.; Radici, E.; Mastaglio, T.W. Measuring sense of presence and user characteristics to predict effective training in an online simulated virtual environment. *Simul. Healthc.* **2014**, *9*, 1–6. [CrossRef] [PubMed]

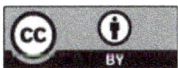

Journal of
Clinical Medicine

MDPI

Article

Application and Validation of Activity Monitors' Epoch Lengths and Placement Sites for Physical Activity Assessment in Exergaming

Jungyun Hwang [1,2,*], Austin Michael Fernandez [1] and Amy Shirong Lu [1,2]

[1] Department of Communication Studies, College of Arts, Media and Design, Northeastern University, Boston, MA 02115, USA; fernandez.au@husky.neu.edu (A.M.F.); a.lu@northeastern.edu (A.S.L.)
[2] Department of Health Sciences, Bouvé College of Health Sciences, Northeastern University, Boston, MA 02115, USA
* Correspondence: j.hwang@northeastern.edu; Tel.: +1-617-373-6331

Received: 11 August 2018; Accepted: 7 September 2018; Published: 11 September 2018

Abstract: We assessed the agreement of two ActiGraph activity monitors (wGT3X vs. GT9X) placed at the hip and the wrist and determined an appropriate epoch length for physical activity levels in an exergaming setting. Forty-seven young adults played a 30-min exergame while wearing wGT3X and GT9X on both hip and wrist placement sites and a heart rate sensor below the chest. Intraclass correlation coefficient indicated that intermonitor agreement in steps and activity counts was excellent on the hip and good on the wrist. Bland-Altman plots indicated good intermonitor agreement in the steps and activity counts on both placement sites but a significant intermonitor difference was detected in steps on the wrist. Time spent in sedentary and physical activity intensity levels varied across six epoch lengths and depended on the placement sites, whereas time spent from a 1-s epoch of the hip-worn monitors most accurately matched the relative exercise intensity by heart rate. Hip placement site was associated with better step-counting accuracy for both activity monitors and more valid estimation of physical activity levels. A 1-s epoch was the most appropriate epoch length to detect short bursts of intense physical activity and may be the best choice for data processing and analysis in exergaming studies examining intermittent physical activities.

Keywords: active video game; accelerometry; physical activity assessment; epoch; placement site; heart rate

1. Introduction

An accelerometer is an electromechanical device used to measure acceleration forces and thereby detect motions [1]. Since accelerometry functions are applicable to wearable activity monitors, accelerometer-based activity monitors have been widely accepted as a useful and practical device for monitoring and tracking physical activity as well as predicting energy expenditure [2]. Further, the use of accelerometer-based activity monitors significantly contributes to the field of physical activity and health, such as the development of physical activity classification [3,4], estimation of the mortality [5], and application for different research settings [6,7]. As such, physical activity assessment must be accurate; thus, researchers have validated accelerometer properties, placements, and/or data processing in regular physical activity settings [2] but seldom in exergaming settings.

Exergaming combines body movements and video gaming and requires bilateral coordination skills of both upper and lower limb movement for different movement patterns (e.g., punching, kicking, jumping) in response to visual cues [8]. Since exergaming increases energy expenditure and achieves moderate-to-vigorous levels of physical activity [9,10], it has been widely implemented in clinical settings [11] as well as in laboratory, home, schools, and the community [12] as an innovative and alternative strategy to promote physical activity and health. To our knowledge, no exergaming studies have processed accelerometry data into quantifiable and interpretable information involving different monitors, placement sites, epoch lengths, or activity cut-points [2]. There is thus an urgent need to validate the use of accelerometry for the assessment of physical activity in exergaming research.

In comparing subjective methods (e.g., diaries, questionnaires) for physical activity assessment, accelerometer-based activity monitors are regarded as the gold standard in detecting steps and quantifying the volume and intensity of physical activity [1]. Such activity monitors have been used in a wide range of applications and in a variety of clinical and research settings [2]. Despite their frequency of usage, validation studies have reported discrepancies in steps or physical activity levels when comparing activity monitors of different brands (e.g., activPAL, Hookie AM20, Polar Active vs. ActiGraph) at different placement sites [7,13,14]; these validation studies have mostly assessed regular physical activities (e.g., walking, running) [15,16] or free-living activities [15,17], but one recent study compared the output of different monitors (pedometer vs. accelerometer) in an exergaming setting [18].

One of the most commonly used activity monitor brands in physical activity research, ActiGraph has developed multiple generations of activity monitors [19]. Researchers have validated different ActiGraph activity monitors—including GT3X vs. GT1M [4], GT1M, GT3X, vs. GT3X+ [20], and recently, GT3X+ vs. GT9X [21]—placed at different sites such as hip vs. wrist [15,22,23] during various physical activities. Although a hip placement site has been validated as an ideal location for accurately measuring steps and physical activity level in regular physical activities [15], the evaluation of multiple placement sites (hip vs. wrist) in exergaming research is needed as more upper limb movements (unlike most regular physical activity) are required for exergaming [8]. In addition, validation studies mainly focusing on young people (from preschoolers to adolescents) have evaluated epoch lengths using different sets of activity cut-points [24–26], which impact the assessment of sedentary behavior and the different levels of physical activity intensity [25,27]. Since the exergaming play we chose to evaluate here features acute bouts of intermittent and spontaneous physical activity, shorter epochs might be a better choice for capturing short bouts of frequently occurring activity [2]. To date, there have been no studies comparing the effect of placement sites and epoch lengths on output especially from exergaming play or in young adults [2]; thus, the most appropriate accelerometer data collection and scoring protocol remains unclear.

Of particular relevance here, studies comparing physical activity levels from different epoch lengths have not validated theses assessments with absolute measures of exercise intensity via indirect calorimetry (e.g., oxygen uptake, metabolic equivalent) or relative measures of exercise intensity via heart rate (HR) monitoring (e.g., %HRmax, %HR reserve (HRR)) [25,26,28,29], which can be used as comparators to determine an appropriate epoch length for the accuracy of physical activity assessment. Whereas either relative or absolute measures can be used for classifying different levels of physical activity intensity [30], the use of relative measures in comparing epoch lengths should be more feasible and effective for such an assessment [4,31]. We believe that studies comparing epochs between activity counts and HR have never been reported, especially in an exergaming setting.

We aimed to examine the agreement of two recent generations of ActiGraph monitors (wGT3X-BT and GT9X Link, referred to below as wGT3X and GT9X, respectively) placed at different sites (hip and wrist). We sought to determine the most appropriate epoch length for physical activity assessment when validated using measurements of relative exercise intensity such as HR in healthy young adults in an exergaming setting. Our findings provide insight into effective data collection strategies for exergaming research, thereby improving the accuracy of physical activity assessment.

2. Materials and Methods

2.1. Participants

We recruited 47 healthy young adults of different ethnic backgrounds and both genders who spoke English from a university in the northeastern region of the United States via web advertisements and flyers. Participants were eligible if they met the following conditions: (1) were between 18 and 25 years old; (2) were free from physical disability (e.g., gait abnormalities); and (3) were not a current or former user of tobacco. Our study was approved by the Institutional Review Board of Northeastern University and all participants signed a written consent form for their participation.

2.2. Study Procedures and Instruments

We used a cross-sectional design and collected data from 22 March 2017 to 21 September 2017. Once a participant arrived at the laboratory, we provided the participant with an orientation on study procedures and potential risks. We measured their weight and height and computed their body mass index (BMI; kg/m^2). We used ActiGraph tri-axial monitors (ActiGraph LLC, Pensacola, FL, USA) including wGT3X (46 × 33 × 15 mm, mass 19 g) and GT9X (35 × 35 × 10 mm, mass 14 g). We rotated and counterbalanced the placement of the ActiGraph monitors to avoid any potential order or placement effects.

Using the ActiLife software v.6.13.2 (ActiGraph LLC, Pensacola, FL, USA), we initialized four ActiGraph tri-axial monitors at a sampling rate of 30 Hz and set the Bluetooth wireless function for a wrist-worn GT9X to integrate with a Polar H7 Bluetooth heart rate sensor (Polar Electro Inc., Lake Success, NY, USA) for continuous heart rate measurement. We positioned a wGT3X with a belt clip and GT9X with an elastic belt at the anterior axillary line of the nondominant hip and another wGT3X with a nylon band and GT9X with a silicone band on the nondominant wrist [14]. We also placed a Polar H7 Bluetooth heart rate sensor on the chest with a soft textile strap.

After we confirmed that all devices worked properly, participants played for three 10-min segments for a total of 30 min. Each segment comprised 2 min of passive rest (standing) followed by 8 min of playing Kung-Fu for Kinect (http://www.kungfuforkinect.com), which involves upper and lower movements via a Kinect sensor on an Xbox One console (Microsoft Inc., Redmond, WA, USA). While playing the exergame, a participant could see his/her own body on the screen and fought enemies using his/her own moves in a 2D fighting adventure environment. When different enemies appeared on the screen, a participant engaged them with a variety of intermittent and spontaneous movement patterns and skills (e.g., jumping, punching, kicking). The intensity level of the exergaming was determined by continuous HR measurement as described above and self-assessment using the Borg rating of perceived exertion (RPE) [32] before and immediately after the 30-min exergaming play. We monitored the play time and recorded the start and end time of each interval on a study checklist.

2.3. Accelerometry Procedure and Data Reduction

The ActiGraph tri-axial monitors measure accelerations from the subject's amplitude (g) and frequency (Hz) of movement in three individual axes (X axis: anterior-posterior, Y axis: vertical, Z axis: medial-lateral). Using the ActiLife software v.6.13.2, we transferred the collected data from the monitors and downloaded the activity counts from the three axes and vector magnitude (VM) obtained from all three axes $(x^2 + y^2 + z^2)^{1/2}$ with six epoch lengths (1, 5, 10, 15, 30, and 60 s). We used the two popular and validated Sasaki and Troiano's activity cut-point sets [3,4] as appropriate for adults to estimate the amount of time spent in sedentary behavior (SB) and light (LPA), moderate (MPA), vigorous (VPA), and very vigorous physical activity (VVPA): (1) Sasaki's cut-points [4] (e.g., a 60 s epoch (counts per minute, CPM): ≤150, 151–2690, 2691–6166, 6167–9642, and >9642) for the categories of SB, LPA, MPA, VPA, and VVPA, respectively, and (2) Troiano's cut-points [3] (e.g., a 60 s epoch (CPM): ≤100, 101–2019, 2020–5998, and ≥5998) for SB, LPA, MPA, and VPA. We combined Sasaki's VVPA with VPA for subsequent data analysis. Sasaki did not report classifications of either SB or LPA;

thus, we used ≤150 and 151–2690 to define these categories, respectively, as 150 CPM may be the most appropriate cut-point to use to define SB for ActiGraph monitors [2,33]. We then converted the dataset into another of five shorter epoch lengths (1, 5, 10, 15, and 30 s) and recalculated the sedentary and physical activity intensity levels for subsequent data analysis. We also summed the step counts calculated from the built-in algorithm of the ActiLife software using a zero-crossing method based on raw accelerations from the vertical axis [1].

We downloaded HR data recorded at every second as a 10-s interval dataset. To compare intensity assessed indirectly via HR with the categories from activity counts in six epoch lengths, we calculated the amount of time spent in SB (<57), LPA (57–63), MPA (64–76), and VPA (>77) based on the categories of relative exercise intensity (%HRmax) [30] after adjusting for age-predicted maximal HR [208 − (0.7 × age)] [34].

2.4. Statistical Data Analyses

We ran statistical data analysis separately for the hip and the wrist. Of the 47 subjects, we analyzed 47 datasets from the wrist but only 45 datasets from the hip for activity counts due to a technical problem with two of the monitors. Additionally, of the 47 subjects, 41 datasets for heart rate were analyzed; five were excluded due to inappropriate data for analysis (namely, logging more than 25 of 30 min at the sedentary level) and a technical problem for one additional monitor.

We used intraclass correlation coefficients (ICC) to examine intermonitor agreement in steps and activity counts using the following categories [35]: poor (<0.5); moderate (0.5–0.75); good (0.75–0.9); and excellent (>0.9). We confirmed this using a Bland-Altman analysis to assess the mean bias and limits of agreement and calculated mean bias % as (GT9X − wGT3X)/mean% [36]. For the Bland-Altman plots and ICC analyses, we used Sasaki's activity cut-points to compare steps, each axis count (CPM), and VM (CPM) between wGT3X and GT9X placed on the hip or the wrist. Additionally, due to the orientation difference of the wGT3X and GT9X monitors when worn on the wrist, we compared data from the Y and X axes in the GT9X to the data from the X and Y axes in the wGT3X, respectively, according to the manufacturer's suggestion (J. MacDonald, written communication, May 2018) (see Supplemental Figure S1). We also performed a repeated measures ANOVA: (1) to assess the mean differences of steps, the three axes' activity counts, and the VM between the monitors; (2) to test for an interaction for time spent in SB and the different levels of physical activity intensity in six epoch lengths with two monitors and two activity cut-point sets; and (3) to compare the mean amount of time spent in SB and different levels of physical activity intensity assessed via HR and activity counts (categorized separately using the two activity cut-point sets) in six epoch lengths averaged from two monitors. When a significant interaction was observed, we performed a Tukey's post hoc test to identify pairwise differences. All statistical data analyses were conducted with IBM SPSS 24.0 (IBM Corp., Armonk, NY, USA). The criterion for significance was $p < 0.05$. Data are presented as mean ± standard deviation.

3. Results

3.1. Descriptive Analysis

Participants (N = 47; 25 males) were, on average, 21.4 ± 2.2 years old, 171.9 ± 10.6 cm in height, and 68.0 ± 16.6 kg in weight, and had a BMI of 23.2 ± 4.7 for body mass index. They consisted of 40.4% Caucasian, 2.1% African American, 44.7% Asian, 6.4% Hispanic/Latino, and 6.4% mixed races or ethnicities. All participants engaged in an approximately 30-min exergaming session. The mean HR during the exergaming was 130.1 ± 22.4 beats/min and the means of RPE before and after the exergaming were 8.3 ± 2.0 and 13.1 ± 2.8, respectively, indicating a moderate intensity level of physical activity.

3.2. Agreement between GT9X and wGT3X Placed on Hip and Wrist

As shown in Table 1, the ICC estimate with a 95% confidence interval indicated excellent agreement in steps, X axis, Y axis, and VM and good agreement in the Z axis between GT9X and wGT3X on the hip placement site, whereas there was good agreement in steps, X axis, Y axis, Z axis, and VM on the wrist placement site.

Table 1. Interclass correlation coefficient between GT9X and wGT3X in steps and activity counts.

		Interclass Correlation Coefficient	95% Confidence Interval
Hip	Steps	0.94	0.89–0.97
	Anterior-posterior (X) axis	0.93	0.88–0.96
	Vertical (Y) axis	0.93	0.87–0.96
	Medial-lateral (Z) axis	0.86	0.77–0.92
	Vector magnitude	0.95	0.92–0.97
Wrist	Steps	0.80	0.66–0.88
	Anterior-posterior (X) axis	0.83	0.71–0.90
	Vertical (Y) axis	0.87	0.77–0.92
	Medial-lateral (Z) axis	0.86	0.77–0.92
	Vector magnitude	0.89	0.81–0.94

The Bland-Altman plots illustrating the agreement between GT9X and wGT3X in steps and tri-axis activity counts with means and a 95% confidence interval are depicted in Figure 1. We found considerable agreement between GT9X and wGT3X on the hip site, as indicated by mean bias differences of 1.1% in steps, −4.0% in X axis, −4.4% in Y axis, −7.4% in Z axis, and −4.2% in VM. We found reasonably good agreements on the wrist, as indicated by mean bias differences of 2.1% in X axis, 0.5% in Y axis, 0.1% in Z axis, and 0.9% in VM; however, there was relatively poor agreement in terms of steps (a mean bias difference of 21.4%) between the monitors.

The step difference between the monitors was significant on the wrist ($F_{1,47} = 73.42$, $p < 0.001$), with steps reported from the GT9X (1418.5 ± 354.1) higher than that from the wGT3X (1144.2 ± 285.9). However, this difference was not significant on the hip ($F_{1,45} = 0.02$, $p = 0.903$), which had similar step counts reported by the GT9X (525.0 ± 310.6) and the wGT3X (522.3 ± 329.3) (Figure 2). There was no significant difference in the X, Y, Z, or VM (CPM) between monitors placed on the wrist and those placed on the hip (Table 2). The wrist-worn monitors produced higher steps (Figure 2), tri-axial counts, and VM than the hip-worn monitors (all, $p < 0.001$) (Table 2).

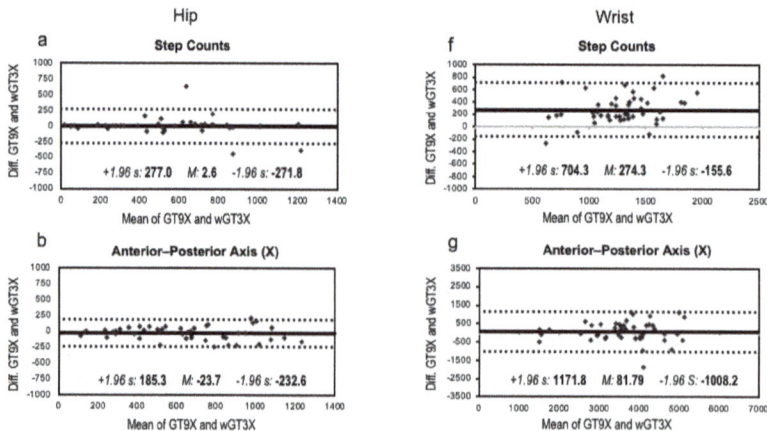

Figure 1. *Cont.*

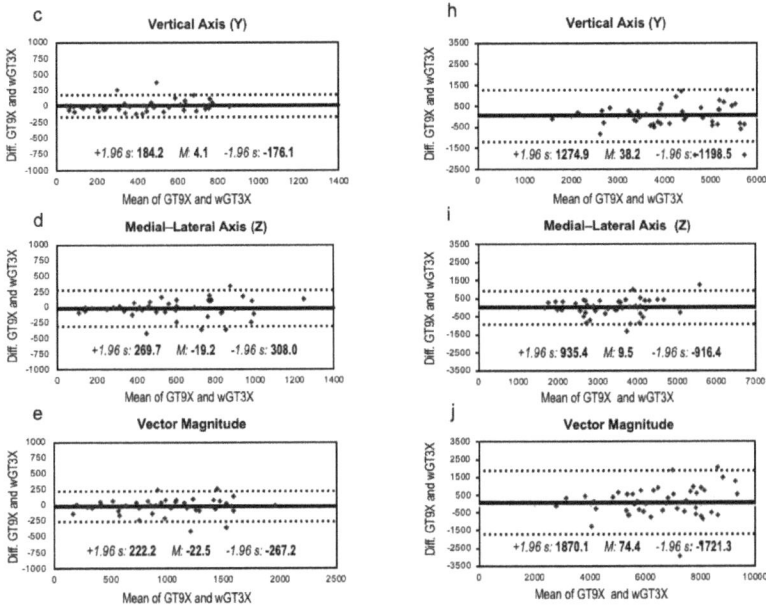

Figure 1. Bland-Altman plots and intraclass correlation (ICC). The solid line represents the mean bias (M), whereas the dotted line indicates the limits of agreement computed as the mean bias plus or minus 1.96 times its standard deviation (s). ICC represents intraclass correlation that measures the agreement of measurements between the GT9X and wGT3X. Data in Figure (a–e) are from the hip-worn monitors, whereas data in Figure (f–j) are from the wrist-worn monitors.

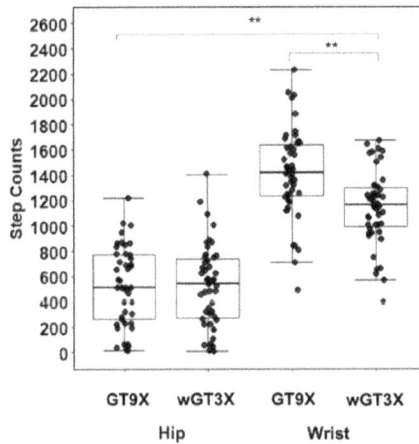

Figure 2. Average step counts. Box plot with scatter represents 25th percentile at bottom and 75th percentile at top with the highest, median, and lowest value. ** $p < 0.001$: higher steps in GT9X vs. wGT3X on the wrist; higher steps in wrist vs. hip.

Table 2. Average of activity counts based on the six epoch lengths.

	wGT3X Hip						GT9X Hip					
	1	5	10	15	30	60	1	5	10	15	30	60
Vertical Axis (Y), Counts	6.8 ±3.9	33.9 ±19.3	67.9 ±38.6	101.9 ±57.9	204.0 ±116.1	407.7 ±232.9	7.0 ±4.2	34.8 ±21.0	69.7 ±42.1	104.6 ±63.1	209.2 ±126.4	419.0 ±253.4
Anterior-Posterior Axis (X), Counts	11.0 ±4.9	55.0 ±24.6	110.1 ±49.3	165.3 ±74.0	330.9 ±148.1	661.9 ±296.6	10.6 ±4.8	53.0 ±23.9	106.0 ±47.7	159.1 ±71.6	318.5 ±143.4	638.0 ±287.6
Medial-Lateral Axis (Z), Counts	9.9 ±4.5	49.4 ±22.7	98.9 ±45.5	148.4 ±68.2	297.2 ±136.6	594.5 ±273.3	9.6 ±4.9	48.2 ±24.4	96.5 ±48.8	144.8 ±73.1	289.8 ±146.5	580.5 ±293.5
Vector Magnitude, Counts	18.8 ±8.0	89.2 ±38.0	175.5 ±74.8	261.1 ±111.5	517.3 ±221.3	1026.2 ±440.0	18.5 ±8.3	87.8 ±39.3	172.6 ±77.2	256.9 ±115.2	508.4 ±228.3	1010.6 ±454.7

	wGT3X Wrist **						GT9X Wrist **					
	1	5	10	15	30	60	1	5	10	15	30	60
Vertical Axis (Y), Counts	71.1 ±19.6	355.6 ±98.0	711.4 ±196.1	1067.5 ±294.5	2137.7 ±589.6	4287.1 ±1184.6	61.0 ±15.9	305.1 ±79.6	610.4 ±159.3	915.9 ±239.1	1833.7 ±478.7	3675.7 ±960.0
Anterior-Posterior Axis (X), Counts	59.6 ±15.6	298.2 ±77.9	596.7 ±155.9	895.4 ±234.1	1793.0 ±468.9	3596.0 ±941.3	71.7 ±20.8	358.8 ±104.3	717.8 ±208.6	1077.1 ±313.0	2156.6 ±626.4	4323.0 ±1254.6
Medial-Lateral Axis (Z), Counts	55.8 ±14.5	279.0 ±72.5	558.3 ±145.1	837.8 ±218.1	1677.7 ±436.5	3364.4 ±877.3	55.9 ±15.6	279.9 ±78.2	559.9 ±156.4	840.2 ±234.8	1682.3 ±469.7	3372.0 ±941.1
Vector Magnitude, Counts	115.9 ±28.2	561.1 ±137.5	1113.0 ±273.7	1663.4 ±410.3	3314.3 ±819.9	6625.0 ±1645.9	117.2 ±30.0	567.7 ±146.5	1125.9 ±291.7	1682.5 ±436.9	3352.3 ±872.7	6698.1 ±1746.1

** $p < 0.001$: higher tri-axial activity counts and vector magnitude in the wrist than the hip.

3.3. Time Spent in Sedentary and Physical Activity Intensity Levels

Since there were no significant interactions between epoch lengths, monitors, and activity cut-point sets, we ran an analysis on the effect of epoch lengths on sedentary and physical activity intensity levels assessed using the two monitors and the two sets of activity cut-points (Figure 3 and Supplemental Table S1). The effect of epoch lengths on activity levels was significant on the hip ($F_{5, 1080}$ = 6.26, p < 0.001), indicating that the shortest epoch (1 s) was significantly related to more time spent in SB (all, p < 0.001), less time spent in LPA (all, p < 0.001) and in MPA (all, p < 0.001) and more time spent in VPA (all, p < 0.001) compared to the other five longer epochs. In addition, the effect of epoch lengths on activity levels was significant on the wrist ($F_{5, 1104}$ = 3.89, p = 0.002), indicating that the shortest epoch was significantly associated with more time spent in SB (all, p < 0.001) and in LPA (all, p < 0.001) and less time spent in MPA (all, p < 0.001) compared to the other five longer epochs. When we categorized physical activity using Sasaki's activity cut-point set, we found that more time was spent in LPA and a shorter time was spent in MPA on the hip ($F_{1, 1080}$ = 32.94, p < 0.001) and the wrist ($F_{1, 1104}$ = 5.76, p = 0.017) compared to our results obtained using Troiano's activity cut-point set. The wGT3X monitor indicated a longer time spent in VPA compared to the GT9X monitor on the wrist ($F_{1, 1104}$ = 4.13, p = 0.042).

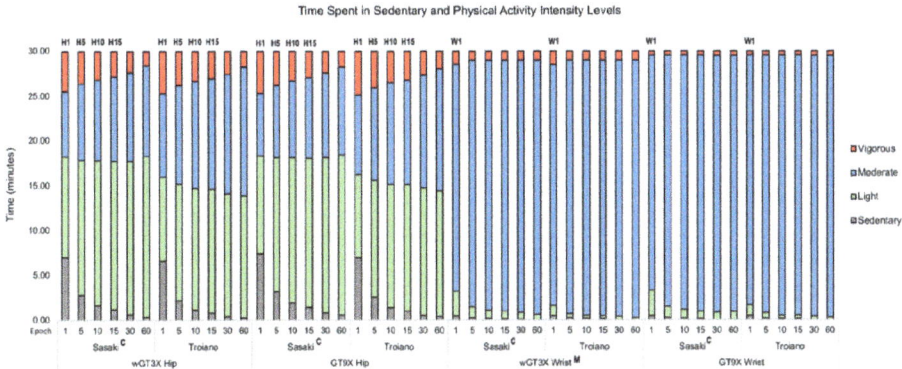

Figure 3. Time spent in sedentary and physical activity intensity levels in epochs. [H1] longer sedentary behavior (SB) and shorter light physical activity (LPA) (1 s vs. other longer five epochs: all, p < 0.001) and shorter moderate physical activity (MPA) and longer vigorous physical activity (VPA) (1 s vs. 10, 15, 30, and 60 s: all, p < 0.001); [H5] longer SB (5 s vs.10, 15, 30, and 60 s: all, p < 0.001), shorter LPA (5 s vs. 60 s: p = 0.039); shorter MPA (5 s vs. 30 and 60 s: p = 0.010 and p < 0.001, respectively), longer VPA (5 s vs. 30 s and 60 s: all, p < 0.001); [H10] longer SB (10 s vs. 60 s: p = 0.012), shorter MPA (10 s vs. 60 s: p = 0.015), longer VPA (10 s vs. 60 s: p < 0.001); [H15] longer VPA (15 s vs. 60 s: p < 0.001); [W1] longer SB (1 s vs. 10, 15, 30, and 60 s: p = 0.038, p = 0.019, p <0.001, and p < 0.001, respectively), longer LPA, and shorter MPA (1 s vs. other five longer epochs: all, p < 0.001); [C] longer LPA and shorter MPA (Sasaki vs. Troiano: all epochs, p < 0.001); [M] longer VPA (wGT3X vs. GT9X, p = 0.021). [H, W, C, and M] are indicated as hip, wrist, cut-point set, and monitor, respectively, while number is presented as epoch length. Data are presented as means in minutes.

3.4. Sedentary and Physical Activity Levels Between Heart Rate and Activity Counts in Epochs

As depicted in Figure 4a,c and in Supplemental Table S2, the time spent (min) in sedentary and physical activity intensity levels for the hip placement site, derived from the two cut-point sets of activity counts, was comparable to the indirect assessment of intensity using HR across six epoch lengths. For instance, the HR-derived measure of SB (7.0 ± 5.6 min) was similar to that determined using a 1-s epoch with both the Sasaki cut-point set (5.9 ± 3.6 min; p = 0.313) and the Troiano cut-point set (5.7 ± 3.6 min; p = 0.159) but differed from that obtained from the longer epoch lengths in either cut-point set (all, $p < 0.001$). The HR-derived measures of LPA (4.6 ± 3.4) were not similar to the intensity level determined using either of the activity cut-point sets across all epoch lengths (all, $p < 0.001$). The HR-derived measures of MPA (9.1 ± 4.7 min) were similar to that determined for all epochs (all, $p > 0.05$) using the Sasaki cut-point set but only for a 1-s epoch (9.8 ± 2.5 min; $p = 0.345$) using the Troiano cut-point set. The HR-derived measures of VPA (6.8 ± 6.3 min) were similar to the activity count intensity measure determined using a 1-s epoch in the Sasaki (5.2 ± 2.8 min; $p = 0.06$) and in the Troiano (5.4 ± 2.9 min; $p = 0.102$) but differed from those determined using the longer epoch lengths (all, $p < 0.001$).

On the wrist placement site (as shown in Figure 4b,d and in Supplemental Table S2), the HR-derived intensity measures of SB, LPA, MPA, and VPA were not comparable to those determined using either cut-point set when compared across all epochs (all, $p < 0.001$, respectively).

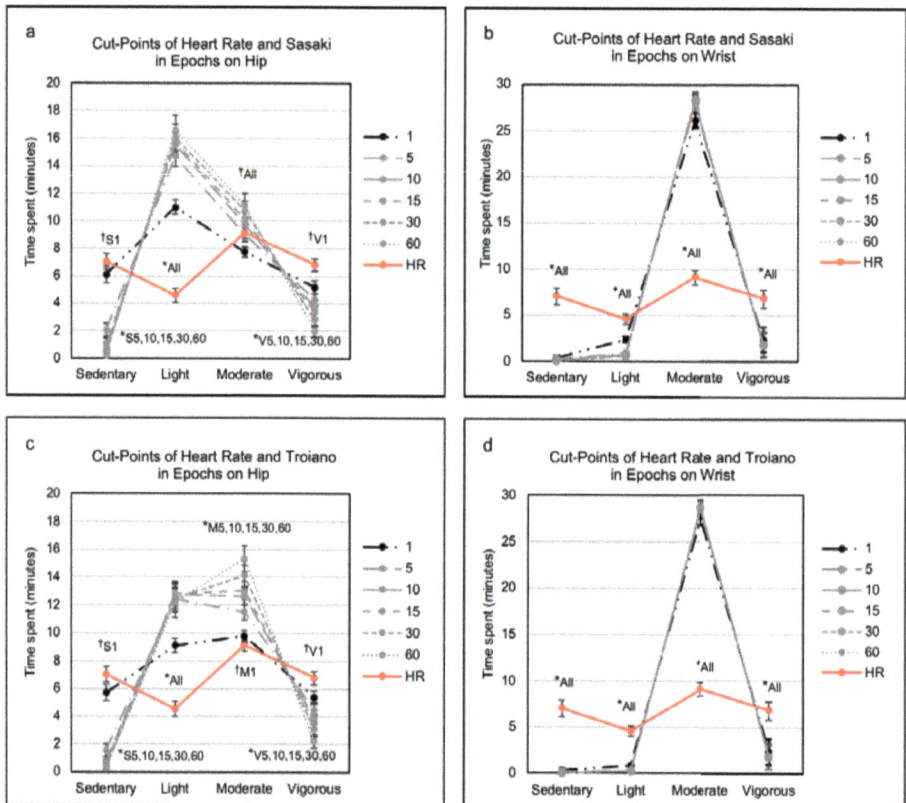

Figure 4. Sedentary and physical activity levels between heart rate and activity counts in epochs. In comparing heart rate, † indicates a nonsignificant difference ($p > 0.05$) with an epoch, whereas * denotes a significant difference ($p < 0.001$) with epochs. The S, M, and V are indicated as sedentary, moderate, and vigorous, respectively, whereas a number and all are represented as an epoch and all epochs, respectively. HR, heart rate. Data are presented as mean ± standard error in minutes.

Additionally, as shown in Supplemental Table S3, there were similar results in sedentary and various physical activity levels at either placement site using either cut-point set when compared separately with GT9X and wGT3X.

4. Discussion

In this study, using an acute bout of exergaming play with two recent generations of ActiGraph monitors, we found that (1) intermonitor differences in steps and activity counts between wGT3X and GT9X were not significant on the hip placement site but were significant in terms of step counts on the wrist placement site; and (2) a 1-s epoch of activity counts obtained from hip-worn activity monitors was the best choice for estimating sedentary and physical activity intensity levels in an exergaming setting when compared with measures of relative exercise intensity using HR. We believe that our work is the first to compare indirect activity intensity measures using HR with activity counts using different epoch lengths, which could be a practical and applicable method for the accuracy of physical activity assessment.

Since newer activity monitor models are continuously being produced by the manufacturers (replacing previous models), researchers have validated outputs (e.g., steps, activity counts) of activity monitors for the accuracy of physical activity assessment. Our results indicated that the differences in steps between wGT3X and GT9X depended on the placement site, although there were strong associations between both monitors on the hip and wrist. More specifically, intermonitor differences for steps between the hip worn-monitors were not significantly different and were generally in good agreement. For these monitors, bias was close to zero, indicating that they were producing similar results, and the 95% limits of agreement were small, suggesting that the hip-worn monitors could be used as an alternative to measure steps. Additionally, there were similar patterns in tri-axial counts, especially on the vertical axis where steps are calculated in the ActiLife step-counting algorithm [1,22].

Our findings are consistent with those of previous studies using other ActiGraph models. These studies showed considerable intermonitor agreement for the vertical axis counts between GT1M and GT3X in young adults during treadmill exercise [4], among GT1M, GT3X, and GT3X+ in children and adolescents with lab-based activities [20], and between the GT3X+ and GT9X in young adults with lab-based activities [21]. However, we observed a relatively poor intermonitor agreement for step counts between the wrist-worn wGT3X and GT9X, as indicated by large and significant intermonitor differences, but reasonably good intermonitor agreement in the vertical and other two axis counts. Some studies have examined possible factors for an intermonitor difference in steps or activity counts. For example, ActiGraph's low-frequency extension filter (the detection of lower amplitude movements) affects the difference in step or activity counts within different generation models (GT3X+ vs. 7164) [37] or in the same models (GT3X+) [38]. In addition, ActiGraph's sampling frequency (the processing of raw acceleration data to activity counts) influences the discrepancy in activity counts within the same models (GT3X+) [39]. Since we used the same sampling frequency (30 Hz) and a normal filter instead of low-frequency extension filter when we compared the wGT3X and the GT9X, the source of the discrepancy in steps between the wrist-worn monitors remains unclear.

A recent study [22] compared step outputs between hip and wrist-worn ActiGraph monitors and between wrist-worn GT3X+ and GT9X monitors during treadmill walking and showed that the discrepancy in tri-axial orientations between GT9X and GT3X+ or other previous ActiGraph monitors might significantly impact step-counting accuracy on the wrist. Further, the ActiGraph step-counting algorithm developed for the hip location might not work for the wrist location [7]. Tudor-Locke et al. [15] examined the accuracy of steps on the hip and wrist placement sites using the same ActiGraph GT3X+ monitors and found the hip site outperformed the wrist site at most treadmill speeds, regardless of the bandpass filter. Moreover, we cannot rule out the possibility that the discrepancy in step counts between the wGT3X and GT9X may be due to differences in individual movement patterns. Since the exergaming we studied requires irregular upper body movements, differences in an individual's arm motion or speed may affect threshold crossing of the acceleration signal, perhaps inducing less step-counting accuracy on the wrist. Additionally, John et al. [22] report that accelerations detected on the wrist were smaller in magnitude than those at the hip during treadmill walking at the same speed, indicating that a wrist-worn monitor would count fewer steps than a hip-worn monitor. However, we found that the wrist-worn GT3X+ monitors resulted in higher steps than hip-worn monitors, which can be explained by the fact that exergaming play involves more arm movements. Thus, when researchers seek to determine the accuracy of step-counting, it is important to take the placement site into consideration. Our result thus suggests that researchers can select either of the two monitors we used here to conduct exergaming research if the devices are placed on the hip.

Of particular importance, we confirmed that epoch lengths differentially influenced assessment of sedentary and different physical activity levels, which is consistent with the previous studies. We found that time spent in SB and physical activity intensity levels varied when assessed using different epoch lengths (1, 5, 10, 15, 30, and 60 s). For instance, as epoch lengths decreased on the hip-worn monitors, estimates of SB and VPA increased while estimates of LPA and MPA decreased. We observed similar patterns in SB and MPA but a different pattern in LPA on the wrist-worn monitors. Our findings here are consistent with those of previous studies showing a varying effect of epoch length with earlier generations of ActiGraph monitors placed on the hip for seven days in a free-living condition. For example, Edwardson and Gorely [26] used single-activity cut-points (i.e., Freedson) and observed that shorter epoch lengths among the four epochs (5, 15, 30, and 60 s) were associated with more time spent in SB and VPA and less time spent in MVPA, MPA, and LPA in children wearing an ActiGraph GT1M monitor on the hip. Banda et al. [25] used multiple activity cut-points (e.g., Evenson, Treuth, Puyan) and showed that shorter epoch lengths among the six epochs (1, 5, 10, 15, 30, and 60 s) were related to more time spent in SB, MPA, and VPA and less time spent in LPA in children wearing the ActiGraph GT3X+ monitor on the hip. Finally, a study examining physical activity levels in middle-aged adults found that an epoch of 4 s among the three epochs (4, 20, and 60 s) was associated with longer time spent in VPA and shorter in LPA [28]. The consistency in findings from the previous studies and our study might be associated with the form and intensity of an intermittent and spontaneous physical activity in which shorter epoch lengths such as a 1-s epoch [25] or a 2-s epoch [29] were the most appropriate epoch length to capture short bouts of vigorous or more intense physical activity. The physical activity form and/or intensity might be comparable to the exergaming play we used, which is characterized by rapid changes from sedentary to intense physical activity occurring frequently in a short period [40]. Taken together, although the results from different epoch lengths vary, shorter epoch lengths may be appropriate for capturing short bouts, especially in more intense physical activity.

However, previous studies examining the effect of epochs on assessment of physical activity levels have not apparently compared relative or absolute measures of exercise intensity [25,26,28], which might attenuate their findings. We compared physical activity intensity based on a cut-point set of HR with each of two cut-point sets of activity counts and found that the amount of time spent in SB, MPA, and VPA with the 1-s epoch length on the hip-worn monitors was similar to that in SB, MPA, and VPA of the HR but that this did not hold for any of the other longer epoch lengths from the hip- or wrist-worn monitors (Figure 4). This is a novel result with respect to previous validations of cut-points of activity counts or raw data (accelerations) against indirect calorimetry (absolute measure) and HR monitoring (relative measure) for physical activity intensity. Previous studies have validated cut-points for physical activity intensity using indirect calorimetry as a gold standard measure of energy expenditure and metabolic equivalent for regular physical activities (e.g., treadmill walking/running) [4,41]. Other studies have used HR monitoring as a relatively less expensive but feasible instrument to support the validation of cut-points with different analytical methods. For instance, Ozemek et al. [42] suggested that activity counts were comparable to heart rate using %HRR at relative moderate (40% HRR) and vigorous (60% HRR) intensities but added that this depended on individual fitness levels. Two studies compared raw data and HR for sedentary activities and different intensity levels of physical activity and showed a strong correlation ($r = 0.97$) [43] and excellent agreement (receiver operating characteristic area under the curve = 0.99) [44]. Thus, measures of indirect calorimetry or HR monitoring can be comparable to intensity assessed using cut-points of activity counts. We found that a 1-s epoch length in conjunction with a hip-worn monitor was the most similar to HR-derived measures and should be the most accurate method for measuring sedentary and various physical activity intensity levels in an exergaming setting.

We should note some important limitations to our results. Based on our statistical methods, we cannot determine the better of the two monitors we tested, but either of the two models of activity monitors can be used interchangeably on the hip placement site. Although hip-worn monitors seemed to be more appropriate for assessing step counts as well as physical activity intensity levels, we cannot generalize our results to other physical activity conditions or other activity monitor brands. Further, even though we demonstrated that a 1-s epoch would be the most appropriate epoch length for detecting short bursts of intense physical activity, it is unclear how an estimate of sedentary and physical activity intensity levels can be comparable to objective measures of energy expenditure [45]. Thus, the fact that we did not use an indirect calorimetry technique as a criterion measure for physical activity intensity [46] may be considered a limitation and therefore may require further investigation.

5. Conclusions

We demonstrated that the activity monitors we used are valid and reliable devices for step-counting accuracy when placed on the hip, and that the hip compared to the wrist is also a more appropriate placement site for accurately measuring levels of physical activity intensity. We suggest that a 1-s epoch is the best choice for data processing and analysis of activity counts for the activity monitors we used in the present study for physical activity assessment. We further recommend that heart rate can be used as a comparator for the validation of cut-points from activity counts. Our findings are applicable in other clinical, research, or school settings focusing on intermittent physical activities similar to exergaming.

Supplementary Materials: The following are available online at http://www.mdpi.com/2077-0383/7/9/268/s1, Figure S1: Orientation of GT9X and wGT3X, Table S1: Time spent on sedentary and physical activity intensity levels in epochs, Table S2: Sedentary and physical activity levels between heart rate and activity counts in epochs with two activity cut-point sets, Table S3: Sedentary and physical activity levels between heart rate and activity counts in epochs with two activity cut-point sets and two activity monitors.

Author Contributions: Conceptualization, J.H. and A.S.L.; Methodology, J.H.; Validation, J.H.; Formal Analysis, J.H.; Investigation, J.H.; Resources, A.S.L.; Data Curation, A.M.F and J.H.; Writing—Original Draft Preparation, J.H.; Writing—Review & Editing, J.H. and A.S.L.; Visualization, J.H.; Supervision, J.H. and A.S.L.; Project Administration, J.H. and A.S.L.; Funding Acquisition, A.S.L.

Funding: This work was supported in part by funding from the National Institute of Diabetes and Digestive and Kidney Diseases (1R01DK109316), The narrative effect of active video games on long-term moderate-to-vigorous physical activity, PI: Amy Shirong Lu.

Acknowledgments: The authors thank the Health Technology Laboratory members, including Mie Hashimoto, MPH, Carlos Andres Hoyos-Cespedes, MPH, Harley Danielle Edge, and Samantha Gutiérrez-Arango for their help with data collection.

Conflicts of Interest: The authors declare no conflict of interest.

References

1. Yang, C.C.; Hsu, Y.L. A review of accelerometry-based wearable motion detectors for physical activity monitoring. *Sensors* **2010**, *10*, 7772–7788. [CrossRef] [PubMed]
2. Migueles, J.H.; Cadenas-Sanchez, C.; Ekelund, U.; Delisle Nystrom, C.; Mora-Gonzalez, J.; Lof, M.; Labayen, I.; Ruiz, J.R.; Ortega, F.B. Accelerometer data collection and processing criteria to assess physical activity and other outcomes: A systematic review and practical considerations. *Sports Med.* **2017**, *47*, 1821–1845. [CrossRef] [PubMed]
3. Troiano, R.P.; Berrigan, D.; Dodd, K.W.; Masse, L.C.; Tilert, T.; McDowell, M. Physical activity in the united states measured by accelerometer. *Med. Sci. Sports Exerc.* **2008**, *40*, 181–188. [CrossRef] [PubMed]
4. Sasaki, J.E.; John, D.; Freedson, P.S. Validation and comparison of actigraph activity monitors. *J. Sci. Med. Sport* **2011**, *14*, 411–416. [CrossRef] [PubMed]

5. Matthews, C.E.; Keadle, S.K.; Troiano, R.P.; Kahle, L.; Koster, A.; Brychta, R.; Van Domelen, D.; Caserotti, P.; Chen, K.Y.; Harris, T.B.; et al. Accelerometer-measured dose-response for physical activity, sedentary time, and mortality in us adults. *Am. J. Clin. Nutr.* **2016**, *104*, 1424–1432. [CrossRef] [PubMed]
6. Troiano, R.P.; McClain, J.J.; Brychta, R.J.; Chen, K.Y. Evolution of accelerometer methods for physical activity research. *Br. J. Sports Med.* **2014**, *48*, 1019–1023. [CrossRef] [PubMed]
7. Bassett, D.R., Jr.; Toth, L.P.; LaMunion, S.R.; Crouter, S.E. Step counting: A review of measurement considerations and health-related applications. *Sports Med.* **2017**, *47*, 1303–1315. [CrossRef] [PubMed]
8. Hwang, J.; Lu, A.S. Narrative and active video game in separate and additive effects of physical activity and cognitive function among young adults. *Sci. Rep.* **2018**, *8*, 11020. [CrossRef] [PubMed]
9. Sween, J.; Wallington, S.F.; Sheppard, V.; Taylor, T.; Llanos, A.A.; Adams-Campbell, L.L. The role of exergaming in improving physical activity: A review. *J. Phys. Act. Health* **2014**, *11*, 864–870. [CrossRef] [PubMed]
10. Smallwood, S.R.; Morris, M.M.; Fallows, S.J.; Buckley, J.P. Physiologic responses and energy expenditure of kinect active video game play in schoolchildren. *Arch. Pediatr. Adolesc. Med.* **2012**, *166*, 1005–1009. [CrossRef] [PubMed]
11. Stanmore, E.; Stubbs, B.; Vancampfort, D.; De Bruin, E.D.; Firth, J. The effect of active video games on cognitive functioning in clinical and non-clinical populations: A meta-analysis of randomized controlled trials. *Neurosci. Biobehav. Rev.* **2017**, *78*, 34–43. [CrossRef] [PubMed]
12. Gao, Z.; Chen, S.; Pasco, D.; Pope, Z. A meta-analysis of active video games on health outcomes among children and adolescents. *Obes. Rev.* **2015**, *16*, 783–794. [CrossRef] [PubMed]
13. Leinonen, A.M.; Ahola, R.; Kulmala, J.; Hakonen, H.; Vaha-Ypya, H.; Herzig, K.H.; Auvinen, J.; Keinanen-Kiukaanniemi, S.; Sievanen, H.; Tammelin, T.H.; et al. Measuring physical activity in free-living conditions-comparison of three accelerometry-based methods. *Front. Physiol.* **2016**, *7*, 681. [CrossRef] [PubMed]
14. Pfister, T.; Matthews, C.E.; Wang, Q.; Kopciuk, K.A.; Courneya, K.; Friedenreich, C. Comparison of two accelerometers for measuring physical activity and sedentary behaviour. *BMJ Open Sport Exerc. Med.* **2017**, *3*, e000227. [CrossRef] [PubMed]
15. Tudor-Locke, C.; Barreira, T.V.; Schuna, J.M., Jr. Comparison of step outputs for waist and wrist accelerometer attachment sites. *Med. Sci. Sports Exerc.* **2015**, *47*, 839–842. [CrossRef] [PubMed]
16. Ellis, K.; Kerr, J.; Godbole, S.; Lanckriet, G.; Wing, D.; Marshall, S. A random forest classifier for the prediction of energy expenditure and type of physical activity from wrist and hip accelerometers. *Physiol. Meas.* **2014**, *35*, 2191–2203. [CrossRef] [PubMed]
17. Ozemek, C.; Kirschner, M.M.; Wilkerson, B.S.; Byun, W.; Kaminsky, L.A. Intermonitor reliability of the gt3x+ accelerometer at hip, wrist and ankle sites during activities of daily living. *Physiol. Meas.* **2014**, *35*, 129–138. [CrossRef] [PubMed]
18. Zeng, N.; Gao, X.; Liu, Y.; Lee, J.E.; Gao, Z. Reliability of using motion sensors to measure children's physical activity levels in exergaming. *J. Clin. Med.* **2018**, *7*, 100. [CrossRef] [PubMed]
19. Wijndaele, K.; Westgate, K.; Stephens, S.K.; Blair, S.N.; Bull, F.C.; Chastin, S.F.; Dunstan, D.W.; Ekelund, U.; Esliger, D.W.; Freedson, P.S.; et al. Utilization and harmonization of adult accelerometry data: Review and expert consensus. *Med. Sci. Sports Exerc.* **2015**, *47*, 2129–2139. [CrossRef] [PubMed]
20. Robusto, K.M.; Trost, S.G. Comparison of three generations of actigraph activity monitors in children and adolescents. *J. Sports Sci.* **2012**, *30*, 1429–1435. [CrossRef] [PubMed]
21. Montoye, A.H.K.; Nelson, M.B.; Bock, J.M.; Imboden, M.T.; Kaminsky, L.A.; Mackintosh, K.A.; McNarry, M.A.; Pfeiffer, K.A. Raw and count data comparability of hip-worn actigraph gt3x+ and link accelerometers. *Med. Sci. Sports Exerc.* **2018**, *50*, 1103–1112. [CrossRef] [PubMed]
22. John, D.; Morton, A.; Arguello, D.; Lyden, K.; Bassett, D. "What is a step?" Differences in how a step is detected among three popular activity monitors that have impacted physical activity research. *Sensors* **2018**, *18*, 1206. [CrossRef] [PubMed]
23. Kamada, M.; Shiroma, E.J.; Harris, T.B.; Lee, I.M. Comparison of physical activity assessed using hip- and wrist-worn accelerometers. *Gait Posture* **2016**, *44*, 23–28. [CrossRef] [PubMed]
24. Trost, S.G.; Loprinzi, P.D.; Moore, R.; Pfeiffer, K.A. Comparison of accelerometer cut points for predicting activity intensity in youth. *Med. Sci Sports Exerc.* **2011**, *43*, 1360–1368. [CrossRef] [PubMed]

25. Banda, J.A.; Haydel, K.F.; Davila, T.; Desai, M.; Bryson, S.; Haskell, W.L.; Matheson, D.; Robinson, T.N. Effects of varying epoch lengths, wear time algorithms, and activity cut-points on estimates of child sedentary behavior and physical activity from accelerometer data. *PLoS ONE* **2016**, *11*, e0150534. [CrossRef] [PubMed]
26. Edwardson, C.L.; Gorely, T. Epoch length and its effect on physical activity intensity. *Med. Sci Sports Exerc.* **2010**, *42*, 928–934. [CrossRef] [PubMed]
27. Nettlefold, L.; Naylor, P.J.; Warburton, D.E.; Bredin, S.S.; Race, D.; McKay, H.A. The influence of epoch length on physical activity patterns varies by child's activity level. *Res. Q. Exerc. Sport* **2016**, *87*, 110–123. [CrossRef] [PubMed]
28. Ayabe, M.; Kumahara, H.; Morimura, K.; Tanaka, H. Epoch length and the physical activity bout analysis: An accelerometry research issue. *BMC Res. Notes* **2013**, *6*, 20. [CrossRef] [PubMed]
29. Baquet, G.; Stratton, G.; Van Praagh, E.; Berthoin, S. Improving physical activity assessment in prepubertal children with high-frequency accelerometry monitoring: A methodological issue. *Prev. Med.* **2007**, *44*, 143–147. [CrossRef] [PubMed]
30. Garber, C.E.; Blissmer, B.; Deschenes, M.R.; Franklin, B.A.; Lamonte, M.J.; Lee, I.M.; Nieman, D.C.; Swain, D.P.; American College of Sports Medicine. American College of Sports Medicine position stand. Quantity and quality of exercise for developing and maintaining cardiorespiratory, musculoskeletal, and neuromotor fitness in apparently healthy adults: Guidance for prescribing exercise. *Med. Sci. Sports Exerc.* **2011**, *43*, 1334–1359. [CrossRef] [PubMed]
31. Rothney, M.P.; Brychta, R.J.; Meade, N.N.; Chen, K.Y.; Buchowski, M.S. Validation of the actigraph two-regression model for predicting energy expenditure. *Med. Sci. Sports Exerc.* **2010**, *42*, 1785–1792. [CrossRef] [PubMed]
32. Borg, G.A. Psychophysical bases of perceived exertion. *Med. Sci. Sports Exerc.* **1982**, *14*, 377–381. [CrossRef] [PubMed]
33. Kozey-Keadle, S.; Libertine, A.; Lyden, K.; Staudenmayer, J.; Freedson, P.S. Validation of wearable monitors for assessing sedentary behavior. *Med. Sci. Sports Exerc.* **2011**, *43*, 1561–1567. [CrossRef] [PubMed]
34. Tanaka, H.; Monahan, K.D.; Seals, D.R. Age-predicted maximal heart rate revisited. *J. Am. Coll. Cardiol.* **2001**, *37*, 153–156. [CrossRef]
35. Koo, T.K.; Li, M.Y. A guideline of selecting and reporting intraclass correlation coefficients for reliability research. *J. Chiropr. Med.* **2016**, *15*, 155–163. [CrossRef] [PubMed]
36. Giavarina, D. Understanding bland altman analysis. *Biochem. Med.* **2015**, *25*, 141–151. [CrossRef] [PubMed]
37. Cain, K.L.; Conway, T.L.; Adams, M.A.; Husak, L.E.; Sallis, J.F. Comparison of older and newer generations of actigraph accelerometers with the normal filter and the low frequency extension. *Int. J. Behav. Nutr. Phys. Act.* **2013**, *10*, 51. [CrossRef] [PubMed]
38. Feito, Y.; Hornbuckle, L.M.; Reid, L.A.; Crouter, S.E. Effect of actigraph's low frequency extension for estimating steps and physical activity intensity. *PLoS ONE* **2017**, *12*, e0188242. [CrossRef] [PubMed]
39. Brond, J.C.; Arvidsson, D. Sampling frequency affects the processing of actigraph raw acceleration data to activity counts. *J. Appl. Physiol.* **2016**, *120*, 362–369. [CrossRef] [PubMed]
40. Moholdt, T.; Weie, S.; Chorianopoulos, K.; Wang, A.I.; Hagen, K. Exergaming can be an innovative way of enjoyable high-intensity interval training. *BMJ Open Sport Exerc. Med.* **2017**, *3*, e000258. [CrossRef] [PubMed]
41. Santos-Lozano, A.; Santin-Medeiros, F.; Cardon, G.; Torres-Luque, G.; Bailon, R.; Bergmeir, C.; Ruiz, J.R.; Lucia, A.; Garatachea, N. Actigraph gt3x: Validation and determination of physical activity intensity cut points. *Int. J. Sports Med.* **2013**, *34*, 975–982. [CrossRef] [PubMed]
42. Ozemek, C.; Cochran, H.L.; Strath, S.J.; Byun, W.; Kaminsky, L.A. Estimating relative intensity using individualized accelerometer cutpoints: The importance of fitness level. *BMC Med. Res. Methodol.* **2013**, *13*, 53. [CrossRef] [PubMed]
43. Aittasalo, M.; Vaha-Ypya, H.; Vasankari, T.; Husu, P.; Jussila, A.M.; Sievanen, H. Mean amplitude deviation calculated from raw acceleration data: A novel method for classifying the intensity of adolescents' physical activity irrespective of accelerometer brand. *BMC Sports Sci. Med. Rehabil.* **2015**, *7*, 18. [CrossRef] [PubMed]
44. Vaha-Ypya, H.; Vasankari, T.; Husu, P.; Suni, J.; Sievanen, H. A universal, accurate intensity-based classification of different physical activities using raw data of accelerometer. *Clin. Physiol. Funct. Imaging* **2015**, *35*, 64–70. [CrossRef] [PubMed]

45. O'Neil, M.E.; Fragala-Pinkham, M.; Lennon, N.; George, A.; Forman, J.; Trost, S.G. Reliability and validity of objective measures of physical activity in youth with cerebral palsy who are ambulatory. *Phys. Ther.* **2016**, *96*, 37–45. [CrossRef] [PubMed]

46. Hwang, J.; Castelli, D.M.; Gonzalez-Lima, F. The positive cognitive impact of aerobic fitness is associated with peripheral inflammatory and brain-derived neurotrophic biomarkers in young adults. *Physiol. Behav.* **2017**, *179*, 75–89. [CrossRef] [PubMed]

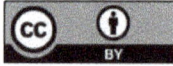

Journal of
Clinical Medicine

MDPI

Article

Impact of Exergaming on Children's Motor Skill Competence and Health-Related Fitness: A Quasi-Experimental Study

Sunyue Ye [1,2,*], Jung Eun Lee [3], David F. Stodden [4] and Zan Gao [5,*]

1   Department of Sports Rehabilitation, College of Physical Education, Longyan University,
    Longyan 364012, China
2   Chronic Disease Research Institute, School of Public Health, School of Medicine, Zhejiang University,
    Hangzhou 310058, China
3   Department of Applied Human Sciences, University of Minnesota, Duluth, MN 55812, USA;
    junelee@d.umn.edu
4   Department of Physical Education, University of South Carolina, Columbia, SC 29208, USA;
    stodden@mailbox.sc.edu
5   School of Kinesiology, University of Minnesota, Minneapolis, MN 55455, USA
*   Correspondence: syye@lyun.edu.cn (S.Y.); gaoz@umn.edu (Z.G.);
    Tel.: +86-135-881-15849 (S.Y.); +1-612-626-4639 (Z.G.)

Received: 23 July 2018; Accepted: 4 September 2018; Published: 7 September 2018

Abstract: This study was designed to examine the effectiveness of a combined exergaming and physical education (PE) program on children's motor skill competence (MSC) and health-related fitness (HRF) as compared to traditional PE. A total of 261 second- and third-grade children (127 boys; 8.25 ± 0.66 years for male; 8.29 ± 0.74 years for female; 73.6% non-Hispanic white) participated in the nine-month study from 2012 to 2013. Children were assigned to one of the two groups: (a) intervention group (125 min of alternating PE and exergaming weekly); and (b) comparison group (125-min weekly PE). MSC was assessed via product scores in two locomotor and two object control skills. HRF included the cardiorespiratory fitness, musculoskeletal fitness, and body mass index (BMI). A multivariate analysis of variance (MANOVA) was performed to analyze the effect of the combined exergaming–PE program on children's MSC and HRF. There were significant group by time interaction effects for BMI, $p < 0.01$, $\eta^2 = 0.20$; musculoskeletal fitness, $p < 0.01$, $\eta^2 = 0.13$; and object control skills (the comparison group demonstrating greater improvement), $p = 0.01$, $\eta^2 = 0.03$. The findings suggest that the combined exergaming program can have a positive effect on children's BMI and musculoskeletal fitness, indicating that exergaming can be an alternative school-based program to supplement traditional PE.

Keywords: active video games; cardiorespiratory fitness; locomotor skills; motor skill competence; musculoskeletal fitness; object control skills

---

1. Introduction

Secular declines in children's health-related fitness (HRF) is a growing concern globally [1–3] and places children at risk for many health issues, including cardiovascular diseases or metabolic syndrome [4], obesity [5], and lower health-related quality of life [6–8]. Similarly, inadequate levels of motor skill competence (MSC) are a concern among health professionals and physical educators [9,10] as the development of MSC is positively linked to children's HRF [11,12] and physical activity (PA) [12,13]. Specifically, competence in fundamental locomotor (e.g., jumping and hopping) and object control (e.g., throwing and kicking) skills is a prerequisite to the development of transitional movement skills [10]. MSC can be enhanced at an early age through targeted intervention, which also is beneficial for overall HRF [14].

Although a body of literature has shown traditional school-based PA programs or physical education (PE) courses can be effective in improving children's HRF [15] and MSC [16,17] in the short term, interventions with long-term sustainability are still needed [15]. To sustain development in children's MSC and HRF, it is critical to design an integrated and fun PA intervention that appeals to children [18]. Exergaming (a.k.a., active video games), a type of video games that requires bodily movement to play the video game, has been shown to increase children's light-to-moderate PA by capitalizing on their interests in games and maintaining PA enjoyment [9,19–21]. Exergaming is one of the innovative and fun ways to motivate children to be active and develop their motor skills [20–22]. For example, exergaming allows children of all skill levels to engage in sport games that they would not be able to unless they have the appropriate skill levels in traditional PE classes. This is also possible because in exergaming, children can still play without needing appropriate equipment for specific sports. A few studies have indicated that integrating exergaming into PE classes contributes to higher levels of children's PA and energy expenditure in both the short- and long-term, possibly due to its fun components [23–26]. While exergaming is an effective means to promote children's PA, evidence on school-based exergaming interventions to promote MSC is lacking [23,27].

Recent studies demonstrated that exergaming has an inconsistent impact on children's MSC in the short term [28,29]. Zeng and Gao, in 2016, concluded in a systematic review that studies that prove exergaming can offer sufficient stimulus for MSC changes were still limited [30]. Moreover, most of these studies examined balance skills or postural stability, with very few addressing the two important categories of MSC in young children [30–32]. Furthermore, no studies have explored the combined effects of exergaming and PE on young children's MSC and HRF across a nine-month school-based intervention. Therefore, this quasi-experimental study was designed to examine the effectiveness of school-based exergaming integration with traditional PE on children's MSC and HRF compared to traditional PE.

2. Materials and Methods

2.1. Participants and Research Setting

A total of 261 second- and third-grade children (8.27 ± 0.70 years; 134 girls; 73.6% non-Hispanic white) from two public elementary schools in southern USA participated in this study across the school year. Due to administrative and logistical reasons, randomization of individual children into either the intervention group or the comparison group was not feasible. Hence, one school served as the intervention school with the other serving as the comparison group. Both public schools were Title I schools (i.e., more than 50% children receive free or reduced-price school meals) in the same school district and were similar in their demographics. The majority of children were from low-income families. Other detailed information about the participants and research setting can be found in a recently published paper [23]. The inclusion criteria for this study were children who were (1) enrolled in a public Title I elementary school; (2) aged 7–9 years; (3) without a diagnosed physical or mental disability according to school records; and (4) able to provide parental consent and child assent. The eligibility of inclusion was verified through demographic information and student records in the schools.

In the intervention school, the exergaming program was integrated into the school's PE curriculum in such a way that exergaming and PE days alternated each week for a combined total of 125 min of biweekly PA; that is, out of 5 days of 25 min classes every two weeks, children's schedules alternated having 3 PE classes in one week and 2 exergaming sessions the following week (Figure 1). A certified PE teacher taught PE and a full-time teacher, trained by the research team, coordinated and supervised children in the exergaming room (i.e., a modified classroom) at the school. In the comparison school, children had 125 min (25 min per class) of PE every two weeks taught by 2 certified teachers. Participants were recruited from 16 classes (average of ≈20 students per class) at the schools, with 8 classes from each school site. The study was approved by the University Institutional Review Board and parental consent and child assent were obtained.

2.2. Procedures

In the intervention school, 12 stations (costing approximately 600 US dollars per station), each equipped with 2 exergaming systems including Wii (Nintendo Co., Ltd., Kyoto, Japan) and Xbox Kinect (Microsoft Corp., Redmond, WA, USA) and a television, were installed in a classroom. Examples of the types of exergaming included were Kinect Ultimate Sports, Just Dance, Wii Sports, and Wii Fit. The variety of games allowed for autonomy in selection and promoted persistent motivation throughout the whole intervention period. A trained teacher supervised their participation of exergaming. Depending on the type of game, either all children participated in an exergaming session simultaneously (i.e., two children/station) or all children participated in one activity (e.g., Just Dance). Children rotated games twice during each session. During PE classes at both schools, a conventional multiactivity curriculum was promoted that mainly included sport- or game-based units and fitness activities [33].

2.3. Measures

Participants demographic information including age and gender was collected using an information sheet filled in by students, with assistance from research staff before intervention.

MSC assessments included performance on four skills (kicking, throwing, standing long jump, and hopping) based on our and other experts' studies [34–38]. We used performance scores of skills to measure children's MSC because the measures are sensitive in discriminating children's competence levels across childhood and align with validated process-oriented assessments of motor skills [34–37]. The maximum speed for kicking (20-cm diameter playground balls) and throwing (using tennis balls) and maximum standing long jump distance were assessed from a total of five trials and used for analysis [38]. Throwing and kicking speed was measured using a radar gun (Stalker Radar, Plano, TX) [38]. For hopping, the average height of a minimum of three hops for each leg was used for analysis [35]. Both standing long jump and hopping performance were calculated based on children's standing height [34,35]. The reliability of these tests (alpha coefficient method) were r = 0.70 ($p < 0.01$) according to a previous study [10].

Cardiorespiratory fitness and musculoskeletal fitness components of children's HRF was measured using the *FITNESSGRAM®*. Trained research staff implemented *FITNESSGRAM®* protocols for the Progressive Aerobic Cardiovascular Endurance Run (PACER), curl-ups, and push-ups [38]. Grip strength was also assessed using a children's grip dynamometer (Lafayette Instrument, Lafayette IN) as an additional indicator of musculoskeletal fitness [39]. The best score of three trials for each hand was averaged and used for data analysis [23]. To assess body composition component of HRF, children's body mass index (BMI) was calculated as the weight in kilograms divided by the height in meters squared. Children's body height and weight were measured using a stadiometer (Seca GmbH, Hamburg, Germany) and digital weight scale (Detecto, Web City, MO, USA), respectively. The validity and reliability of all of these measures have been noted in previous studies [34,35,38–40]. Baseline MSC and HRF tests were measured in September of 2012 and post-tests were conducted in May of 2013.

2.4. Data Analysis

The demographic characteristics of participants were described through a descriptive analysis. Missing data of one or some indices of MSC and HRF were imputed by the expectation maximization (EM) method, although participants with missing data for all indices were excluded. All indices of MSC and HRF scores were normalized and then converted to standard T-scores (T-score = 50 + 10 * Z-score). Performance scores for the MSC tests were grouped according to locomotor and object control separately. The locomotor skill score was the mean T-scores for both standing long jump and hopping, while object control skill score was defined as the mean score of kicking and throwing T-scores. In regard to HRF, the musculoskeletal fitness score was calculated as the mean of the T-scores of grip strength, push-ups, and curl-ups.

T-tests and paired T-tests were conducted to observe any differences in all variables of interest between the comparison and intervention groups and between the pre- and post-intervention tests, respectively. Since there were significant between-group differences in baseline scores of PACER (higher in comparison group) and BMI (higher in intervention group), as well as curl-up (higher in comparison group), the difference in scores between pre- and post-tests for each variable were set as the outcome variable. In order to explore the effects of intervention on children's MSC and HRF over time, a multivariate analysis of variance (MANOVA) was conducted. All descriptive and inferential statistical analyses were conducted using SPSS 20.0 (IBM Corp., Armonk, NY, USA) and the significance level was set at 0.05 for all statistical analyses.

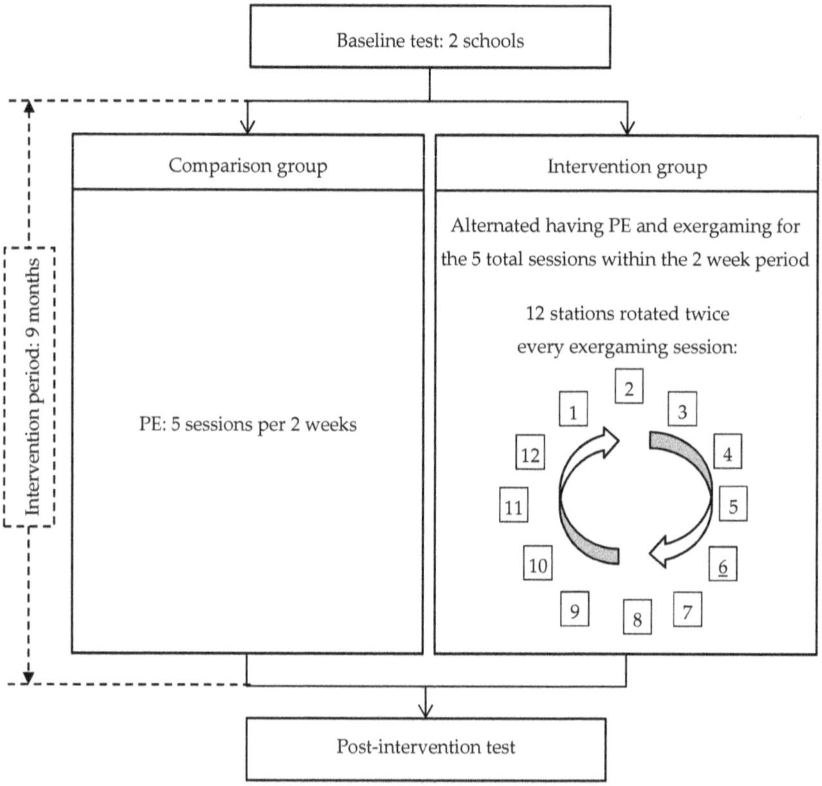

Figure 1. Study design and intervention flow.

3. Results

Eleven children were removed from the study from pre-test to post-test due to missing data for all indices of MSC and HRF ($n = 10$) or being an outlier ($n = 1$). Baseline demographic characteristics of participants are shown in Table 1. Children's mean age was 8.27 years, and 75% of the sample was non-Hispanic white. The intervention effects on children's MSC and HRF are described in Table 2. Significant group by time interaction effects were revealed for HRF and MSC variables including: musculoskeletal fitness, $F (1, 250) = 38.33$, $p < 0.01$, $\eta^2 = 0.13$; BMI, $F (1, 250) = 61.39$, $p < 0.01$, $\eta^2 = 0.20$; and object control skills, $F (1, 250) = 6.77$, $p = 0.01$, $\eta^2 = 0.03$. While children in the comparison group displayed significantly higher cardiorespiratory fitness scores (PACER) than children in the intervention group at both baseline and post-tests ($p < 0.01$), the comparison and intervention groups both demonstrated increase over time in their cardiorespiratory fitness ($p < 0.01$). Likewise, the decline in intervention children's BMI demonstrated a significant difference from the increased BMI in the comparison group. In addition, the between-group difference in the change scores of children's musculoskeletal fitness was significant, favoring the intervention group.

Table 1. Demographic characteristics of participants in baseline and post-intervention.

Variables *	Baseline			Post-Intervention		
	Comparison (n = 115)	Intervention (n = 135)	p Value [‡]	Comparison (n = 115)	Intervention (n = 135)	p Value [‡]
Age (years)	8.41 (0.71)	8.14 (0.67)	0.002	/	/	/
Girls (counts) [†]	59 (51.3)	70 (51.9)	0.931	/	/	/
White American (counts) [†]	69 (60.0)	118 (87.4)	<0.001	/	/	/
Height (cm)	131.77 (7.59)	129.46 (6.83)	0.012	132.73 (7.24)	132.80 (7.19)	0.942
Weight (kg)	30.77 (9.12)	31.69 (8.69)	0.417	33.73 (9.65)	32.95 (9.72)	0.524
Motor skill competence						
Kicking (m/s)	10.95 (1.79)	11.06 (2.46)	0.691	12.06 (1.87)	11.84 (1.92)	0.360
Throwing (m/s)	14.10 (3.82)	14.55 (3.35)	0.317	14.74 (3.87)	14.48 (3.69)	0.586
Standing long jump (%)	0.93 (0.15)	0.93 (0.17)	0.979	0.93 (0.15)	0.91 (0.17)	0.390
Hops (%)	0.64 (0.12)	0.62 (0.14)	0.190	0.67 (0.12)	0.70 (0.14)	0.124
Health-related fitness						
PACER (laps)	22.92 (11.15)	14.04 (7.08)	<0.001	26.87 (13.24)	20.67 (9.30)	<0.001
Grip strength (kg)	13.90 (2.96)	14.50 (3.48)	0.143	12.86 (3.66)	16.22 (4.01)	<0.001
Push-ups (counts)	7.47 (6.26)	6.24 (6.07)	0.116	9.32 (6.47)	8.65 (6.23)	0.409
Curl-ups (counts)	34.60 (26.57)	23.49 (21.86)	<0.001	18.58 (18.93)	21.33 (19.65)	0.262
BMI (kg/cm^2)	17.60 (3.78)	18.72 (3.67)	0.019	18.88 (3.89)	18.42 (3.87)	0.346

Note: * All values are the mean, with standard deviation in brackets; [†] Frequencies (percentage); [‡] Student's T-test for continuous variables and chi-squared test for categorical variables; Standing long jump (%): standing long jump (cm) divided by body height (cm); Hops (%): hops (cm) divided by body height (cm); PACER: progressive aerobic cardiovascular endurance run; BMI: body mass index.

Table 2. Baseline and post-intervention motor skill competence and health-related fitness descriptive and inferential statistics.

Tests	Conditions	Baseline T-Scored Mean (SD)	Post-Test T-Scored Mean (SD)	Diff. Mean (SD)	F	p	η^2
MSC							
Locomotor	Intervention (n = 135)	49.34 (7.23)	50.11 (7.21)	0.77 (4.64)	1.03	0.311	0.00
	Comparison (n = 115)	49.77 (6.68)	49.98 (6.68)	0.20 (4.16)			
Object control	Intervention (n = 135)	49.02 (9.21)	50.87 [‡] (9.01)	1.85 (5.51)	6.77	0.010	0.03
	Comparison (n = 115)	48.20 (8.45)	51.73 [‡] (8.66)	3.54 (4.59)			
HRF							
PACER	Intervention (n = 135)	44.23 [†] (6.33)	49.00 [‡] (8.56)	4.77 (6.40)	1.77	0.184	0.01
	Comparison (n = 115)	52.21 (9.95)	55.69 [‡] (11.84)	3.48 (8.93)			
Musculoskeletal fitness	Intervention (n = 135)	49.37 (6.74)	51.25 [‡] (7.08)	1.88 (5.19)	38.33	<0.001	0.13
	Comparison (n = 115)	50.83 (7.64)	48.30 [‡] (6.08)	−2.53 (6.08)			
Body mass index	Intervention (n = 135)	50.81 * (9.76)	50.01 [†] (10.31)	−0.80 (4.33)	61.39	<0.001	0.20
	Comparison (n = 115)	47.83 (10.06)	51.24 [‡] (10.35)	3.41 (4.12)			

Note: Musculoskeletal fitness: represents the compiled score for grip strength, curl-ups, and push-ups tests; SD: standard deviation; MSC: motor skill competence; Locomotor: combining standing long jump and hops; Object control: combining kicking and throwing; HRF: health-related fitness; PACER: progressive aerobic cardiovascular endurance run; Musculoskeletal fitness: combining grip strength, push-ups, and curl-ups; Diff.: difference between the baseline and post-test. T test was conducted to observe the difference between comparison and intervention groups at the baseline. * $p < 0.05$ compared with comparison group; [†] $p < 0.01$ compared with comparison group; [‡] $p < 0.01$ compared with baseline.

In terms of children's MSC, significant improvement effects over time were revealed in children's object control skills in both the intervention and comparison groups ($p < 0.01$), with the comparison group demonstrating greater improvement, $F (1, 250) = 6.77$, $p = 0.01$, $\eta^2 = 0.03$, compared to the intervention group. Slight improvement in the locomotor skills of children was observed in the intervention and comparison groups over time; however, these changes in score were not significant.

4. Discussion

As an innovative technology and potential tool for capturing and maintaining children's interest and motivation to be physically active and fit [41], exergaming has been integrated into a traditional PE curriculum within the school day [24,25]. However, the impact of exergaming on children's motor skills is not well understood. Our findings indicate that an integrated school-based exergaming/PE program demonstrated greater overall positive benefits on children's muscle strength and BMI, compared to traditional PE only. This impact on fitness may be due to: (1) more light and moderate PA in exergaming compared to fitness activities offered in PE classes, which could lead to body weight improvement in children [42], and (2) specificity of fitness exergames (i.e., Wii Fit and Just Dance) offered in the intervention group, which can improve children's some musculoskeletal fitness. Playing games from the Wii system may have improved children's grip strength through use of the controllers [43]. Previous evidence has illustrated controversy on the notion that exergaming provides sufficient PA intensity to improve children's HRF [19]. Specifically, some literature did not support the capability of exergaming to improve children's physical fitness or to provide health benefits [19,27,44,45], while other literature suggests exergaming can promote health benefits associated with maintenance of weight status and increased cardiorespiratory fitness [46,47]. The inconsistent findings might be owed to the setting in which exergames were played (e.g., laboratory, home, or school), types of the games, duration/dose, and intervention fidelity [48–50]. Previous studies have shown that the following factors are important in enhancing children's motivation, ultimately leading to appropriate improvement in their HRF: (a) presence of the supervision of specialist teachers; (b) appropriate organization behavior management; and (c) including a variety of PA programs [16,51,52]. Thus, we speculate that adequate supervision and consistent incorporation of different types of exergames offered to children led to greater increases in musculoskeletal fitness, as most of the previous relevant studies have intervened through only one type of exergame [20,49,53,54].

Our findings in children's MSC only partially supported the other portion of our hypothesis. When examining locomotor skills data, there was no significant difference in changes of score between the comparison and the intervention group, suggesting little impact of exergames on children's hopping and standing long jump. While the comparison group demonstrated significantly greater improvement in object control skills as compared to the intervention group across the school year, the effect size was small ($\eta^2 = 0.03$). The significant increase in object control skills in the traditional PE groups may be indicative of having more overall time spent in performing object control skills in a more ecologically valid setting (e.g., more time spent in PE). Specifically, no Wii or Xbox games provide opportunities for actual kicking and throwing activities. Games noted within exergaming games (e.g., Wii Sports and Kinect Ultimate Sports) do not necessarily demand that individuals demonstrate their highest level of throwing (e.g., primarily using elbow extension and wrist flexion in the Wii baseball game). Thus, the virtual games promoted in exergaming may not demand the same type of movement execution and effort to promote skill development to the same degree as traditional practice experiences.

In the present study, kicking skills of children in the intervention group increased over time; however, their standing long jump decreased at the end of the program. It appears that development of the standing long jump (locomotor skills) through semi-structured exergaming is more challenging than acquiring kicking skills (object control skills). Indeed, in two recent studies [31,55], similar findings were shown. The researchers tested the efficacy of six 50-min sessions of active video games (AVGs) on 6–10-year-olds' actual and perceived objective motor skills. Not only did they not find any significant differences between the control and intervention groups on both outcomes, they also did not find any improvement in the skills between typically developing children and children with autism spectrum disorder. The authors suggested that the play nature of AVGs may not provide adequate practice of the correct movements that are required to perform the skills [31,55]. Similarly, Pedersen et al., in their study in which they examined the effects of 30-min Nintendo Wii tennis games in improving reaction time for contralateral arm movement in children aged 7–12 years, revealed that these short bouts of exergaming sessions did not enhance children's motor processing speed (reaction time) [56]. Reaction time may not be directly related to the performance of object control skills measured in the current study; however, it is a good indicator of how children's object control skills would be applied in more advanced sport skill settings.

On the contrary, other studies have shown that the use of exergaming could be a feasible and pleasant approach to improve elementary school or nontypically-developing children's gross motor skills [32,57]. In one of these studies, an eight-week long exergaming intervention was found effective in improving children's object control skills. In this case, however, the effectiveness of the intervention in enhancing the skills was due to the selection and implementation of exergames (i.e., Baseball mini games; NBA Baller Beats, Bowling, and Soccer mini games; Xbox Kinect) that were specifically geared toward developing the same six objective control skills, namely throwing, kicking, catching, dribbling, rolling, and striking. Based on these findings of previous literature, we speculate that the lack of games that would provide opportunities for children to practice throwing and kicking skills could have been one of the reasons why we did not observe improvement in object control skills in the current study.

Another important point to note may be the quality of play, to which Howie and her colleagues attributed the ineffectiveness of an exergaming (Xbox 360 with Kinect) intervention on children's motor coordination (MABC-2) [58]. In this home-based exergaming intervention study for the clinical pediatric population, the authors mention motivation–outcome trade-off, which describes how self-selected games may increase children's motivation to play longer, but not necessarily the quality of play that leads to motor skill improvement. The study suggests the importance of finding a challenging point for each individual and adhering to the game to experience motor skill improvement, instead of switching games that they favor. We speculate that this may be very much aligned to our findings in current study. Children in this present study could have played longer and at higher intensities to increase their HRF; however, not at high enough quality to contribute to improvement in object control skills.

In our previous study, in which we examined the effect of an exergaming program in increasing children's PA, we did not see any significant increase in their PA levels [23]. However, significant exergaming effects on children's HRF were observed in our current study. It is plausible that these inconsistent results between the two studies are due to several possible reasons. First, measurement of children's PA was limited to school time, not whole days (24 h), which could not reflect actual total levels of daily PA. Second, increase in children's HRF may not be due to total PA levels, but more due to other factors such as dietary intake, basic metabolic rate, and intensity of exercise. Third, it is possible that exergaming had a beneficial effect in current study because it was combined with PE. In this case, PE can provide opportunities that exergaming cannot offer and lead to greater effects of intervention than the effects that would be brought by PE or exergaming alone. However, further studies are warranted to explore the potential interactions.

This study was conducted in a real-world setting, examining the effects of a combination of exergaming and traditional PE, and including both HRF and MSC as outcome variables, which are the strengths of this study. However, the study is not without limitations. First, our study did not implement random recruitment or random assignment, which limits the generalizability. Second, it is also difficult to define the independent effect of exergaming on the outcomes as our intervention had both PE and exergaming sessions. Third, flexibility, which is one of the five HRF components, was not included in our HRF outcomes, and this study could improve by implementing a follow-up measurement to avoid potential seasonal effects on children's HRF/MSC and to explore the durability of children's interest in exergaming. Moreover, children in our study could have been exposed to a "Hawthorne Effect", as teachers and research assistants were observing them at the time of testing. Children could have modified their behavior (e.g., making much more effort in physical activity) in response to their awareness of being observed or intervened. In addition, there might have been some motivational issues in children in the comparison group at the curl-ups testing, as the post-test score plummeted from the baseline. Examining our data, a good number of children who scored high in the baseline did not do as well in their post-test, which might have influenced the overall musculoskeletal fitness score in the comparison group. Lastly, the information about energy expenditure was not collected during the exergaming and PE sessions.

5. Conclusions

A well-implemented class combining exergaming and traditional PE can be beneficial in developing children's musculoskeletal fitness and BMI compared to the sole traditional PE class. Considering the potential benefits of exergaming in stimulating children's interest in PA and developing HRF [59], integration of an exergaming component into PE is partly recommended. However, when exergaming is implemented, several things should be taken into consideration. The structure of the exergaming may depend on the goal of the program, whether it be promotion of PA, enhancement of HRF, or/and improvement in MSC. If practitioners are in pursuit of children's MSC, the traditional PE classes may be a better choice than exergaming. Future studies with randomization and long-term design are needed to confirm our results.

Author Contributions: S.Y. and J.E.L. drafted the manuscript. Z.G. and D.F.S. designed and conducted the research and helped revise the manuscript. S.Y. analyzed data and had primary responsibility for the final content. All authors read and approved the final manuscript.

Funding: This study was funded by a grant from the National Institute of Child and Human Development (1R15HD071514-01A1) and China Postdoctoral Science Foundation (2017M621903).

Acknowledgments: The authors would like to thank the research assistants who helped with data collection and students and teachers who cooperated with data collection.

Conflicts of Interest: The authors declare no conflict of interest.

References

1. Roriz de Oliveira, M.S.; Seabra, A.; Garganta, R.; Ribeiro Maia, J.A. Decennial trend in passing rates of health-related physical fitness in children from Maia county, northern Portugal. *Ann. Hum. Biol.* **2012**, *39*, 453.
2. Albon, H.M.; Hamlin, M.J.; Ross, J.J. Secular trends and distributional changes in health and fitness performance variables of 10–14-year-old children in New Zealand between 1991 and 2003. *Br. J. Sport Med.* **2010**, *44*, 263–269. [CrossRef] [PubMed]
3. Zhu, Z.; Yang, Y.; Kong, Z.X.; Zhang, Y.M.; Zhuang, J. Prevalence of physical fitness in Chinese school-aged children: Findings from the 2016 physical activity and fitness in China-the Youth Study. *J. Sport Health Sci.* **2017**, *6*, 395–403. [CrossRef]
4. Smith, J.J.; Eather, N.; Morgan, P.J.; Plotnikoff, R.C.; Faigenbaum, A.D.; Lubans, D.R. The health benefits of muscular fitness for children and adolescents: A systematic review and meta-analysis. *Sports Med.* **2014**, *44*, 1209–1223. [CrossRef] [PubMed]
5. Casonatto, J.; Fernandes, R.A.; Batista, M.B.; Cyrino, E.S.; Coelho-e-Silva, M.J.; de Arruda, M.; Ronque, E.R.V. Association between health-related physical fitness and body mass index status in children. *J. Child Health Care* **2016**, *20*, 294–303. [CrossRef] [PubMed]
6. Gu, X.L.; Chang, M.; Solmon, M.A. Physical activity, physical fitness, and health-related quality of life in school-aged children. *J. Teach. Phys. Educ.* **2016**, *35*, 117–126. [CrossRef]
7. Venckunas, T.; Emeljanovas, A.; Mieziene, B.; Volbekiene, V. Secular trends in physical fitness and body size in Lithuanian children and adolescents between 1992 and 2012. *J. Epidemiol. Commun. Health* **2017**, *71*, 181–187. [CrossRef] [PubMed]
8. Dos Santos, F.K.; Prista, A.; Gomes, T.N.Q.F.; Daca, T.; Madeira, A.; Katzmarzyk, P.T.; Maia, J.A.R. Secular trends in physical fitness of Mozambican school-aged children and adolescents. *Am. J. Hum. Biol.* **2015**, *27*, 201–206. [CrossRef] [PubMed]

9. Soltani, P.; Vilas-Boas, J.P. Sport Exergames for physical education. In *Encyclopedia of Information Science and Technology*, 4th ed.; IGI Global: Calgary, AB, Canada, 2018; pp. 7358–7367.

10. Barnett, L.M.; Van Beurden, E.; Morgan, P.J.; Brooks, L.O.; Beard, J.R. Does childhood motor skill proficiency predict adolescent fitness? *Med. Sci. Sport Exerc.* **2008**, *40*, 2137–2144. [CrossRef] [PubMed]

11. Re, A.H.N.; Cattuzzo, M.T.; Santos, F.M.C.; Monteiro, C.B.M. Anthropometric characteristics, field test scores and match-related technical performance in youth indoor soccer players with different playing status. *Int. J. Perform. Anal. Sport* **2014**, *14*, 482–492.

12. Lima, R.A.; Pfeiffer, K.; Larsen, L.R.; Bugge, A.; Moller, N.C.; Anderson, L.B.; Stodden, D.F. Physical activity and motor competence present a positive reciprocal longitudinal relationship across childhood and early adolescence. *J. Phys. Act. Health* **2017**, *14*, 440–447. [CrossRef] [PubMed]

13. Haga, M.; Gisladottir, T.; Sigmundsson, H. The relationship between motor competence and physical fitness is weaker in the 15-16 yr. adolescent age group than in younger age groups (4–5 yr. and 11–12 yr.). *Percept. Mot. Skill* **2015**, *121*, 900–912. [CrossRef] [PubMed]

14. Wick, K.; Leeger-Aschmann, C.S.; Monn, N.D.; Radtke, T.; Ott, L.V.; Rebholz, C.E.; Cruz, S.; Gerber, N.; Schmutz, E.A.; Puder, J.J.; et al. Interventions to promote fundamental movement skills in childcare and kindergarten: A systematic review and meta-analysis. *Sports Med.* **2017**, *47*, 2045–2068. [CrossRef] [PubMed]

15. Lai, S.K.; Costigan, S.A.; Morgan, P.J.; Lubans, D.R.; Stodden, D.F.; Salmon, J.; Barnett, L.M. Do school-based interventions focusing on physical activity, fitness, or fundamental movement skill competency produce a sustained impact in these outcomes in children and adolescents? A systematic review of follow-up studies. *Sports Med.* **2014**, *44*, 67–79. [CrossRef] [PubMed]

16. Tompsett, C.; Sanders, R.; Taylor, C.; Cobley, S. Pedagogical approaches to and effects of fundamental movement skill interventions on health outcomes: A systematic review. *Sports Med.* **2017**, *47*, 1795–1819. [CrossRef] [PubMed]

17. Morgan, P.J.; Barnett, L.M.; Cliff, D.P.; Okely, A.D.; Scott, H.A.; Cohen, K.E.; Lubans, D.R. Fundamental movement skill interventions in youth: A systematic review and meta-analysis. *Pediatrics* **2013**, *132*, E1361–E1383. [CrossRef] [PubMed]

18. Butt, J.; Weinberg, R.S.; Breckon, J.D.; Claytor, R.P. Adolescent physical activity participation and motivational determinants across gender, age, and race. *J. Phys. Act. Health* **2011**, *8*, 1074–1083. [CrossRef] [PubMed]

19. Kari, T. Promoting physical activity and fitness with exergames: Updated systematic review of systematic reviews. In *Transforming Gaming and Computer Simulation Technologies across Industries*; IGI Global: Calgary, AB, Canada, 2017; pp. 225–245.

20. Chen, H.; Sun, H.C. Effects of active videogame and sports, play, and active recreation for kids physical education on children's health-related fitness and enjoyment. *Games Health J.* **2017**, *6*, 312–318. [CrossRef] [PubMed]

21. Pasco, D.; Roure, C.; Kermarrec, G.; Pope, Z.; Gao, Z. The effects of a bike active video game on players' physical activity and motivation. *J. Sport Health Sci.* **2017**, *6*, 25–32. [CrossRef]

22. Barnett, L.M.; Bangay, S.; McKenzie, S.; Ridgers, N.D. Active gaming as a mechanism to promote physical activity and fundamental movement skill in children. *Front. Public Health* **2013**, *1*, 74. [CrossRef] [PubMed]

23. Gao, Z.; Pope, Z.; Lee, J.E.; Stodden, D.; Roncesvalles, N.; Pasco, D.; Huang, C.C.; Feng, D. Impact of exergaming on young children's school day energy expenditure and moderate-to-vigorous physical activity levels. *J. Sport Health Sci.* **2017**, *6*, 11–16. [CrossRef]

24. Chukhlantseva, N. Integration of active videogames in physical training of school students. *Sci. Educ.* **2017**, *4*, 14–20. [CrossRef]

25. Arajuo, J.G.E.; Batista, C.; Moura, D.L. Exergames in physical education: A systematic review. *Movimento* **2017**, *23*, 529–542.

26. Staiano, A.E.; Beyl, R.A.; Hsia, D.S.; Katzmarzyk, P.T.; Newton, R.L. Twelve weeks of dance exergaming in overweight and obese adolescent girls: Transfer effects on physical activity, screen time, and self-efficacy. *J. Sport Health Sci.* **2017**, *6*, 4–10. [CrossRef] [PubMed]

27. Norris, E.; Hamer, M.; Stamatakis, E. Active video games in schools and effects on physical activity and health: A systematic review. *J. Pediatr.* **2016**, *172*, 40–46. [CrossRef] [PubMed]

28. Barnett, L.M.; Ridgers, N.D.; Reynolds, J.; Hanna, L.; Salmon, J. Playing active video games may not develop movement skills: An intervention trial. *Preve. Med. Rep.* **2015**, *2*, 673–678. [CrossRef] [PubMed]

29. Hulteen, R.M.; Johnson, T.M.; Ridgers, N.D.; Mellecker, R.R.; Barnett, L.M. Children's movement skills when playing active video games. *Percept. Mot. Skill* **2015**, *121*, 767–790. [CrossRef] [PubMed]
30. Zeng, N.; Gao, Z. Effects of exergaming on fundamental movement skills among children and young adults: A systematic review. In *Gaming: Trends, Perspectives and Impact on Health*; Nova Science Publishers: Hauppauge, NY, USA, 2016; pp. 41–58.
31. Edwards, J.; Jeffrey, S.; May, T.; Rinehart, N.J.; Barnett, L.M. Does playing a sports active video game improve object control skills of children with autism spectrum disorder? *J. Sport Health Sci.* **2017**, *6*, 17–24. [CrossRef]
32. Vernadakis, N.; Papastergiou, M.; Zetou, E.; Antoniou, P. The impact of an exergame-based intervention on children's fundamental motor skills. *Comput. Educ.* **2015**, *83*, 90–102. [CrossRef]
33. Metzler, M. *Instructional Models for Physical Education*; Holocomb Hathaway: Scottsdale, AZ, USA, 2005.
34. Lane, A.P.; Molina, S.L.; Tolleson, D.A.; Langendorfer, S.J.; Goodway, J.D.; Stodden, D.F. Developmental sequences for the standing long jump landing: A pre-longitudinal screening. *J. Mot. Learn. Dev.* **2018**, *6*, 114–129. [CrossRef]
35. Nesbitt, D.R.; Molina, S.; Sacko, R.; Robinson, L.; Brian, A.; Stodden, D.F. Examining the feasibility of supine-to-stand as a measure of functional motor competence. *J. Mot. Learn. Dev.* **2018**, in press. [CrossRef]
36. Stodden, D.F.; Langendorfer, S.J.; Fleisig, G.S.; Andrews, J.R. Kinematic constraints associated with the acquisition of overarm throwing part I: Step and trunk actions. *Res. Q. Exerc. Sport* **2006**, *77*, 417–427. [CrossRef] [PubMed]
37. Stodden, D.F.; Langendorfer, S.J.; Fleisig, G.S.; Andrews, J.R. Kinematic constraints associated with the acquisition of overarm throwing part II: Upper extremity actions. *Res. Q. Exerc. Sport* **2006**, *77*, 428–436. [CrossRef] [PubMed]
38. Stodden, D.F.; Gao, Z.; Goodway, J.D.; Langendorfer, S.J. Dynamic relationships between motor skill competence and health-related fitness in youth. *Pediatr. Exerc. Sci.* **2014**, *26*, 231–241. [CrossRef] [PubMed]
39. Pate, R.R.; Blimkie, C.; Castelli, D.; Corbin, C.B.; Daniels, S.R.; Kohl, H.W.; Malina, R.M.; Sacheck, J.; Stodden, D.F.; Whitt-Glover, M.; et al. Fitness measures and health outcomes in youth. In *Institute of Medicine*; Pillsbury, L., Oria, M., Pate, R., Eds.; National Academies Press: Washington, DC, USA, 2012.
40. Wind, A.E.; Takken, T.; Helders, P.J.M.; Engelbert, R.H.H. Is grip strength a predictor for total muscle strength in healthy children, adolescents, and young adults? *Eur. J. Pediatr.* **2010**, *169*, 281–287. [CrossRef] [PubMed]
41. Finco, M.D.; Reategui, E.; Zaro, M.A.; Sheehan, D.D.; Katz, L. Exergaming as an alternative for students unmotivated to participate in regular physical education classes. *IJGBL* **2015**, *5*, 1–10. [CrossRef]
42. Sween, J.; Wallington, S.F.; Sheppard, V.; Taylor, T.; Llanos, A.A.; Adams-Campbell, L.L. The role of exergaming in improving physical activity: A review. *J. Phys. Act. Health* **2014**, *11*, 864–870. [CrossRef] [PubMed]
43. Salem, Y.; Gropack, S.J.; Coffin, D.; Godwin, E.M. Effectiveness of a low-cost virtual reality system for children with developmental delay: A preliminary randomised single-blind controlled trial. *Physiotherapy* **2012**, *98*, 189–195. [CrossRef] [PubMed]
44. Gao, Z. Fight fire with fire? Promoting physical activity and health through active video games. *J. Sport Health Sci.* **2017**, *6*, 1–3. [CrossRef]
45. Gao, Z.; Zhang, T.; Stodden, D. Children's physical activity levels and psychological correlates in interactive dance versus aerobic dance. *J. Sport Health Sci.* **2013**, *2*, 146–151. [CrossRef]
46. Maddison, R.; Mhurchu, C.N.; Jull, A.; Prapavessis, H.; Foley, L.S.; Jiang, Y.N. Active video games: The mediating effect of aerobic fitness on body composition. *Int. J. Behav. Nutr. Phys.* **2012**, *9*, 54. [CrossRef] [PubMed]
47. Gao, Z.; Chen, S.; Pasco, D.; Pope, Z. A meta-analysis of active video games on health outcomes among children and adolescents. *Obes. Rev.* **2015**, *16*, 783–794. [CrossRef] [PubMed]
48. Christison, A.L.; Evans, T.A.; Bleess, B.B.; Wang, H.P.; Aldag, J.C.; Binns, H.J. Exergaming for health: A randomized study of community-based exergaming curriculum in pediatric weight management. *Games Health J.* **2016**, *5*, 413–421. [CrossRef] [PubMed]
49. Naugle, K.E.; Naugle, K.M.; Wikstrom, E.A. Cardiovascular and affective outcomes of active gaming: Using the Nintendo Wii as a cardiovascular training tool. *J. Strength Cond. Res.* **2014**, *28*, 443–451. [CrossRef] [PubMed]

50. Foley, L.; Jiang, Y.N.; Mhurchu, C.N.; Jull, A.; Prapavessis, H.; Rodgers, A.; Maddison, R. The effect of active video games by ethnicity, sex and fitness: Subgroup analysis from a randomised controlled trial. *Int. J. Behav. Nutr. Phys.* **2014**, *11*, 46. [CrossRef] [PubMed]

51. Hardy, L.L.; O'Hara, B.J.; Rogers, K.; St George, A.; Bauman, A. Contribution of organized and nonorganized activity to children's motor skills and fitness. *J. School Health* **2014**, *84*, 690–696. [CrossRef] [PubMed]

52. Laitakari, J.; Vuori, I.; Oja, P. Is long-term maintenance of health-related physical activity possible? An analysis of concepts and evidence. *Health Educ. Res.* **1996**, *11*, 463–477. [CrossRef] [PubMed]

53. Sabel, M.; Sjolund, A.; Broeren, J.; Arvidsson, D.; Saury, J.M.; Gillenstrand, J.; Emanuelson, I.; Blomgren, K.; Lannering, B. Effects of physically active video gaming on cognition and activities of daily living in childhood brain tumor survivors: A randomized pilot study. *Neuro-Oncol. Pract.* **2017**, *4*, 98–110. [CrossRef]

54. Gao, Z. Motivated but not active: The dilemmas of incorporating interactive dance into gym class. *J. Phys. Act. Health* **2012**, *9*, 794–800. [CrossRef] [PubMed]

55. Johnson, T.M.; Ridgers, N.D.; Hulteen, R.M.; Mellecker, R.R.; Barnett, L.M. Does playing a sports active video game improve young children's ball skill competence? *J. Sci. Med. Sport* **2016**, *19*, 432–436. [CrossRef] [PubMed]

56. Pedersen, S.J.; Cooley, P.D.; Cruickshank, V.J. Caution regarding exergames: A skill acquisition perspective. *Phys. Educ. Sport Pedagog.* **2017**, *22*, 246–256. [CrossRef]

57. Page, Z.E.; Barrington, S.; Edwards, J.; Barnett, L.M. Do active video games benefit the motor skill development of non-typically developing children and adolescents: A systematic review. *J. Sci. Med. Sport* **2017**, *20*, 1087–1100. [CrossRef] [PubMed]

58. Howie, E.K.; Campbell, A.C.; Abbott, R.A.; Straker, L.M. Understanding why an active video game intervention did not improve motor skill and physical activity in children with developmental coordination disorder: A quantity or quality issue? *Res. Dev. Disabil.* **2017**, *60*, 1–12. [CrossRef] [PubMed]

59. Baranowski, T. Exergaming: Hope for future physical activity? or blight on mankind? *J. Sport Health Sci.* **2017**, *6*, 44–46. [CrossRef]

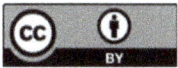

Journal of
Clinical Medicine

MDPI

Article

Association between Air Quality and Sedentary Time in 3270 Chinese Adults: Application of a Novel Technology for Posture Determination

Yiqun Ma [1], Bing Yuan [2], Shuhui Fan [1], Yizhou Luo [1] and Xu Wen [1,*]

[1] Department of Sport & Exercise Science, College of Education, Zhejiang University, Hangzhou 310028, China; mayiqun@zju.edu.cn (Y.M.); fsh1130@zju.edu.cn (S.F.); luoyizhou@zju.edu.cn (Y.L.)
[2] Information Technology Center, Zhejiang University, Hangzhou 310028, China; yuanbing@zju.edu.cn
* Correspondence: wenxu@zju.edu.cn; Tel.: +86-571-8827-3691

Received: 18 July 2018; Accepted: 2 September 2018; Published: 6 September 2018

Abstract: This study investigated the association between ambient air quality and sedentary time in Chinese adults. The participants were 3270 Chinese users (2021 men and 1249 women) of wrist-worn activity trackers. The data of participants' daily activities were collected from July 2015 to October 2015. A novel algorithm based on raw accelerometer data was employed to determine sedentary time. Personal data, including sex, age, weight and height, were self-reported by the participants. Data of air quality, ambient temperature and weather were collected from the data released by the China National Environmental Monitoring Centre and the China Central Meteorological Observatory and matched in accordance with the Global Positioning System and time information. Multilevel regression analyses were conducted to investigate the association between air quality and sedentary time and adjusted for gender, age, region, body mass index, weather, temperature, weekday/weekend and monitored wake time per day. Better air quality index levels and lower concentrations of fine particulate matter were significantly associated with approximately 20 and 45 min reduction in sedentary time, respectively. Poor air quality appears to be an independent factor associated with prolonged sedentary time in Chinese adults.

Keywords: sedentary behaviour; air quality; socio-ecological model; wrist-worn activity tracker

1. Introduction

Sedentary behaviour is defined as any waking behaviour with a sitting, reclining or lying posture that requires an energy expenditure ≤ 1.5 metabolic equivalents [1]. It is a distinct concept from physical inactivity, which refers to an insufficient physical activity level to meet the present physical activity recommendations [1]. Sufficient moderate- to vigorous-intensity physical activity (MVPA) means that an individual is not physically inactive but cannot guarantee the individual from accumulating a large amount of sedentary time. Several studies have reported that the negative health consequences of prolonged sedentary time may include obesity, type 2 diabetes and cardiovascular diseases (e.g., coronary heart disease, myocardial infarction and stroke) [2–4]. These consequences are suggested to be independent of those attributable to the lack of physical activity [5–7]. Moreover, strong evidence suggests that people who engage in high amounts of sedentary behaviour can be at increased risk of mortality regardless of their level of MVPA [6,8,9]. Although a study based on 155,054 Chinese adults showed that 81.3% of the men and 88.5% of the women were physically inactive [10], few studies have reported the sedentary time of Chinese adults. Therefore, given the limited data on sedentary behaviour in Chinese adults and the usually negative health consequences of sedentariness, investigations of sedentary time in China should be made, and correlates should be clarified to help design, tailor and evaluate sedentary behaviour interventions.

A socio-ecological model is widely applied in the conceptualisation of factors influencing sedentary behaviour [11–13]. This socio-ecological approach assumes that multiple levels of influence, including intrapersonal, interpersonal, organisational, environmental and policy, exist, thus emphasising the interrelationships between individuals and the social, physical and policy environments [13]. A large number of factors in the model, particularly individual correlates, have been verified by numerous empirical studies [12,14]. In terms of physical environmental factors, type of residence [15,16], density [17] and proximity [18] of green spaces; neighbourhood walkability [19,20]; and season [21] have been reported to be related to sedentary behaviour. To date, however, the associations between other physical environmental factors such as air quality with sedentary behaviour have not yet been sufficiently investigated.

Although air quality has generally improved in China, the current situation of air pollution in the country is still a cause for concern. In 2016, the annual mean concentration of fine particulate matter (PM$_{2.5}$) was 47 µg/m^3 [22], which is 14.8% higher than the Chinese primary standard (40 µg/m^3) [23] and 213.33% higher than the American secondary standard (15 µg/m^3) [24]. Although the detrimental impact of air pollution on human health has been universally proven [25,26], knowledge about its effect on health behaviour is limited.

Several studies have investigated the association between air pollution and physical inactivity. These studies have shown that poor air quality may lead to decreased physical activity. Using data from the Behavioural Risk Factor Surveillance System (BRFSS), Wen et al. examined the relationship between air quality index (AQI) media alerts and changes in outdoor activities amongst people with asthma and showed that media alerts may be associated with self-reported decreases in outdoor activities [27]. Two other cross-sectional studies based on data from the BRFSS indicated that increased levels of air pollution are related to reduced leisure-time physical activity amongst American adults [28,29]. This result was confirmed by a retrospective study in the United States, in which ambient PM$_{2.5}$ air pollution was observed to be associated with a modest but measurable increase in the leisure-time physical inactivity of individuals [30]. Similar findings amongst Chinese adults have been made. By analysing the data collected from 153 users of an exercise app and the AQI during the same period, Hu et al. concluded that people's participation in outdoor exercise was impeded by air pollution severity [31]. Cohort studies of university retirees [32] and university students [33] living in Beijing, China, also revealed the same conclusions.

Despite the abundant literature concerning the relationship between air quality and decreased physical activity, we only found one empirical study involving the association between air quality and sedentary behaviour. In a population-based mail survey of 1332 Australian adults, researchers examined the associations between physical activity and sedentary behaviour with multiple individual-level and environmental-level variables; one of their findings was that air pollution was significantly associated with increased sedentary time [34].

Considerable attention has been paid on the measurement of sedentary behaviour. Subjective methods, including self-report or proxy-report questionnaire, are widely applied in studies of sedentary behaviour; however, the validity and reliability of these responses are subject to recall error and social desirability bias [35]. For objective methods, accelerometers can be used to estimate the total time and breaks of sedentary behaviour [36], which are based on movement detection but are traditionally considered to be poorly able to distinguish amongst different postures, therefore misestimating the real sedentary time [37]. Accelerometers are also typically hip-worn devices, which leads to lower wear compliance than wrist-worn devices [38]. Sedentary Sphere, a novel algorithm, was developed to analyse data from wrist-worn triaxial accelerometers and determine postures, leading to better compliance in large samples [39]. By using the method, the direction of the activity monitor and the wrist position could be determined based on the gravitational component of the acceleration data. In brief, posture is determined according to the angle of arm elevation and the intensity of activities. For instance, if arm elevation is higher than 15° below the horizontal position and the intensity of activity is light or moderate, the data indicate a seated or reclining position and could be identified as sedentary behaviours. This method was found to be valid in measuring sedentary time [40]. Moreover, as Sedentary Sphere is mainly based on the direction of the gravity component rather than the magnitude of accelerations, it could be applied to estimate sedentary time with different brands of wrist-worn accelerometers in different studies [41]. In addition, the cost of commercial activity monitors with Sedentary Sphere is lower than that of professional monitors, such as activPAL, therefore allowing a relatively larger sample size.

In the present study, a popular brand of activity tracker named Bong II (which is a light, convenient and wrist-worn triaxial accelerometer with Sedentary Sphere algorithm) was used to determine whether the sedentary time of Chinese adults is associated with ambient air quality. We hypothesised that people would spend more sedentary time in days with bad air quality than in days with good air quality.

2. Methods

2.1. Participants

In this study, researchers contacted several manufacturers of wrist-worn accelerometers, introduced the research plan and sought for research cooperation. Hangzhou Gongke Technology Co., Ltd., the manufacturer of the Bong II accelerometer, agreed to participate. With the assistance of the manufacturer, an informed consent form that introduced the objective and content of the research as well as the benefits of participating in the study was sent to approximately 20,000 customers via the Internet. The participants would receive a personal sedentary behaviour report for free. Only users who endorsed the informed consent form were recruited to this study. The data were collected from the Bong II activity monitors and transmitted to the company via the Internet. Personal information, including age, sex, height and weight, was self-reported on the App of Bong II by participants when they first used the product. Researchers were unable to access the data until privacy information (name, address, telephone number, email, etc.) of participants was deleted.

A total of 4604 Chinese users of Bong II were recruited. The data of participants' daily activities were collected from July 2015 to October 2015. The inclusion criteria were as follows: (1) participants aged 18 years or older; (2) wearing time ≥18 h/day; (3) wear duration ≥4 consecutive days; and (4) data of Global Positioning System (GPS) and air quality are available. The data of 3270 participants were finally included in the analysis. Figure 1 shows the number of participants in each province. The abbreviated names of provinces are in accordance to the authority file released by the Ministry of Industry and Information Technology of China [42]. The research protocol was reviewed and approved by the Ethics Committee of College of Education at Zhejiang University.

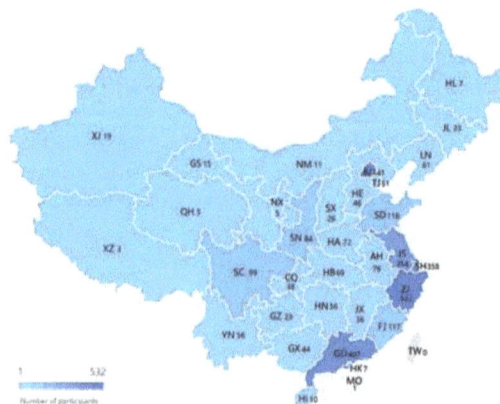

Figure 1. Distribution of participants.

2.2. Measurement of Sedentary Behaviour

The sedentary time was measured using Bong II. It is 14 g in weight, 4 cm in length, 2 cm in width and 0.9 cm in thickness; it has an adjustable wristband and will not interfere with the participants' activities. The product is waterproof, and the participants were encouraged to wear it on the nondominant wrist for 24 h a day. The price of Bong II is approximately 20 dollars.

The monitor has a triaxial accelerometer with a sampling frequency of 100 Hz and an output data rate of 1 to 15 s epoch based on the type of activities. The Bong software 2.0 was used to convert the raw 100 Hz files to 15 s epoch files containing x, y and z vectors (mean acceleration over the epoch, retaining the gravity vector) and vector magnitude values (summed over the epoch, corrected for gravity).

The algorithm applied in this study came from Sedentary Sphere, the efficacy of which has been proven valid and reliable for the classification of posture from a wrist-worn triaxial accelerometer in adults [39,41]. The details of the method were mentioned in previous studies [39,41]. Briefly, Sedentary Sphere follows a principle based on arm elevation to identify postures. If the data plotted on Sedentary Sphere in latitudes of elevation are greater than 15° below the horizontal position, this finding indicates that the wrist is elevated. Meanwhile, if the vector magnitude of the acceleration data suggests low intensity of activities, then a sitting or reclining posture can be identified. Meanwhile, if the data plotted on Sedentary Sphere in latitudes of elevation are less than 15° below the horizontal position during low physical activity level, then a standing position is indicated.

The 15 s epoch files were imported into the custom-built Excel spreadsheet developed by Leicester-Loughborough Diet, Lifestyle and Physical Activity Biomedical Research Unit [43], enabling the calculation of the most likely posture with the data of wrist triaxial accelerometers. The validity of measuring sedentary time in free-living adults by a wrist-worn triaxial accelerometer with Sedentary Sphere has been confirmed in several studies given the consistency of its results with those of activPAL, a small lightweight triaxial accelerometer generally considered to be the 'gold standard' in identifying sedentary behaviour [39–41,44,45]. The intraclass correlation coefficient (ICC) was reported to be 0.80 (95% confidence interval, 0.68–0.88) [40].

In the preliminary research on the reliability and validity of the activity tracker, 32 undergraduate students (18 males and 14 females) were required to wear the activity tracker on their nondominant wrist and activPAL on their right thigh for seven consecutive days in free-living settings, and the ICC between the sedentary time measured by the monitor and activPAL was 0.78 (95% confidence interval, 0.68–0.86) with a mean bias of +18 min. In a laboratory setting, the participants performed a series of required activities, and the accuracy of the wrist-worn activity tracker in classifying lying, sitting and upright activities was 89%. The sensitivity and specificity were 91.8% and 86.3%, respectively.

2.3. Air Quality

Daily data of air quality were collected from the data released by the China National Environmental Monitoring Centre and matched in accordance with GPS and time information recorded by the activity tracker. Data of air quality include the daily AQI used by the Chinese government [23], the 24 h average concentrations of particulate matter with aerodynamic diameters less than 10 and 2.5 μm (PM_{10} and $PM_{2.5}$) and the daily maximum 8 h average concentrations of ozone (O_3).

The AQI was initially divided into six categories according to the recommendation of the Ministry of Environmental Protection of China: excellent (AQI = 0–50), good (AQI = 51–100), lightly polluted (AQI – 101–150), moderately polluted (AQI = 151–200), heavily polluted (AQI = 201–300) and severely polluted (AQI > 300). However, the three most-polluted categories were combined into one because of the paucity of heavily polluted and severely polluted days. Therefore, in this analysis, the AQI was finally divided into four categories as follows: excellent (AQI = 0–50), good (AQI = 51–100), lightly polluted (AQI = 101–150) and moderately and heavily polluted (AQI > 150). Concentrations of air pollutants were also divided into four categories in accordance with the AQI.

2.4. Covariates

Age was divided into four categories (18–29, 30–39, 40–49 and above 50). Height and weight were used to determine body mass index (BMI) levels.

Given the evidence that air pollution differs between weekends and weekdays [46] and sedentariness may also differ in a similar pattern [47], a weekday/weekend classification was listed in the potential covariates. The region is also a possible covariate. Thus, provinces were divided into the north and south by a most widely accepted boundary in China, which is intensively applied in studies investigating the regional differences [48,49].

Daily data of ambient temperature and weather were obtained from the China Central Meteorological Observatory and matched in accordance with GPS and time information. The temperature was categorised into quartiles. Weathers were divided into sunny, cloudy and overcast and rainy days.

As variations in wearing time of the activity tracker and wake time are likely to cause differences in recorded sedentary time, monitored wake time was added as a covariate in the analyses.

2.5. Statistical Analysis

Two-level linear regression analyses were conducted to investigate the association of air quality and sedentary time. The records of each participant in each day were nested within individuals. Between days, the association between air quality and sedentary behaviour was anticipated to exhibit temporal autocorrelation. Thus, the repeated covariance type was set as first-order autoregressive structure. We used restricted maximum likelihood estimation of variance components.

Firstly, a null model was conducted to determine the necessity of multilevel analysis. Secondly, we investigated the unadjusted and adjusted associations between sedentary time and individual factors, including age, gender, BMI and region, and other potential covariates, such as weather, temperature and weekday/weekend classification. Finally, both unadjusted and adjusted associations between sedentary time and air quality were investigated. The full model included all variables mentioned above. All statistical analyses were conducted using IBM SPSS Statistics v20.0 with a significance level of $p = 0.05$.

3. Results

3.1. Sedentary Time and Potential Covariates

The descriptive characteristics of 3270 included participants are shown in Table 1. A total of 2021 males and 1249 females were included in this study. The mean age was 30.54 years with a range from 18 years to 86 years. The majority of participants had a normal weight. The mean monitored duration was 11.43 days, longer than the required monitored time in most previous studies [50–53]. A person-day means a monitored day of a participant, and a total of 37,361 person-days were recorded, which is the sum of the numbers of monitored days of all participants. The mean sedentary time in males was 585.56 min/day, slightly higher than 562.65 min/day in females.

Table 1. Descriptive information of the study participants.

	Total	Male	Female	t/χ^2	p
Number of participants (%)	3270 (100)	2021 (61.8)	1249 (38.2)	-	-
Person-day	37,361	23,225	14,136	-	-
Wearing time/day, hour; mean (SD)	22.69 (0.98)	22.67 (1.00)	22.71 (0.94)	−4.69 ***	0.000
Monitored duration, day; mean (SD)	11.43 (4.15)	11.49 (4.11)	11.32 (4.20)	1.17	0.244
Age group (%)					
18–29	1763 (53.9)	1089 (53.9)	674 (54.0)		
30–39	1171 (35.8)	723 (35.8)	448 (35.9)	4.86	0.182
40–49	247 (7.6)	145 (7.2)	102 (8.2)		
Above 50	89 (2.7)	64 (3.2)	25 (2.0)		

Table 1. *Cont.*

	Total	Male	Female	t/χ^2	p
BMI level (%)					
Underweight	757 (23.1)	376 (18.6)	381 (30.5)		
Normal	2175 (66.5)	1386 (68.6)	789 (63.2)	104.04 ***	0.000
Overweight	327 (10.0)	258 (12.8)	69 (5.5)		
Obese	11 (0.3)	1 (0.0)	10 (0.8)		
Sedentary time/day, minute; mean (SD)	576.89 (146.93)	585.56 (149.22)	562.65 (141.94)	14.84 ***	0.000

*** $p < 0.001$.

The mean sedentary time per day was 585.56 min (standard deviation (SD): 149.22) in men and 562.65 min (SD: 141.94) in women based on the data collected by the activity tracker. Chinese adults spent nearly 10 h per day on sedentary behaviour. Table 2 shows the associations between sedentary time and potential covariates. The results show that significant association exists between gender and sedentary time (min/day). In the adjusted models, women spent approximately 25 min lesser sedentary time than men ($p = 0.000$). Weather is also significantly associated with sedentary time. On rainy days, sedentary time was 6.73 min longer than sunny days and 5.84 min longer than cloudy and overcast days ($p = 0.003$ and 0.002, respectively). Moreover, sedentary time was 47.43 min longer in weekdays compared with weekends ($p = 0.000$).

Table 2. Associations between sedentary time (minutes) and potential covariates.

		Unadjusted			Adjusted [1]		
		Estimate (SE)	95% CI	p	Estimate (SE)	95% CI	p
Age	18–29	12.51 (9.88)	−6.86, 31.89	0.205	9.76 (10.81)	−11.45, 30.96	0.367
	30–39	4.04 (10.00)	−15.57, 23.64	0.686	0.54 (10.91)	−20.87, 21.94	0.961
	40–49	−6.73 (11.27)	−28.83, 15.37	0.550	−7.40 (12.32)	−31.58, 16.77	0.548
	≥50 (ref)	-	-	-	-	-	-
Gender	Female	−21.90 (3.29) ***	−28.35, −15.45	0.000	−24.69 (3.71) ***	−31.96, −17.43	0.000
	Male (ref)	-	-	-	-	-	-
BMI	Underweight	−13.36 (28.67)	−69.57, 42.85	0.641	−53.87 (33.49)	−119.53, 11.79	0.108
	Normal	−12.95 (28.54)	−68.92, 43.00	0.650	−60.57 (33.36)	−125.99, 4.85	0.070
	Overweight	−11.19 (28.93)	−67.91, 45.53	0.699	−60.02 (33.78)	−126.27, 6.22	0.076
	Obese (ref)						
Region	North	−5.77 (3.50)	−12.63, 1.10	1.00	−6.51 (4.12)	−14.60, 1.58	0.115
	South (ref)	-	-	-	-	-	-
Weather	Sunny	−8.04 (2.30) ***	−12.55, −3.52	0.000	−6.73 (2.28) **	−11.24, −2.23	0.003
	Cloudy and overcast	−3.67 (1.89)	−7.39, 0.05	0.053	−5.84 (1.88) **	−9.53, −2.16	0.002
	Rain (ref)	-	-	-	-	-	-
Weekday/ weekend	Weekdays	48.57 (1.44) ***	45.74, 51.39	0.000	47.43 (1.69) ***	44.12, 50.74	0.000
	Weekends (ref)	-	-	-	-	-	-
Temperature	<20	2.95 (3.18)	−3.27, 9.18	0.353	−0.57 (3.49)	−7.42, 6.28	0.870
	20–22.1	10.51 (2.76) ***	5.09, 15.92	0.000	5.54 (3.06)	−0.47, 11.55	0.071
	22.1–25	6.12 (2.51) *	1.20, 11.05	0.015	4.13 (2.76)	−1.29, 9.54	0.135
	≥25 (ref)	-	-	-	-	-	-

[1] The adjusted model included all seven variables. * $p < 0.05$, ** $p < 0.01$, *** $p < 0.001$

3.2. Air Quality and Sedentary Time

The ambient air quality during monitored days is presented in Table 3. $PM_{2.5}$, PM_{10} and O_3 are the major air pollutants in China. The mean concentrations of $PM_{2.5}$ at 24 h, PM_{10} at 24 h, and O_3 at 8–24 h are 38.69, 64.02 and 124.43 µg/m^3, which are higher than the national primary limits (10.54%, 28.04% and 24.43%, respectively) [23]. In the majority of the monitored days, the air quality was excellent (31.3%) and good (51.1%). However, several of the monitored days were still lightly polluted (16.5%) and moderately and heavily polluted (1.2%).

Table 3. Descriptive statistics of air quality [1].

AQI Categories, Days (%)	
Excellent (AQI = 0–50)	11,680 (31.3)
Good (AQI = 50–100)	19,088 (51.1)
Lightly polluted (AQI = 100–150)	6155 (16.5)
Moderately and heavily polluted (AQI > 150)	438 (1.2)
$PM_{2.5}$ Levels, Days (%)	
0–35 $\mu g/m^3$	18,594 (49.8)
35–75 $\mu g/m^3$	16,485 (44.1)
75–115 $\mu g/m^3$	2112 (5.7)
>115 $\mu g/m^3$	170 (0.5)
PM_{10} Levels, Days (%)	
0–50 $\mu g/m^3$	13,087 (35.0)
50–150 $\mu g/m^3$	23,630 (63.2)
150–250 $\mu g/m^3$	626 (1.7)
>250 $\mu g/m^3$	18 (0.0)
O_3 Levels, Days (%)	
0–160 $\mu g/m^3$	23,960 (64.1)
160–200 $\mu g/m^3$	7716 (20.7)
200–300 $\mu g/m^3$	5423 (14.5)
>300 $\mu g/m^3$	262 (0.7)

[1] The classification of AQI and concentrations of air pollutants are according to the Ambient Air Quality Standards in China.

Table 4 reports both unadjusted and adjusted associations between sedentary time and air quality. The results indicate a significant association between sedentary time and air quality. In days with excellent, good and lightly polluted air quality, people spent approximately 20 min lesser sedentary time than in moderately and heavily polluted days (Table 4). The sedentary time in days when the concentration of $PM_{2.5}$ is above 115 $\mu g/m^3$ was approximately 45 min longer than in other days with lower concentration of $PM_{2.5}$.

Table 4. Associations between air quality and sedentary time (minutes).

		Unadjusted			Adjusted [1]		
		Estimate (SE)	95% CI	*p*	Estimate (SE)	95% CI	*p*
AQI	Excellent	−12.21 (6.56)	−25.08, 0.65	0.063	−19.20 (8.63) *	−34.91, −3.49	0.017
	Good	−17.44 (6.51) **	−30.20, −4.69	0.007	−22.92 (7.94) **	−38.48, −7.35	0.004
	Lightly polluted	−9.10 (6.48)	−21.79, 3.60	0.160	−21.28 (7.91) **	−36.78, −5.78	0.007
	Moderately and heavily polluted (ref)	-	-	-	-	-	-
$PM_{2.5}$	0–35 $\mu g/m^3$	−36.80 (10.64) ***	−57.65, −15.94	0.001	−45.35 (12.21) ***	−69.29, −21.41	0.000
	35–75 $\mu g/m^3$	−36.77 (10.63) ***	−57.61, −15.93	0.001	−45.74 (12.19) ***	−69.64, −21.84	0.000
	75–115 $\mu g/m^3$	−33.13 (10.80) **	−54.29, −11.96	0.002	−45.54 (12.35) ***	−69.74, −21.33	0.000
	>115 $\mu g/m^3$ (ref)	-	-	-	-	-	-
PM_{10}	0–50 $\mu g/m^3$	−32.81 (32.87)	−97.24, 31.62	0.318	−32.59 (32.60)	−96.49, 31.31	0.318
	50–150 $\mu g/m^3$	−36.31 (32.85)	−100.68, 28.07	0.269	−35.65 (32.57)	−99.48, 28.18	0.274
	150–250 $\mu g/m^3$	−26.47 (32.92)	−90.99, 38.06	0.421	−31.07 (32.66)	−95.08, 32.94	0.341
	>250 $\mu g/m^3$ (ref)	-	-	-	-	-	-
O_3	0–160 $\mu g/m^3$	−3.74 (8.25)	−19.83, 12.34	0.648	−6.17 (10.57)	−26.89, 14.55	0.560
	160–200 $\mu g/m^3$	−2.68 (8.30)	−18.94, 13.58	0.747	−6.14 (10.63)	−26.98, 14.69	0.563
	200–300 $\mu g/m^3$	3.93 (8.16)	−12.05, 19.92	0.629	−5.53 (10.50)	−26.11, 15.04	0.598
	>300 $\mu g/m^3$ (ref)	-	-	-	-	-	-

[1] Adjusted for gender, weather, temperature, weekday/weekend and monitored wake time per day. * $p < 0.05$, ** $p < 0.01$, *** $p < 0.001$.

4. Discussion

The objective of this study was to investigate the association between air quality and sedentary time in Chinese adults, providing evidence for future environmental risk assessment and health behaviour intervention. A wrist-worn activity tracker with an algorithm modified from Sedentary Sphere was utilised to monitor sedentary time. Multilevel analyses were conducted with adjustment for individual factors, temperature, weather and weekday/weekend classification.

The results indicated that air quality was independently associated with sedentary time in Chinese adults. This finding corresponds to several previous studies to some extent. For example, Hu et al. reported that people's participation in outdoor exercise decreases as air pollution severity increases [31], and Salmon et al. determined that air pollution was significantly associated with an increase in sedentary time [34]. This result also supported the assumption of the socio-ecological model that air quality is an important physical environmental correlate of sedentary behaviour [11]. There are several possible explanations for this finding. Directly, air pollutant inhalation would impair vascular and lung function and decrease exercise performance [54,55], leading to less active time. Indirectly, smog appearance [30], media alerts [27] and mood [13] could play an intermediary role in this relationship. When the ambient air quality is poor, people may cancel their plans of outdoor activity and instead stay indoors sedentarily because of concerns about the potential negative effects of air pollution on health [56]. Further studies are needed to explore more plausible mechanisms.

The finding suggests that better AQI levels were significantly associated with approximately 20 min reduction in sedentary time, and lower levels of $PM_{2.5}$ pollution were associated with approximately 45 min reduction in sedentary time. We compared these magnitudes of effects with those of several other environmental factors of sedentary time in previous studies. Compared with long day length and good weather conditions, short day length and poor weather conditions, including high precipitation and low temperatures, were associated with 15 min longer sedentary time [57]. Notably, women living in medium- and high-walkable neighbourhoods reported significantly 14 and 17 min less TV viewing time per day compared with those residing in low-walkable neighbourhoods [19]. This comparison indicated that the magnitude of the effect of air quality may be equal to or larger than some other factors at the environmental level.

According to the results of this study, people tend to prolong their sedentary time in moderately and heavily polluted days. Therefore, in these days, it is particularly necessary to remind people not to spend too much time on sedentary behaviour and perform more other indoor activities. Given that air quality is an important factor of sedentary time, the government and the public should make efforts to reduce air pollution not only for its direct impairment on health [25,26] but also for its association with unhealthy behaviours. However, considering that the exact amount of sedentary time a person would have to reduce in order to achieve meaningful health benefits is still unclear due to the preference to categorisation of sedentary time in previous studies [58], further studies are needed to investigate whether the magnitudes of effects of improved air quality are large enough to help people gain a significantly decreased mortality.

Admittedly, this study presents limitations. Firstly, the map (Figure 1) shows that the sample is not balanced amongst provinces. The majority of participants were in the east and the middle. Thus, the sample might not be entirely representative for the entire country. However, participants were from 33 out of 34 provinces, autonomous regions and municipalities of China, and the majority of Chinese population reside in the east and the middle [59]. Thus, the participants in this study could still reflect the current situation of Chinese adults to some extent. Secondly, although the sample size was relatively large, the monitored days were unevenly distributed in each air quality level. Moreover, buyers of the wrist-worn activity tracker could share several common characteristics, such as socio-economic status and exercise habits, such that the participants are not entirely representative of all Chinese citizens. In addition, this study is unable to distinguish contexts of sedentary behaviour, such as occupational, traffic-related and leisure sedentariness, which limits further analyses. Finally, one limitation of Sedentary Sphere is that its classification accuracy for sitting postures was reported to be approximately 60%, with the majority of misclassifications occurring during the sitting postures that did not involve any accompanying hand movement [39,41]. However, although the accuracy rate of Sedentary Sphere is lower than that of activPAL and ActiGraph, the effects of this weakness can be attenuated if the sample size is sufficient. Regardless, the relationship between air quality and sedentary behaviour requires further investigation with the assistance of novel data processing technologies.

The strengths of this study lay in its novel posture determination algorithm, relatively large sample size, well-matched air quality data and multilevel analyses. Firstly, instead of determining sedentary time merely based on energy expenditure, Sedentary Sphere was applied and assisted in estimating sedentary time. In addition, the affordable cost of this commercial wrist-worn activity tracker with acceptable validity allowed a relatively large sample size in our study. A total of 3270 participants from 33 of 34 provinces in China were included in the analysis. However, only few previous studies applied this novel technology. The application of Sedentary Sphere in the current study showed its potential to expand more possibilities for future studies. Moreover, in previous studies investigating the relationship between air quality and physical activity, self-reported physical activity data were commonly matched to monthly average air quality parameters. By contrast, in the current study, daily data of sedentary time and parameters of 24 h air quality where sedentary behaviours occurred were accurately matched, leading to better precision. Besides, unlike previous studies [27–29,31], we used multilevel modelling including a within-subject component, which increases the power of this study and helps make more causal interpretations.

5. Conclusions

Air quality appears to be an important factor associated with sedentary time of Chinese adults. People spent significantly longer sedentary time in moderately and heavily polluted days than in other days with better air quality.

Author Contributions: X.W. conceived and designed the study, collected the data, oversaw the data analysis and edited the manuscript. Y.M. played a role in data analyses and wrote the manuscript. B.Y. played a large role in data collection and data analysis. S.F. and Y.L. helped write the manuscript.

Funding: This research was funded by the Fundamental Research Funds for the Central Universities of China.

Acknowledgments: The authors thank Hangzhou Gongke Technology Co., Ltd. and all the participants for their support in this study.

Conflicts of Interest: The authors declare no conflict of interest.

References

1. Tremblay, M.S.; Aubert, S.; Barnes, J.D.; Saunders, T.J.; Carson, V.; Latimercheung, A.E.; Chastin, S.F.M.; Altenburg, T.M.; Mai, J.M.C. Sedentary behavior research network (SBRN)—Terminology consensus project process and outcome. *Int. J. Behav. Nutr. Phys. Act.* **2017**, *14*, 75. [CrossRef] [PubMed]
2. Hu, F.B.; Li, T.Y.; Colditz, G.A.; Willett, W.C.; Manson, J.E. Television watching and other sedentary behaviors in relation to risk of obesity and type 2 diabetes mellitus in women. *JAMA* **2003**, *289*, 1785–1791. [CrossRef] [PubMed]
3. Maher, C.A.; Mire, E.; Harrington, D.M.; Staiano, A.E.; Katzmarzyk, P.T. The independent and combined associations of physical activity and sedentary behavior with obesity in adults: Nhanes 2003–2006. *Obesity* **2013**, *21*, E730–E737. [CrossRef] [PubMed]
4. Owen, N.; Bauman, A.; Brown, W. Too much sitting: A novel and important predictor of chronic disease risk? *Br. J. Sports Med.* **2009**, *43*, 81–83. [CrossRef] [PubMed]
5. Shilpa, D.; Liza, S. Sedentary behavior and physical activity are independent predictors of successful aging in middle-aged and older adults. *J. Aging Res.* **2012**, *2012*, 190654.
6. Biswas, A.; Oh, P.I.; Faulkner, G.E.; Bajaj, R.R.; Silver, M.A.; Mitchell, M.S.; Alter, D.A. Sedentary time and its association with risk for disease incidence, mortality, and hospitalization in adults: A systematic review and meta-analysis. *Ann. Intern. Med.* **2015**, *162*, 123–132. [CrossRef] [PubMed]

7. Inoue, S.; Sugiyama, T.; Takamiya, T.; Oka, K.; Owen, N.; Shimomitsu, T. Television viewing time is associated with overweight/obesity among older adults, independent of meeting physical activity and health guidelines. *J. Epidemiol.* **2012**, *22*, 50–56. [CrossRef] [PubMed]
8. Dunstan, D.W.; Barr, E.G. Television viewing time and mortality: The australian diabetes, obesity and lifestyle study (AusDiab). *Circulation* **2010**, *122*, 384–391. [CrossRef] [PubMed]
9. Grøntved, A.; Hu, F.B. Television viewing and risk of type 2 diabetes, cardiovascular disease, and all-cause mortality a meta-analysis. *JAMA* **2011**, *305*, 2448–2455. [CrossRef] [PubMed]
10. Zhang, Y.; Jiang, C.; Wang, M.; Zou, J. Characteristics of the chinese population whose physical exercise is "only sedentariness" in leisure time. *Shandong Sports Sci. Technol.* **2015**, *37*, 104–109.
11. Owen, N.; Sugiyama, T.; Eakin, E.E.; Gardiner, P.A.; Tremblay, M.S.; Sallis, J.F. Adults' sedentary behavior determinants and interventions. *Am. J. Preventive Med.* **2011**, *41*, 189–196. [CrossRef] [PubMed]
12. Rhodes, R.E.; Mark, R.S.; Temmel, C.P. Adult sedentary behavior: A systematic review. *Am. J. Preventive Med.* **2012**, *42*, e3–e28. [CrossRef] [PubMed]
13. O'Donoghue, G.; Perchoux, C.; Mensah, K.; Lakerveld, J.; Van der Ploeg, H.; Bernaards, C.; Chastin, S.F.; Simon, C.; O'Gorman, D.; Nazare, J.A. A systematic review of correlates of sedentary behaviour in adults aged 18–65 years: A socio-ecological approach. *BMC Public Health* **2016**, *16*, 163. [CrossRef] [PubMed]
14. Prince, S.A.; Reed, J.L.; McFetridge, C.; Tremblay, M.S.; Reid, R.D. Correlates of sedentary behaviour in adults: A systematic review. *Obesity Rev. Off. J. Int. Assoc. Study Obesity* **2017**, *18*, 915–935. [CrossRef] [PubMed]
15. Van Uffelen, J.G.; Heesch, K.C.; Brown, W. Correlates of sitting time in working age australian women: Who should be targeted with interventions to decrease sitting time? *J. Phys. Act. Health* **2012**, *9*, 270–287. [CrossRef] [PubMed]
16. Uijtdewilligen, L.; Twisk, J.W.; Singh, A.S.; Chinapaw, M.J.; Van Mechelen, W.; Brown, W.J. Biological, socio-demographic, work and lifestyle determinants of sitting in young adult women: A prospective cohort study. *Int. J. Behav. Nutr. Phys. Act.* **2014**, *11*, 7. [CrossRef] [PubMed]
17. Storgaard, R.L.; Hansen, H.S.; Aadahl, M.; Glumer, C. Association between neighbourhood green space and sedentary leisure time in a danish population. *Scand. J. Public Health* **2013**, *41*, 846–852. [CrossRef] [PubMed]
18. Astell-Burt, T.; Feng, X.; Kolt, G.S. Greener neighborhoods, slimmer people? Evidence from 246,920 australians. *Int. J. Obesity* **2014**, *38*, 156–159. [CrossRef] [PubMed]
19. Sugiyama, T.; Salmon, J.; Dunstan, D.W.; Bauman, A.E.; Owen, N. Neighborhood walkability and TV viewing time among australian adults. *Am. J. Prev. Med.* **2007**, *33*, 444–449. [CrossRef] [PubMed]
20. Kozo, J.; Sallis, J.F.; Conway, T.L.; Kerr, J.; Cain, K.; Saelens, B.E.; Frank, L.D.; Owen, N. Sedentary behaviors of adults in relation to neighborhood walkability and income. *Health Psychol. Off. J. Div. Health Psychol. Am. Psychol. Assoc.* **2012**, *31*, 704–713. [CrossRef] [PubMed]
21. Rich, C.; Griffiths, L.J.; Dezateux, C. Seasonal variation in accelerometer-determined sedentary behaviour and physical activity in children: A review. *Int. J. Behav. Nutr. Phys. Act.* **2012**, *9*, 49. [CrossRef] [PubMed]
22. Ministry of Ecology and Environment of the People's Republic of China: Daily Report on Air Quality of Cities in China. Available online: http://www.mep.gov.cn/hjzli/dqwrfz/dqwrfzxdjh/ (accessed on 29 May 2018).
23. Ministry of Ecology and Environment of the People's Republic of China. Ambient Air Quality Standards. Available online: http://kjs.mep.gov.cn/hjbhbz/bzwb/dqhjbh/dqhjzlbz/201203/t20120302_224165.shtml (accessed on 29 May 2018).
24. United States Environmental Protection Agency: National Ambient Air Quality Standards. Available online: https://www.epa.gov/criteria-air-pollutants/naaqs-table (accessed on 29 May 2018).
25. Mannucci, P.M.; Harari, S.; Martinelli, I.; Franchini, M. Effects on health of air pollution: A narrative review. *Intern. Emerg. Med.* **2015**, *10*, 657–662. [CrossRef] [PubMed]
26. World Health Organization. Ambient (Outdoor) Air Quality and Health. Available online: http://www.who.int/mediacentre/factsheets/fs313/en/ (accessed on 30 May 2018).
27. Wen, X.J.; Balluz, L.; Mokdad, A. Association between media alerts of air quality index and change of outdoor activity among adult asthma in six states, brfss, 2005. *J. Community Health* **2009**, *34*, 40–46. [CrossRef] [PubMed]
28. Roberts, J.D.; Voss, J.D.; Knight, B. The association of ambient air pollution and physical inactivity in the united states. *PLoS ONE* **2014**, *9*, e90143. [CrossRef] [PubMed]

29. Wen, X.J.; Balluz, L.S.; Shire, J.D.; Mokdad, A.H.; Kohl, H.W., III. Association of self-reported leisure-time physical inactivity with particulate matter 2.5 air pollution. *J. Environ. Health* **2009**, *72*, 40–44. [PubMed]

30. An, R.; Xiang, X. Ambient fine particulate matter air pollution and leisure-time physical inactivity among us adults. *Public Health* **2015**, *129*, 1637–1644. [CrossRef] [PubMed]

31. Hu, L.; Zhu, L.; Xu, Y.; Lyu, J.; Imm, K.; Yang, L. Relationship between air quality and outdoor exercise behavior in china: A novel mobile-based study. *Int. J. Behav. Med.* **2017**, *24*, 1–8. [CrossRef] [PubMed]

32. Yu, H.; An, R.; Andrade, F. Ambient fine particulate matter air pollution and physical activity: A longitudinal study of university retirees in beijing, china. *Am. J. Health Behav.* **2017**, *41*, 401. [CrossRef] [PubMed]

33. Yu, H.; Miao, Y.; Gordon, S.P.; Zhang, R. The association between ambient fine particulate air pollution and physical activity: A cohort study of university students living in beijing. *Int. J. Behav. Nutr. Phys. Act.* **2017**, *14*, 136. [CrossRef] [PubMed]

34. Salmon, J.; Owen, N.; Crawford, D.; Bauman, A.; Sallis, J.F. Physical activity and sedentary behavior: A population-based study of barriers, enjoyment, and preference. *Health Psychol. Off. J. Div. Health Psychol. Am. Psychol. Assoc.* **2003**, *22*, 178–188. [CrossRef]

35. Adams, S.A.; Matthews, C.E.; Ebbeling, C.B.; Moore, C.G.; Cunningham, J.E.; Fulton, J.; Hebert, J.R. The effect of social desirability and social approval on self-reports of physical activity. *Am. J. Epidemiol.* **2005**, *161*, 389–398. [CrossRef] [PubMed]

36. Matthews, C.E.; Chen, K.Y.; Freedson, P.S.; Buchowski, M.S.; Beech, B.M.; Pate, R.R.; Troiano, R.P. Amount of time spent in sedentary behaviors in the United States, 2003–2004. *Am. J. Epidemiol.* **2008**, *167*, 875–881. [CrossRef] [PubMed]

37. Atkin, A.J.; Gorely, T.; Clemes, S.A.; Yates, T.; Edwardson, C.; Brage, S.; Salmon, J.; Marshall, S.J.; Biddle, S.J. Methods of measurement in epidemiology: Sedentary behaviour. *Int. J. Epidemiol.* **2012**, *41*, 1460–1471. [CrossRef] [PubMed]

38. Freedson, P.S.; John, D. Comment on "estimating activity and sedentary behavior from an accelerometer on the hip and wrist". *Med. Sci. Sports Exerc.* **2013**, *45*, 962–963. [CrossRef] [PubMed]

39. Rowlands, A.V.; Olds, T.S.; Hillsdon, M.; Pulsford, R.; Hurst, T.L.; Eston, R.G.; Gomersall, S.R.; Johnston, K.; Langford, J. Assessing sedentary behavior with the geneactiv: Introducing the sedentary sphere. *Med. Sci. Sports Exerc.* **2014**, *46*, 1235–1247. [CrossRef] [PubMed]

40. Pavey, T.G.; Gomersall, S.R.; Clark, B.K.; Brown, W.J. The validity of the geneactiv wrist-worn accelerometer for measuring adult sedentary time in free living. *J. Sci. Med. Sport* **2016**, *19*, 395–399. [CrossRef] [PubMed]

41. Rowlands, A.V.; Yates, T.; Olds, T.S.; Davies, M.; Khunti, K.; Edwardson, C.L. Sedentary sphere: Wrist-worn accelerometer-brand independent posture classification. *Med. Sci. Sports Exerc.* **2016**, *48*, 748–754. [CrossRef] [PubMed]

42. Ministry of Industry and Information Technology of People's Republic of China: China Internet Domain Name System. Available online: http://www.miit.gov.cn/n1146295/n1652858/n1652930/n4509607/c6072462/content.html (accessed on 30 May 2018).

43. Leicester-Loughborough Diet, Lifestyle and Physical Activity Biomedical Research Unit. Sedentary Sphere: A Method for the Analysis, Identification and Visual Presentation of Raw Acceleration Data from Triaxial Accelerometers (Geneactiv, Activinsights, Cambs, UK). Available online: http://www.ll.dlpa.bru.nihr.ac.uk/Sedentary_Sphere-5483.html (accessed on 23 August 2018).

44. Davies, G.; Reilly, J.J.; McGowan, A.J.; Dall, P.M.; Granat, M.H.; Paton, J.Y. Validity, practical utility, and reliability of the activpal in preschool children. *Med. Sci. Sports Exerc.* **2012**, *44*, 761–768. [CrossRef] [PubMed]

45. Dowd, K.P.; Harrington, D.M.; Donnelly, A.E. Criterion and concurrent validity of the activpal professional physical activity monitor in adolescent females. *PLoS ONE* **2012**, *7*, e47633. [CrossRef] [PubMed]

46. Marr, L.C.; Harley, R.A. Spectral analysis of weekday-weekend differences in ambient ozone, nitrogen oxide, and non-methane hydrocarbon time series in california. *Atmos. Environ.* **2002**, *36*, 2327–2335. [CrossRef]

47. Clemens, D.; Nicole, G.; Wirth, M.D.; Hand, G.A.; Shook, R.P.; Stephanie, B.; Blair, S.N. The association of physical activity during weekdays and weekend with body composition in young adults. *J. Obesity* **2016**, *2016*, PMC4855007. [CrossRef] [PubMed]

48. Wu, D. A study on north-south differences in economic growth. *Geogr. Res.* **2001**, *20*, 238–246.

49. Chen, Z. Regional development difference from the south to the north in east and middle China. *Geogr. Res.* **1999**, *18*, 80–87.

50. Vallance, J.K.; Boyle, T.; Courneya, K.S.; Lynch, B.M. Accelerometer-assessed physical activity and sedentary time among colon cancer survivors: Associations with psychological health outcomes. *J. Cancer Surviv. Res. Pract.* **2015**, *9*, 404–411. [CrossRef] [PubMed]

51. Walker, R.G.; Obeid, J.; Nguyen, T.; Ploeger, H.; Proudfoot, N.A.; Bos, C.; Chan, A.K.; Pedder, L.; Issenman, R.M.; Scheinemann, K.; et al. Sedentary time and screen-based sedentary behaviors of children with a chronic disease. *Pediatr. Exerc. Sci.* **2015**, *27*, 219–225. [CrossRef] [PubMed]

52. Healy, G.N.; Wijndaele, K.; Dunstan, D.W.; Shaw, J.E.; Salmon, J.; Zimmet, P.Z.; Owen, N. Objectively measured sedentary time, physical activity, and metabolic risk: The australian diabetes, obesity and lifestyle study (Ausdiab). *Diabetes Care* **2008**, *31*, 369–371. [CrossRef] [PubMed]

53. Matthews, C.E.; Ainsworth, B.E.; Thompson, R.W.; Bassett, D.R., Jr. Sources of variance in daily physical activity levels as measured by an accelerometer. *Med. Sci. Sports Exerc.* **2002**, *34*, 1376–1381. [CrossRef] [PubMed]

54. Rundell, K.W.; Caviston, R. Ultrafine and fine particulate matter inhalation decreases exercise performance in healthy subjects. *J. Strength Cond. Res.* **2008**, *22*, 2. [CrossRef] [PubMed]

55. Cutrufello, P.T.; Rundell, K.W.; Smoliga, J.M.; Stylianides, G.A. Inhaled whole exhaust and its effect on exercise performance and vascular function. *Inhal. Toxicol.* **2011**, *23*, 658. [CrossRef] [PubMed]

56. Qian, X.; Xu, G.; Li, L.; Shen, Y.; He, T.; Liang, Y.; Yang, Z.; Zhou, W.W.; Xu, J. Knowledge and perceptions of air pollution in ningbo, china. *BMC Public Health* **2016**, *16*, 1138. [CrossRef] [PubMed]

57. Wu, Y.T.; Luben, R.; Wareham, N.; Griffin, S.; Jones, A.P. Weather, day length and physical activity in older adults: Cross-sectional results from the european prospective investigation into cancer and nutrition (EPIC) norfolk cohort. *PLoS ONE* **2017**, *12*, e0177767. [CrossRef] [PubMed]

58. Rezende, L.F.M.; Rey-López, J.P.; Matsudo, V.K.R.; Luiz, O.C. Sedentary behavior and health outcomes among older adults: A systematic review. *BMC Public Health* **2014**, *14*, 333. [CrossRef] [PubMed]

59. National Bureau of Statistics of China. China Statistical Yearbook 2015. Available online: http://www.stats.gov.cn/tjsj/ndsj/2015/indexch.htm (accessed on 18 July 2018).

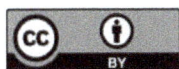

Journal of
Clinical Medicine

MDPI

Article

Safety and Lack of Negative Effects of Wearable Augmented-Reality Social Communication Aid for Children and Adults with Autism

Ned T. Sahin [1,2,*] , Neha U. Keshav [1] , Joseph P. Salisbury [1] and Arshya Vahabzadeh [1,3]

[1]   Brain Power, LLC, Cambridge, MA 02142, USA; neha@brain-power.com (N.U.K.);
     joey@brain-power.com (J.P.S.); arshya@brain-power.com (A.V.)
[2]   Department of Psychology, Harvard University, Cambridge, MA 02138, USA
[3]   Psychiatry Academy, Massachusetts General Hospital, Boston, MA 02114, USA
*   Correspondence: sahin@post.harvard.edu; Tel.: +1-6173318401

Received: 21 June 2018; Accepted: 21 July 2018; Published: 30 July 2018

Abstract: There is a growing interest in the use of augmented reality (AR) to assist children and adults with autism spectrum disorders (ASD); however, little investigation has been conducted into the safety of AR devices, such as smartglasses. The objective of this report was to assess the safety and potential negative effects of the *Empowered Brain system*, a novel AR smartglasses-based social communication aid for people with ASD. The version of the Empowered Brain in this report utilized Google Glass (Google, Mountain View, CA, USA) as its hardware platform. A sequential series of 18 children and adults, aged 4.4 to 21.5 years (mean 12.2 years), with clinically diagnosed ASD of varying severity used the system. Users and caregivers were interviewed about the perceived negative effects and design concerns. Most users were able to wear and use the Empowered Brain ($n = 16/18$, 89%), with most of them reporting no negative effects ($n = 14/16$, 87.5%). Caregivers observed no negative effects in users ($n = 16/16$, 100%). Most users (77.8%) and caregivers (88.9%) had no design concerns. This report found no major negative effects in using an AR smartglasses-based social communication aid across a wide age and severity range of people with ASD. Further research is needed to explore longer-term effects of using AR smartglasses in this population.

Keywords: Autism; autism spectrum disorder; augmented reality; technology; Google Glass; social communication; safety; smartglasses; digital health; Amazon; Amazon Web Services; Google

1. Introduction

Autism Spectrum Disorder (ASD) is a neurodevelopmental disorder affecting 1 in 68 children in the United States [1] and is characterized by social communication impairment as well as the presence of a restricted and/or repetitive range of interests and behaviors [2]. The rising prevalence of ASD has increased the demand for educational and behavioral services, often exhausting these limited resources [3,4]. There has been considerable interest in the development and study of technology-aided approaches for the social, cognitive, and behavioral challenges related to ASD [5–7]. Technology-aided approaches may be especially suitable for people with ASD given that some of these individuals may show a natural propensity to utilize digital tools [8], display a fondness for electronic media [9], express a preference for standardized and predictable interactions [8], enjoy game-like elements [10], and/or favor computer-generated speech [11]. However, technology may also have negative effects in some people with ASD. Individuals may develop problematic video game use [12], and can become agitated or disruptive when attempting to disengage from video games [12]. Anecdotally, many caregivers describe meltdowns and other episodes of behavioral dysregulation in children with ASD when attempting to stop them playing on smartphone and/or tablets [13].

Evidence suggests that a broad range of technology-aided interventions, such as those using computer programs and virtual reality (VR), may be effective for people with ASD [5]. Technology-based interventions have been found to be beneficial for improving a wide range of skills and behaviors, including aiding social and emotional skills [14,15], communication ability [15], academics [16], employment proficiencies [6], and challenging behaviors [14]. Additionally, teaching of socio-emotional skills to children and adolescents with ASD is important, as it can help them prepare for the workplace [6,17]. This is a key consideration, as the current rates of unemployment and underemployment among people with ASD are high [18], and the social demand of job and job interviews have been identified as a key challenge [19].

There is particular interest in interventions that help users learn while continuing to interact with the people and environment around them. Learning socio-emotional skills in real life settings (such as in social skills groups) may increase the chance that these behaviors will generalize to the challenges of daily life [20]. Augmented reality (AR) is a technology that holds considerable promise in this regard, allowing users to see and interact with the real world around them, while virtual objects and audio guidance are provided through a visual overlay and audio speakers (Figure 1A,B). In contrast, current VR headsets place users and their senses into an entirely virtual world, while simultaneously removing their ability to see and sense real-world stimuli, hazards, and social situations around them (Figure 1C). In contrast to VR headsets, AR allows users to see their real-world environment, allowing them to navigate an environmental hazard more readily, or to socially engage with another person. Nonetheless, AR incorporates many of the features of VR that are thought to make VR technology well suited to the creation of learning tools for people with ASD [21], including being a primarily visual and auditory experience, being able to individualize the experience, promoting generalization and decreasing rigidity through subtle, gradual modifications of the experience [21].

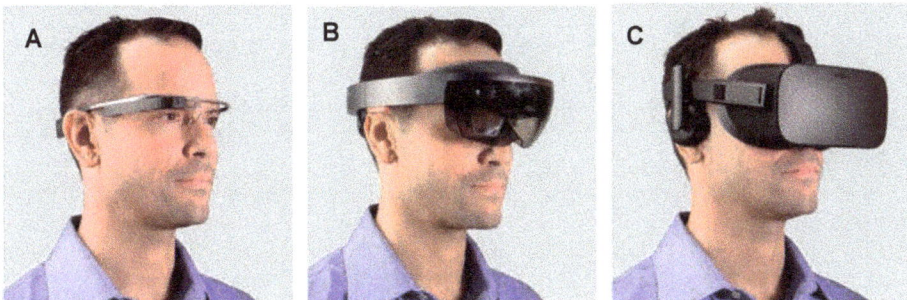

Figure 1. Head-worn Computers or Displays Vary in Size, Weight, and Face-Obstruction. (**A**) Glass Explorer Edition (originally known as Google Glass): AR smartglasses with a fully stand-alone onboard computer (weight 42 grams). (**B**) Microsoft Hololens: AR headset with a fully stand-alone onboard computer and depth camera (weight 579 grams). (**C**) Oculus Rift: VR headset display, which must be tethered continuously to a powerful computer to drive it (weight 470 grams). VR headsets and some AR devices are large, heavy, and block the social world considerably. Image depicts the study author, NTS.

AR experiences can also be easily modified and personalized for each individual, an important consideration given that many people with ASD exhibit intense interest in a restricted range of topics and may experience extreme distress if changes to their routine/environment occur [2]. AR experiences are also not restricted solely to real-world limitations on time, space, and resources. For instance, users may have the opportunity to interact with objects or experiences from historical or fantasy worlds, or a simplified and cartoon-like interaction, where the sensory and perceptual experiences may be reduced in complexity and/or magnitude.

Most ASD-related research into AR has focused on the use of smartphone- and/or tablet-based apps. While research has been limited, AR apps on smartphones/tablets have been shown to improve selective and sustained attention [22], attention to social cues [23], the ability to understand emotions and facial expressions in storybook characters [23], and navigating the physical world when attempting to find employment opportunities [24]. However, smartphone-based AR may carry with it a risk of negative effects, including grip and postural strain, minor falls, and falls leading to major trauma and blindness [25,26].

While AR has been investigated as an educational medium for ASD children for at least a decade [27], minimal research has been conducted into the safety of head-mounted AR in ASD populations. This has potential implications, as head-mounted AR, in particular, smartglasses, may offer advantages compared to smartphone- or tablet-based AR and may be the optimal future platform for AR [28,29]. The generalized use of AR smartglasses may still be in its infancy, but the use of such devices will be fueled by their ability to improve social interactions and relationships, making life more efficient, and provide enjoyment and fun to the user [30]. AR smartglasses may also be beneficial tools for clinical research. AR smartglasses contain a wide array of sensors. These are intended to allow for basic features, such as gesture-based control of the devices (to make up for the lack of keyboards and traditional input devices). However, we have shown that these sensors can also be used creatively to collect quantitative data that may help assess brain function [31]. Analysis of quantitative data from sensors in smart-devices may help to advance digital phenotyping of neurobehavioral conditions [31]. To our knowledge, we have published the first reports on the use of AR smartglasses in children with ASD [31–36].

Even in VR, about which there are many more reports in the literature, there are very few reports on people with ASD using modern VR headsets [37,38]. Therefore, it would be useful to understand how children and adults with ASD respond to AR smartglasses, particularly when the smartglasses function as an assistive device loaded with specialized assistive social and behavioral coaching software [31]. Of primary importance in assessing a new assistive technology is the assessment of (a) the safety of such an approach and (b) any potential negative effects.

There are both human and device factors that make it conceivable that even commercially-available AR technology could elicit concerns regarding safety or negative effects when applied as an assistive technology for this special population.

Firstly, in regard to human factors, it has been widely reported that people with ASD have a range of sensory [2,39], motor [40], and cognitive challenges [41,42], as well as strong negative reactions to transitions [43]. More specifically, atypical reactivity to sensory inputs, such as touch, sound, temperature, and sight, is a diagnostic criterion of ASD [2], affecting up to 93% of people with the condition [44]. Altered sensory reactivity is also highly heterogeneous in the ASD population. Each member of this diverse spectrum may be affected across several senses with hyper- or hypo-sensitivities, representing a complex matrix of sensory subtypes [39]. It is therefore important to determine whether individuals can safely use smartglasses for an extended period and to monitor how they respond to visual, auditory, and vibrotactile cues, delivered through the device.

Secondly, there may be safety concerns because ASD is often associated with altered motor movements, such as repetitive behaviors (a "core" symptom of ASD) [2] or impairments of motor coordination [40]. It is thus important to assess if such motor challenges may lead to falls or injury when people with ASD utilize AR smartglasses [40].

Thirdly, people with ASD may differ in their ability to remain attentive and focus on using smartglasses as part of social communication training, especially given the high rate of comorbidity between ASD and attention deficit hyperactivity disorder [45]. Some individuals may find themselves becoming distracted when using AR or in the process of becoming familiar with using AR while simultaneously navigating the real world [46].

These attentional difficulties may compound the motor coordination challenges in ASD, as mentioned above, increasing the potential of AR smartglasses use to cause falls and/or trips.

Additionally, over 30% of children with ASD demonstrate wandering/elopement behavior, and it would be prudent to investigate any technology that would affect their perception, attention, and ability to avoid hazards [47].

Finally, people with ASD may face major challenges in coping with transitions in activities [2,48] and have demonstrated oppositional defiant behaviors and aggression when asked to stop playing video games [12] or stop using a piece of technology [13]. This suggests a possible risk of meltdown when an AR session is ended, though it remains to be seen whether stopping the use of smartglasses results in less difficulty than when stopping the use of a smartphone or tablet (which may be more engrossing or cognitively demanding).

Instruction manuals for AR smartglasses are an additional indication that there may be device-related factors that result in risks. For instance, the Microsoft HoloLens manual identifies the potential side effects as nausea, motion sickness, dizziness, disorientation, headache, fatigue, eye strain, dry eyes, and seizures [49], although their occurrence among users with ASD has not been studied. There is evidence that Google Glass can reduce the visual field of users' right eye, although this effect seems mostly attributable to the frame of the glasses [50].

Few studies have investigated how these new AR devices may impact the perceptual abilities of regular users, raising concerns that some individuals may become distracted, have altered reaction times, misjudge hazards in the real-world, and/or experience altered distance and speed perception [46].

AR may share a subset of the risks of VR, and VR research has reported potential side effects that include eye strain, headache, and disorientation during the use of a VR headset [51]. However, there have been continuous advances in VR technology, and a recent study noted that people with ASD experienced relatively few negative effects when using a VR headset of the modern generation [38].

Assessing negative effects in people with ASD is not a simple undertaking, given that these individuals have challenges in communicating their experiences. It is therefore important to explicitly ask for their feedback, and seek feedback from their caregivers to have a more comprehensive method for detecting any negative effects.

2. Aims of Research

Given the potential for AR smartglasses to be used in people with ASD, and yet the uncertainty as to whether this technology would be safe in this population, we studied a specific AR smartglasses technology in 18 children and adults with ASD. The system used in this study was the *Empowered Brain, previously called the Brain Power Autism system (BPAS)* (Brain Power, LLC, Cambridge, MA, USA) [31].

2.1. The Empowered Brain System

The Empowered Brain is a social communication aid that consists of AR smartglasses with apps that allow children and adults with ASD to coach themselves on important socio-emotional and cognitive skills [31,32]. The typical session length of a Empowered Brain intervention is 10 min in duration, and a session is typically conducted once or twice a day.

Users of the Empowered Brain learn life skills through gamified interactions and a combination of intrinsic and extrinsic rewards for successfully completing tasks. In certain situations, such as coaching of appropriate face-directed gaze and emotion recognition, the Empowered Brain is designed to be used while the user is interacting with another person. The system was designed using serious game principles and an iterative process, where continuous feedback from people with ASD, clinicians, neuroscientists, educators, caregivers, design specialists, and engineers helped to develop the system that was used in this report. Additionally, the facial affective analytics component of the Empowered Brain was developed in partnership with Affectiva, an emotion artificial intelligence company. Other artificial intelligence functions of the Empowered Brain (deep learning and machine learning) have been developed through a partnership with Amazon (Seattle, WA, USA). The work was also made possible by Google, Inc., (Mountain View, CA, USA), now known as Alphabet, Inc.,

(Mountain View, CA, USA), who provided substantial hardware as well as guidance in engineering. Engineering guidance, including how best to develop apps that would be accessible to a diverse set of users, was provided, in part, through the Glass Enterprise Partnership Program.

The Empowered Brain is designed to be accessible to people with ASD and to minimize potential negative effects. A number of elements were used to achieve this, including, but not limited to, the use of calming tones and emotional artificial intelligence, the minimization of audio and visual sensory load, graduated transitions between learning segments, and the modification of the functionality of the tactile input surfaces of the smartglasses. In this study, we focused on understanding the safety and potential negative effects that children and adults with ASD may experience as they use AR smartglasses that are delivering cognitive and social self-coaching apps.

2.2. Technical Specifications of Empowered Brain

The Empowered Brain in this report is based on Google Glass Explorer Edition (Google Glass XE) (Figure 1A) [52]. Google Glass XE are titanium-framed smartglasses, with a high resolution right-sided monocular optical display. Google Glass EE contains a 5-megapixel camera, and can record video at 720p [52]. Audio is generated through a bone conduction transducer on the right side of the smartglasses. It has a lithium ion battery with a capacity of 670 mAH. Battery life in medical settings has been documented as being between 8.5–10 h, although it may be significantly shortened when running high demand applications [53]. The Empowered Brain combines Google Glass XE with a series of apps that help to coach social and emotional skills (summary in Table 1 and [31]).

Table 1. Intervention focus of Empowered Brain Software Applications.

Empowered Brain App	ASD-Related Challenge	Educational Element	Software Element	Interactivity
Face2Face	Reduced attention to faces	Increased attention to human faces	AR guidance of user to the face of facilitator using game-like interface, guidance arrows and cartoon-like masks.	Requires live facilitator to be present. Face of facilitator is utilized by app.
Emotion Charades	Difficulty in recognizing facial emotions of others	Improved ability to recognize human facial emotions	App detects human face and identifies emotion displayed. User tilts head corresponding to emotion on human face. Head movement is detected by Empowered Brain (Google Glass) sensors.	Two-person interaction, requires facilitator to be present. Facial emotions of facilitator are utilized by app.
Transition Master	Difficulty in handling change of physical environment	Enhanced ability to handle environment/task transitions	App presents user with 360-degree visual image of another environment. User explores environment through head movements that are detected by Empowered Brain sensors.	No interactive facilitator required. User can interact with the environment alone.

2.3. Face2Face

Human faces are the richest source of socially salient information on humans, information that is crucial to successful social functioning [54]. People with ASD have been found to have a wide range of impairments to their ability to attend to faces, recognize facial emotions, and demonstrate neurotypical patterns of socially-related eye gaze [55–59]. The Empowered Brain includes the Face2Face app, a game-like software that uses a range of strategies to coach users to attend to human faces (Figure 2).

The user, while wearing the Empowered Brain with Face2Face running, sits in front of a human partner who will help to facilitate the interaction. The Face2Face app is able to detect the presence of a human face in its visual field.

Face2Face determines where the user is looking relative to the partner's face, and generates a series of AR elements in the user's field of view (Figure 2). These AR elements, such as guidance arrows and cartoon-like masks, are designed to guide the user to look towards the partner's face if attention is lost. The guidance arrows help to direct the user towards the partner's face, dynamically lengthening and shortening in accordance with the user's head movements. The cartoon-like mask is overlaid over the partner's face to improve the attention and motivation of the user to move their head in the direction of the face. The cartoon-like mask becomes more translucent as the user moves to look closer to the partner's face. Based on the user's performance, points are awarded, and the user can 'level up', unlocking further cartoon-like elements. Short auditory tones that correspond with various game events are present throughout the experience, and are delivered through the bone conduction transducer on the right side of the Empowered Brain smartglasses.

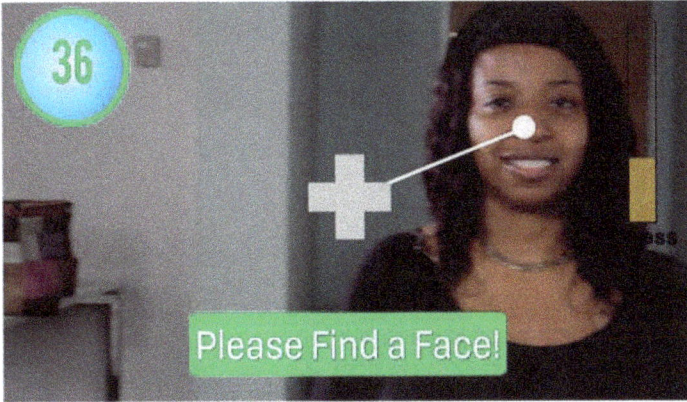

Figure 2. Face2Face module. Representative screen-capture image demonstrating a moment of what a Face2Face user experiences. Face2Face is one of the apps or modules of the Empowered Brain wearable system. This module includes artificial intelligence that finds and tracks faces, and is designed to make an engaging video game-like experience out of learning to direct one's gaze toward a partner when conversing. Through the computer screen of the wearable smartglasses headset (such as Google Glass), the user gets feedback that encourages face-directed gaze. For instance, in the moment represented here, the user is guided to redirect attention back to the partner's face via tones, visual words, and a dynamic arrow (drawing on "universal design for learning" by engaging multiple alternative senses and channels of reinforcement simultaneously). When mutual gaze is re-established, the user continues to earn points, stars, and temporary cartoon facemasks for achievement levels.

2.4. Emotion Charades

The Empowered Brain also includes Emotion Charades, an app that helps to teach human facial emotions through a game-like experience. Emotion Charades, like Face2Face, requires a partner to be present. The focus of the experience is the human-human interaction, with game providing motivation, a semi-scripted paradigm within which to interact, and tracking of progress over time. Emotion Charades, the Empowered Brain can not only detect a human face, but also identify the emotional expression that is being displayed through emotion artificial intelligence technology (Affectiva, Boston, MA, USA). Once an emotion has been detected by the device, two different AR emojis are presented to the user via the private optical display on Glass (Figure 3). One emoji corresponds to the facial expression of emotion that the partner is displaying, while the other does not. The user is asked to identify the correct emoji using a simple left or right head tilt. The head movements are detected by the software using in-built motion sensors of the headset. A correct choice triggers on-screen visual and verbal rewards and an auditory cue. Like Face2Face, short audio cues, corresponding to different game events, are delivered via the bone conduction transducer.

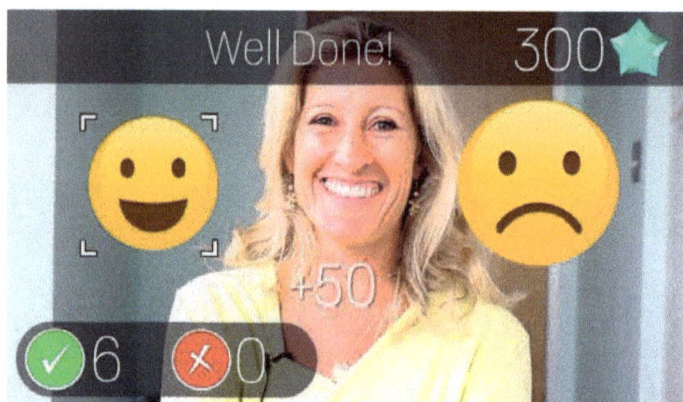

Figure 3. Emotion Charades **module**. Snapshot of what appears on the smartglasses screen during a representative moment during the Emotion Charades module. The moment depicted is immediately after the user has correctly chosen the "happy" emoticon as the one that represents the emotional expression on the face of the partner. The user gets multi-sensory automated feedback, and additionally the partner is cued to give the user specific prompts and mini-exercises to reinforce increasing levels of processing of the target emotions.

2.5. Transition Master

The Empowered Brain system also incorporates Transition Master, an app that can familiarize a user with a new environment by allowing her or him to interact with and view a 360-degree image of the physical location, as displayed by the optical display of the smartglasses (Figure 4). Transition Master is designed to help users with changes in environment. Many people with ASD commonly experience extreme distress during a change of activity or environment [2]. In the app, the 360-degree image of the "new" location is shown on the optical display. The 360-degree view dynamically changes in real-time with the head movements of the user. Transition Master, unlike Face2Face or Emotion Charades, does not require another person to be a facilitator, or to present a stimulus to the user. Auditory cues and sounds are provided during the experience. The user can tap the headset to transport to other linked rooms or areas when viewing a door, hallway, or other way one would naturally move though the space in reality.

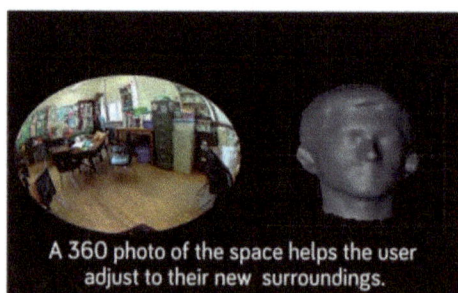

Figure 4. Transition Master Module. Spherical, immersive images can readily be taken of a new place such as a new classroom, or stressful environments such as a crowded or noisy mall or restaurant. These images are displayed by the Empowered Brain headset, offering the user exposure to an unfamiliar setting or context and the ability to practice navigating the environment before visiting it in person.

3. Methods

The methods and procedures of this study were approved by Asentral, Inc., Institutional Review Board, an affiliate of the Commonwealth of Massachusetts Department of Public Health. The study (2015-405A) was performed in accordance with relevant guidelines and regulations. The study was conducted in accordance with the Declaration of Helsinki.

User Recruitment

A sequential sample of 18 children and adults with ASD were recruited from a database of individuals who completed a web-based signup form, expressing interest in our study (mean age 12.2 years, range: 4.4–21.5 years; Table 2). Users included males and females, both verbal and non-verbal, and represented a wide range of ASD severity levels. Caregivers confirmed that the participants had received a professional ASD diagnosis.

Table 2. Demographics of Study Participants.

Demographics		
Number of Participants	18	
Age (mean ± SD)	12.2 ± 5.2	Range = 4.4 years–21.5 years
Participant gender	Male: 16 (88.9%)	Female: 2 (11.1%)
Verbal or nonverbal	Verbal: 16 (88.9%)	Nonverbal: 2 (11.1%)
Social Communication Questionnaire (SCQ) Score (mean ± SD)	18.8 ± 6.75	Range = 6–28

A Social Communication Questionnaire (SCQ) was completed for all users, with scores ranging from 6 to 28, with an average of 18.8. The SCQ is a validated way to obtain diagnostic and screening information about ASD [60,61]. Information regarding sensory symptoms was available in 14 of the 18 users, with the majority of those users having sensory challenges ($n = 13/14$, 92%).

Written and informed consent was obtained from all adult research participants and from the parents/legal guardians of all minors. Participants between 7 and 17 years-old additionally provided written consent, when appropriate. Every user was accompanied by a caregiver, and participants and caregivers could exit the session at any time and for any reason. Written and informed consent was obtained from all adults and the parents/legal guardians of all minors for the publication of their identifiable images. Consent was obtained for video and audio recording of the sessions. No compensation was offered to any participant or caregiver for taking part in the study, although reimbursement for their parking expenses was offered.

4. Exclusions

Individuals who had expressed interest via the website signup, but who had a known history of epilepsy or seizure disorder, were not enrolled in this study. Participants who had an uncontrolled or severe medical or mental health condition that would make participation in the study very difficult were also not enrolled. Two individuals were excluded due to the above criteria.

Data Collection Procedure

All testing was undertaken in a controlled research environment, and each participant (user) was accompanied to the session by their caregiver. Each user–caregiver dyad was tested separately. A total of 18 user–caregiver dyads participated in the below intervention; 2 were excluded due to meeting the exclusion criteria, stated above.

Each user and caregiver was asked to sit on chairs facing one another (Figure 5). A doctoral level clinical researcher oriented users and caregivers to the Empowered Brain hardware [Google Glass XE (Figure 1A)]. Users who could physically wear the smartglasses for at least one minute were allowed to proceed to testing the different Empowered Brain social and cognitive coaching apps (Table 1). The users and caregivers interacted with each other through a series of gamified experiences on the Empowered Brain.

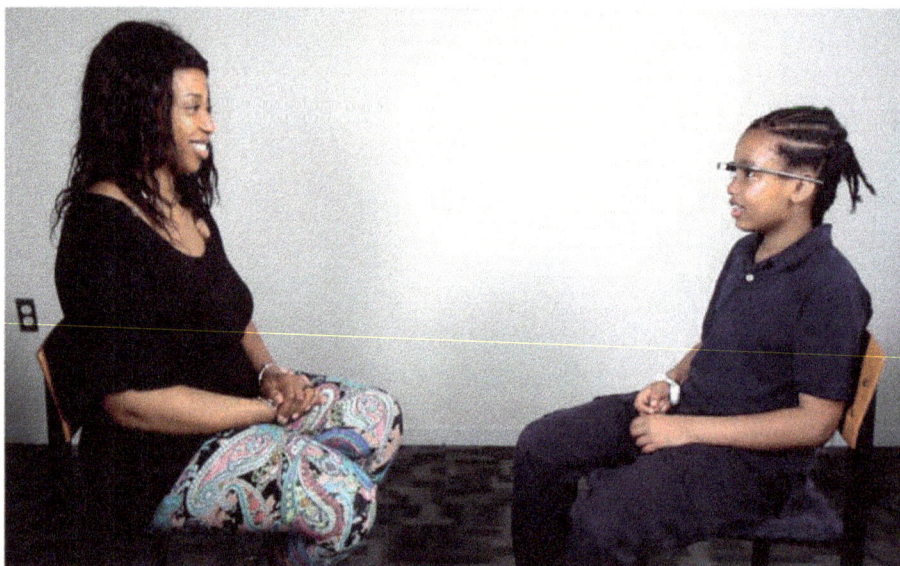

Figure 5. Empowered Brain User-Caregiver Setup. In each session, the participant and caregiver sit facing one another, promoting a 'heads-up' social interaction while trialing the apps. Written and informed consent has been obtained for the publication of these images from the depicted adult and from the parents/legal guardians of the minor.

The experiences were semi-structured in nature, with a total session duration of 60–90 min. The level of variability in the session length, required to use the range of apps, was reflective of the considerable range of ASD severity in the user group. After orientation and an assessment of tolerability, users were able to use Transition Master, then Face2Face, followed by Emotion Charades (Figure 6). Each user experienced each app for approximately 10 min (Figure 7). As previously noted, the Empowered Brain has been designed to be used in 10 min sessions, either once or twice a day. The relatively long duration of testing, relative to real-world use, was chosen in order to more robustly assess the response of users to the technology.

The smartglasses were taken off the user by staff or the caregiver, as required, for the purpose of repositioning, if the Empowered Brain application was to be changed or if there were user/caregiver usability questions.

Following the experience with the system, structured interviews were conducted with users and their caregivers. In the structured interviews, users and caregivers were asked to identify any perceived negative effects of using the system, and could raise concerns or give comments about the design of the smartglasses hardware as well as the apps.

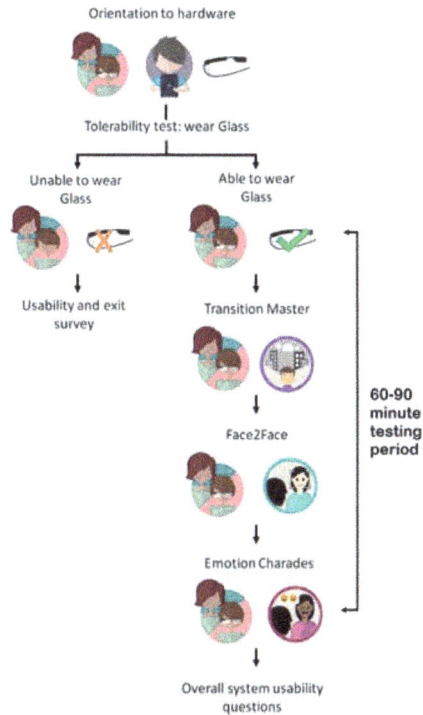

Figure 6. Outline of Phases of Study, including orientation to hardware, initial tolerability test of 1-min duration, followed by 60–90 min multi-module testing period.

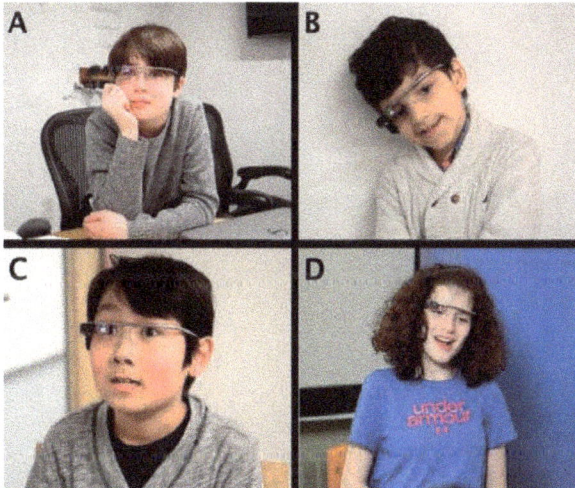

Figure 7. (**A–D**) Smartglasses Platform in Use. Four representative trial participants (**A–D**) wearing the Empowered Brain. This version of the Empowered Brain used the Glass Explorer Edition device (originally known as Google Glass). Written and informed consent has been obtained from the parents/legal guardians of the minors for the publication of these images.

5. Results

Sixteen of the 18 users (89%) tolerated wearing Empowered Brain smartglasses for at least one minute. The two users who did not tolerate this initial testing did not use Empowered Brain apps. While the two users and their caregivers did not report any adverse effects, the users did not express an interest in wearing the Empowered Brain or continuing the testing session. It was noted that both users were non-verbal, and were relatively young, aged 5.5 and 5.8 years. Of the remaining users, 14 out of 16 users (87.5%), and 16 out of 16 caregivers (100%), reported no minor negative effects, and 100% of caregivers and users reported no major negative effects (Table 3; Figure 8).

Table 3. Negative Effects. Issues reported by users or caregivers during the testing session are reported below.

Negative Effects	User (%, *n*)	Caregiver (%, *n*)	Notes
Gastrointestinal (nausea, vomiting)	0%, 0	0%, 0	None reported
Ophthalmic (eye strain, dry eyes, changes in vision)	6.3%, 1	0%, 0	Eye strain complaint, user took 20 s break and continued without further complaint
Motor (trips, falls, abnormal motor movements)	0%, 0	0%, 0	None reported
Behavioral (tantrums, meltdowns)	0%, 0	0%, 0	None reported
Dermatologic (skin injury or burns, skin irritation)	0%, 0	0%, 0	None reported
Any complaint of discomfort	6.3%, 1	0%, 0	Nose pieces initially caused one user discomfort.
Minor neurological (headache, dizziness)	6.3%, 1	0%, 0	One complaint of dizziness.
Major neurological (seizures, dystonia, loss of consciousness)	0%, 0	0%, 0	None reported

All Negative Effects of the Empowered Brain System As Reported by 18 Children and Adults with Autism After minimum of 1-hour sessions

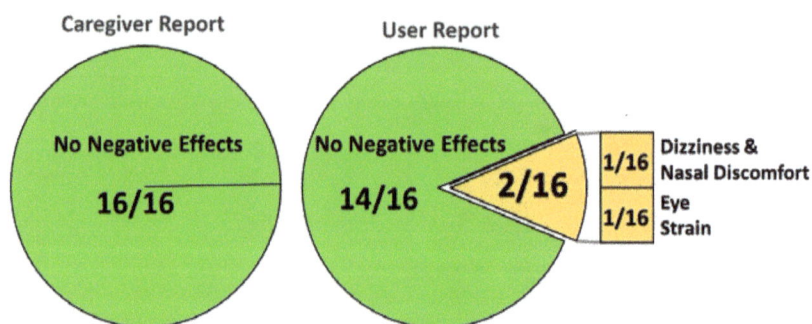

Figure 8. All Reported Negative Effects of the Empowered Brain System. Two users reported a total of three negative effects. One user experienced dizziness and nasal discomfort, and one user experienced eye strain. Caregivers reported that they observed no negative effects on users.

Negative effects were determined inductively. The three instances of negative effects were reported by two users. The effects were all mild in nature, transitory in duration, and did not result in session termination. The reported negative effects were one case of dizziness, one case of eye strain, and one instance of initial nasal bridge discomfort. The caregiver of the user experiencing dizziness later explained that the effect may have been related to the user not wearing his/her prescription glasses, and that s/he had previously experienced similar dizziness when s/he had tried a modern VR headset. This same user also experienced initial discomfort with the nose pads, but resolved the discomfort by adjusting the placement of the smartglasses. The user who had complained of eye strain resolved the issue with a 20-s break in testing.

In users who passed the initial tolerability test, the majority of users and their caregivers did not have any design concerns about the system (75% and 87.5% respectively) (Table 3). The only design concern highlighted by users and caregivers was that the smartglasses became warm to the touch during use, although this did not result in any negative effects (Table 4).

Table 4. Design concerns. Design concerns reported by users and by caregivers, including concerns raised spontaneously during or following testing session, as well as those mentioned in response to direct questions about design during structured interviews following testing sessions.

Design Concerns	User (%, *n*)	Caregiver (%, *n*)	Notes
Smartglasses (hardware)	25%, 4	12.5%, 2	Users and caregivers reported the smartglasses becoming warm after continued use
Applications (software)	0%, 0	0%, 0	None reported

6. Discussion

The safety and effects of AR smartglasses in children and adults with ASD is an important but poorly researched area, especially given the potential benefits of this technology. People with ASD who use AR smartglasses could potentially experience negative effects due to a range of known device-related factors and ASD-related human factors. ASD-related human factors include challenges in sensory, motor, attentional, and transition-related processes. Device-related factors, as per manufacturer warnings about side effects, include dizziness, headache, and seizures.

This paper explored the use of the Empowered Brain, a novel technological system that uses AR smartglasses to deliver social and cognitive coaching to children and adults with ASD. The focus was on exploring the safety and negative effects of using this technology across a broad age and severity range of children and adults with clinically diagnosed ASD. The duration of use of the Empowered Brain was between 60–90 min, considerably longer than the length of the 10-min intervention that the Empowered Brain has been created to deliver. Additionally, the practicalities of conducting this research involved circumstances that the authors believe could have made the experience more difficult for users than would have been the case had they tested/used the AR smartglasses in a more naturalistic home setting. During the day of testing, users and caregivers were exposed to novel surroundings by attending the research center and being asked to undertake a number of environmental transitions prior to the testing, and users had the additional sensory load of being video and audio recorded while using the Empowered Brain.

In this context our results are encouraging, and suggest that the majority of people with ASD can use these AR smartglasses without reporting any major negative effects. Of the 16 users who managed to wear and use the Empowered Brain ($n = 16/18$), neither caregivers nor users reported negative effects in 14 cases ($n = 14/16$, 87.5%). In the two individuals who reported negative effects, there were three reported issues: One case of dizziness, one case of eye strain, and one instance of initial nasal bridge discomfort. These negative effects were mild in nature, temporary, and did not lead to the user or caregiver stopping the session. It is important to note that these negative effects were not reported by the caregiver, but rather the participant, further justifying the explicit interviewing of people with ASD in order to understand their experience of this technology. Our participant sample included individuals who had a considerable ASD-related symptom load and those whose symptoms at the time of testing would fall below the typical cut-offs used for ASD-screening via the SCQ. The mean SCQ score of our participants was, however, markedly higher than previously used screening cut-offs. As we previously noted, two individuals were not able to, or did not show interest in, wearing/using the Empowered Brain. This small, but clinically important, group of participants were non-verbal, relatively young and were not reported to have had any negative effects. This may suggest that the technology may be more suited to people with higher-functioning ASD and that some individuals with ASD may struggle to utilize current AR smartglasses, particularly in a research environment.

The participants' caregivers suggested that an acclimation period to the physical wearing of smartglasses would likely improve the participants' reaction to the system.

This study tested the use of this particular technology for a prolonged single intervention session, between 6–9 times the length of the anticipated session length of 10 min. However, the study did not explore the longitudinal use of the technology outside of a controlled research environment. The study was conducted in a controlled research environment, as this allows for a more accurate assessment of participant and caregiver behavior and responses. However, many individuals with ASD receive therapeutic and educational interventions, over a prolonged period of time, in a variety of settings, such as their schools and homes. In this regard, it would be useful to conduct similar research that would incorporate longitudinal assessments in these ecologically valid environments.

The relative lack of negative effects in this AR paradigm is an important finding across such a wide age and severity range of people with ASD, and it indirectly supports recent research demonstrating minimal negative effects when modern VR headsets were used by people with ASD [38]. It was reassuring to see that no major negative effects were reported and, additionally, that no behavioral problems, such as tantrums or meltdowns, occurred when users were asked to stop using the smartglasses during adjustments or application switches, especially given earlier outlined concerns regarding the potential for distress relating to transitions involving technology. Despite the majority of users having sensory sensitivities, there were no concerns regarding sensory-related negative experiences during the use of the Empowered Brain. There were also no falls or motor issues encountered during this study, although our experimental methodology and intervention did not require users to stand, walk, or otherwise demonstrate motor, gait, or balance activities that could be deemed to be a stress test of such activities in this population. Users and caregivers were seated during the experience, and this approach may have intrinsically reduced the risk of falls. AR technologies that require users to attend to the software, while simultaneously requiring users to engage in complex physical and cognitive real-world tasks would need to be more rigorously evaluated. Our prior research has suggested that the use of smartglasses technology alone, without AR, can be used to safely assess balance and complex body movement [1]. Therefore, our findings may not be generalizable to situations where users would be required to engage in notable motor activity in combination with a task-related cognitive load.

There were no design concerns by the majority of caregivers and users. Design concerns were raised by two caregivers and four users, who noticed a feeling of warmth from the external side of the hardware after extended use. However, this did not result in any reported negative effects. User acceptance of design is an important part of any assistive technology experience, so it was useful to know that users and caregivers had few concerns about the design and use of the Empowered Brain.

There remains a critical need to conduct further research to understand the feasibility and safety associated with new emerging technologies, especially those that may be used in vulnerable populations, such as ASD. The use of AR smartglasses may have considerable potential as an augmentative technology in helping people with ASD, particularly when they are shown to be usable and safe in the ASD population and supported by robust evidence of efficacy. While our results suggest that this particular combination of hardware and software is largely devoid of negative effects, our findings may not be generalizable to systems based on other types of AR smartglasses or software apps. Therefore, our findings should not be considered evidence that all AR technologies and software are safe in ASD populations but should rather be considered preliminary evidence that carefully designed technology with user involvement can allow for the safe delivery of specific AR-related interventions.

Additionally, while this report does not identify any short term adverse events, as with any technology, further research is warranted to explore the positive and negative effects of longer term repeated use.

Author Contributions: N.T.S. is the inventor of the Empowered Brain. N.T.S., J.P.S., N.U.K., and A.V. designed and undertook the intervention. The writing of this report was led by A.V., and all authors contributed.

J. Clin. Med. **2018**, *7*, 188

Funding: This work was supported by the Office of the Assistant Secretary of Defense for Health Affairs, through the Autism Research Program under Award No. W81XWH 17-1-0449. Early work to transform smartglasses into biomedical sensors was supported in part by the United States Army Medical Research and Materiel Command under Contract No. W81XWH-14-C-0007 (awarded to TIAX, LLC). Opinions, interpretations, conclusions, and recommendations are those of the authors and are not necessarily endorsed by the Department of Defense.

Acknowledgments: The authors thank Google, Inc., (Mountain View, CA, USA) for a generous grant and also the Glass team at X (formerly Google X) for technical guidance on Glass software development. The authors also thank Amazon and Amazon Web Services for support, guidance, and access to pre-release artificial intelligence tools. The authors are also grateful to Affectiva for their emotion artificial intelligence technology that has helped to enable this work. This work was supported by the Office of the Assistant Secretary of Defense for Health Affairs, through the Autism Research Program under Award No. W81XWH 17-1-0449. Early work to transform smartglasses into biomedical sensors was supported in part by the United States Army Medical Research and Materiel Command under Contract No. W81XWH-14-C-0007 (awarded to TIAX, LLC). Opinions, interpretations, conclusions, and recommendations are those of the authors and are not necessarily endorsed by the Department of Defense.

Conflicts of Interest: This report was supported by Brain Power, a neurotechnology company that develops a range of artificially intelligent wearable technologies. Brain Power has engineering and technical partnerships with major technology companies and also receives funding support from Federal and Congressional sources.

Abbreviations

AR   Augmented Reality
ASD   Autism Spectrum Disorder
BPAS   Brain Power Autism System
SCQ   Social Communication Questionnaire
VR   Virtual Reality

References

1. Autism and Developmental Disabilities Monitoring Network Surveillance Year 2010 Principal Investigators; Centers for Disease Control and Prevention (CDC). Prevalence of autism spectrum disorder among children aged 8 years-autism and developmental disabilities monitoring network, 11 sites, United States, 2010. *Morb. Mortal. Wkly Rep. Surveill. Summ.* **2014**, *63*, 1–21.
2. Association, A.P. *Diagnostic and Statistical Manual of Mental Disorders (DSM-5®)*; American Psychiatric Pub: Washington, DC, USA, 2013.
3. Kogan, M.D.; Strickland, B.B.; Blumberg, S.J.; Singh, G.K.; Perrin, J.M.; van Dyck, P.C. A national profile of the health care experiences and family impact of autism spectrum disorder among children in the United States, 2005–2006. *Pediatrics* **2008**, *122*, e1149–e1158. [CrossRef] [PubMed]
4. Boyle, C.A.; Boulet, S.; Schieve, L.A.; Cohen, R.A.; Blumberg, S.J.; Yeargin-Allsopp, M.; Visser, S.; Kogan, M.D. Trends in the prevalence of developmental disabilities in US children, 1997–2008. *Pediatrics* **2011**, *127*, 1034–1042. [CrossRef] [PubMed]
5. Grynszpan, O.; Weiss, P.L.; Perez-Diaz, F.; Gal, E. Innovative technology-based interventions for autism spectrum disorders: A meta-analysis. *Autism* **2014**, *18*, 346–361. [CrossRef] [PubMed]
6. Walsh, E.; Holloway, J.; McCoy, A.; Lydon, H. Technology-Aided Interventions for Employment Skills in Adults with Autism Spectrum Disorder: A Systematic Review. *Rev. J. Autism Dev. Disord.* **2017**, *4*, 12–25. [CrossRef]
7. Didehbani, N.; Allen, T.; Kandalaft, M.; Krawczyk, D.; Chapman, S. Virtual reality social cognition training for children with high functioning autism. *Comput. Hum. Behav.* **2016**, *62*, 703–711. [CrossRef]
8. Golan, O.; Baron-Cohen, S. Systemizing empathy: Teaching adults with Asperger syndrome or high-functioning autism to recognize complex emotions using interactive multimedia. *Dev. Psychopathol.* **2006**, *18*, 591–617. [CrossRef] [PubMed]
9. Shane, H.C.; Albert, P.D. Electronic screen media for persons with autism spectrum disorders: Results of a survey. *Rev. J. Autism Dev. Disord.* **2008**, *38*, 1499–1508. [CrossRef] [PubMed]
10. Mayes, S.D.; Calhoun, S.L. Analysis of WISC-III, Stanford-Binet: IV, and academic achievement test scores in children with autism. *Rev. J. Autism Dev. Disord.* **2003**, *33*, 329–341. [CrossRef]
11. Schlosser, R.W.; Blischak, D.M. Is there a role for speech output in interventions for persons with autism? A review. *Focus Autism Other Dev. Disabil.* **2001**, *16*, 170–178. [CrossRef]

12. Mazurek, M.O.; Engelhardt, C.R. Video game use and problem behaviors in boys with autism spectrum disorders. *Res. Autism Spectrum Disord.* **2013**, *7*, 316–324. [CrossRef]
13. Samuel, A. Personal Technology and the Autistic Child: What One Family Has Learned: Wall Street Journal. 2017. Available online: http://www.wsj.com/articles/personal-technology-and-the-autistic-child-what-one-family-has-learned-1466993100 (accessed on 4 July 2018).
14. Ramdoss, S.; Machalicek, W.; Rispoli, M.; Mulloy, A.; Lang, R.; O'Reilly, M. Computer-based interventions to improve social and emotional skills in individuals with autism spectrum disorders: A systematic review. *Dev. Neurorehabil.* **2012**, *15*, 119–135. [CrossRef] [PubMed]
15. Ramdoss, S.; Lang, R.; Mulloy, A.; Franco, J.; O'Reilly, M.; Didden, R.; Lancioni, G. Use of computer-based interventions to teach communication skills to children with autism spectrum disorders: A systematic review. *J. Behav. Educ.* **2011**, *20*, 55–76. [CrossRef]
16. Pennington, R.C. Computer-assisted instruction for teaching academic skills to students with autism spectrum disorders: A review of literature. *Focus Autism Other Dev. Disabil.* **2010**, *25*, 239–248. [CrossRef]
17. Wainer, A.L.; Ingersoll, B.R. The use of innovative computer technology for teaching social communication to individuals with autism spectrum disorders. *Res. Autism Spectrum Disord.* **2011**, *5*, 96–107. [CrossRef]
18. Shattuck, P.T.; Narendorf, S.C.; Cooper, B.; Sterzing, P.R.; Wagner, M.; Taylor, J.L. Postsecondary education and employment among youth with an autism spectrum disorder. *Pediatrics* **2012**, *129*, 1042–1049. [CrossRef] [PubMed]
19. Hurlbutt, K.; Chalmers, L. Employment and adults with Asperger syndrome. *Focus Autism Other Dev. Disabil.* **2004**, *19*, 215–222. [CrossRef]
20. Reichow, B.; Steiner, A.M.; Volkmar, F. Cochrane review: Social skills groups for people aged 6 to 21 with autism spectrum disorders (ASD). *Evid.-Based Child Health Cochrane Rev. J.* **2013**, *8*, 266–315. [CrossRef] [PubMed]
21. Strickland, D. Virtual reality for the treatment of autism. *Stud. Health Technol. Inform.* **1997**, *44*, 81–86. [PubMed]
22. Escobedo, L.; Tentori, M.; Quintana, E.; Favela, J.; Garcia-Rosas, D. Using augmented reality to help children with autism stay focused. *IEEE Pervasive Comput.* **2014**, *13*, 38–46. [CrossRef]
23. Chen, C.-H.; Lee, I.-J.; Lin, L.-Y. Augmented reality-based video-modeling storybook of nonverbal facial cues for children with autism spectrum disorder to improve their perceptions and judgments of facial expressions and emotions. *Comput. Hum. Behav.* **2016**, *55*, 477–485. [CrossRef]
24. McMahon, D.; Cihak, D.F.; Wright, R. Augmented reality as a navigation tool to employment opportunities for postsecondary education students with intellectual disabilities and autism. *J. Res. Technol. Educ.* **2015**, *47*, 157–172. [CrossRef]
25. Radu, I.; Guzdial, K.; Avram, S. (Eds.) An Observational Coding Scheme for Detecting Children's Usability Problems in Augmented Reality. In Proceedings of the 2017 Conference on Interaction Design and Children, Stanford, CA, USA, 27–30 June 2017; ACM: New York, NY, USA, 2017.
26. Franchina, M.; Sinkar, S.; Ham, B.; Lam, G.C. A blinding eye injury caused by chasing Pokemon. *Med. J. Aust.* **2017**, *206*, 384. [CrossRef] [PubMed]
27. Richard, E.; Billaudeau, V.; Richard, P.; Gaudin, G. (Eds.) Augmented reality for rehabilitation of cognitive disabled children: A preliminary study. In Proceedings of the Virtual Rehabilitation, Venice, Italy, 27–29 September 2007.
28. Monkman, H.; Kushniruk, A.W. (Eds.) A see through future: Augmented reality and health information systems. *Stud. Health Technol. Inform.* **2015**, *208*, 281–285.
29. Salisbury, J.P.; Keshav, N.U.; Sossong, A.D.; Sahin, N.T. Concussion Assessment with Smartglasses: Validation Study of Balance Measurement toward a Lightweight, Multimodal, Field-Ready Platform. *JMIR mHealth uHealth* **2018**, *6*, 15. [CrossRef] [PubMed]
30. Rauschnabel, P.A.; Brem, A.; Ro, Y. *Augmented Reality Smart Glasses: Definition, Conceptual Insights, and Managerial Importance*; Unpublished Working Paper; The University of Michigan-Dearborn, College of Business: Dearborn, MI, USA, 2015.
31. Liu, R.; Salisbury, J.P.; Vahabzadeh, A.; Sahin, N.T. Feasibility of an Autism-Focused Augmented Reality Smartglasses System for Social Communication and Behavioral Coaching. *Front. Pediatr.* **2017**, *5*, 145. [CrossRef] [PubMed]

32. Keshav, N.U.; Salisbury, J.P.; Vahabzadeh, A.; Sahin, N.T. Social Communication Coaching Smartglasses: Well Tolerated in a Diverse Sample of Children and Adults With Autism. *JMIR Mhealth Uhealth.* **2017**, *5*, e140. [CrossRef] [PubMed]
33. Sahin, N.T.; Keshav, N.U.; Salisbury, J.P.; Vahabzadeh, A. Second Version of Google Glass as a Wearable Socio-Affective Aid: Positive School Desirability, High Usability, and Theoretical Framework in a Sample of Children with Autism. *JMIR Hum. Factors* **2018**, *5*, e1. [CrossRef] [PubMed]
34. Vahabzadeh, A.; Keshav, N.U.; Salisbury, J.P.; Sahin, N.T. Improvement of Attention-Deficit/Hyperactivity Disorder Symptoms in School-Aged Children, Adolescents, and Young Adults with Autism via a Digital Smartglasses-Based Socioemotional Coaching Aid: Short-Term, Uncontrolled Pilot Study. *JMIR Ment. Health* **2018**, *5*, e25. [CrossRef] [PubMed]
35. Sahin, N.T.; Abdus-Sabur, R.; Keshav, N.U.; Liu, R.; Salisbury, J.P.; Vahabzadeh, A. Case Study of a Digital Augmented Reality Intervention for Autism in School Classrooms: Associated with Improved Social Communication, Cognition, and Motivation as rated by Educators and Parents. *Front. Educ.* **2018**, *3*, 57.
36. Longitudinal Socio-Emotional Learning Intervention for Autism via Smartglasses: Qualitative School Teacher Descriptions of Practicality, Usability, and Efficacy in General and Special Education Classroom Settings. Available online: https://psyarxiv.com/xpduy/ (accessed on 30 July 2018).
37. Newbutt, N.; Sung, C.; Kuo, H.J.; Leahy, M.J. The acceptance, challenges, and future applications of wearable technology and virtual reality to support people with autism spectrum disorders. In *Recent Advances in Technologies for Inclusive Well-Being*; Springer: Berlin, Germany, 2017; pp. 221–241.
38. Newbutt, N.; Sung, C.; Kuo, H.-J.; Leahy, M.J.; Lin, C.-C.; Tong, B. Brief report: A pilot study of the use of a virtual reality headset in autism populations. *J. Autism Dev. Disord.* **2016**, *46*, 3166–3176. [CrossRef] [PubMed]
39. Ausderau, K.K.; Sideris, J.; Little, L.M.; Furlong, M.; Bulluck, J.C.; Baranek, G.T. Sensory subtypes and associated outcomes in children with autism spectrum disorders. *Autism Res.* **2016**, *9*, 1316–1327. [CrossRef] [PubMed]
40. Fournier, K.A.; Hass, C.J.; Naik, S.K.; Lodha, N.; Cauraugh, J.H. Motor coordination in autism spectrum disorders: A synthesis and meta-analysis. *J. Autism Dev. Disord.* **2010**, *40*, 1227–1240. [CrossRef] [PubMed]
41. Howlin, P.; Savage, S.; Moss, P.; Tempier, A.; Rutter, M. Cognitive and language skills in adults with autism: A 40-year follow-up. *J. Child Psychol. Psychiatry* **2014**, *55*, 49–58. [CrossRef] [PubMed]
42. Landry, O.; Al-Taie, S. A meta-analysis of the Wisconsin Card Sort Task in autism. *J. Autism Dev. Disord.* **2016**, *46*, 1220–1235. [CrossRef] [PubMed]
43. Sevin, J.A.; Rieske, R.D.; Matson, J.L. A Review of Behavioral Strategies and Support Considerations for Assisting Persons with Difficulties Transitioning from Activity to Activity. *Rev. J. Autism Dev. Disord.* **2015**, *2*, 329–342. [CrossRef]
44. McCormick, C.; Hepburn, S.; Young, G.S.; Rogers, S.J. Sensory symptoms in children with autism spectrum disorder, other developmental disorders and typical development: A longitudinal study. *Autism* **2016**, *20*, 572–579. [CrossRef] [PubMed]
45. Ronald, A.; Simonoff, E.; Kuntsi, J.; Asherson, P.; Plomin, R. Evidence for overlapping genetic influences on autistic and ADHD behaviours in a community twin sample. *J. Child Psychol. Psychiatry* **2008**, *49*, 535–542. [CrossRef] [PubMed]
46. Sabelman, E.E.; Lam, R. The real-life dangers of augmented reality. *IEEE Spectrum* **2015**, *52*, 48–53. [CrossRef]
47. Rice, C.E.; Zablotsky, B.; Avila, R.M.; Colpe, L.J.; Schieve, L.A.; Pringle, B.; Blumberg, S.J. Reported wandering behavior among children with autism spectrum disorder and/or intellectual disability. *J. Pediatr.* **2016**, *174*, 232.e2–239.e2. [CrossRef] [PubMed]
48. Dettmer, S.; Simpson, R.L.; Myles, B.S.; Ganz, J.B. The use of visual supports to facilitate transitions of students with autism. *Focus Autism Other Dev. Disabil.* **2000**, *15*, 163–169. [CrossRef]
49. Microsoft. Health & Safety. 2017. Available online: https://www.microsoft.com/en-us/hololens/legal/health-and-safety-information (accessed on 2 September 2017).
50. Ianchulev, T.; Minckler, D.S.; Hoskins, H.D.; Packer, M.; Stamper, R.; Pamnani, R.D.; Koo, E.Y. Wearable technology with head-mounted displays and visual function. *JAMA* **2014**, *312*, 1799–1801. [CrossRef] [PubMed]
51. LaViola, J.J., Jr. A discussion of cybersickness in virtual environments. *ACM SIGCHI Bull.* **2000**, *32*, 47–56. [CrossRef]

52. Google. Google Glass Tech Specs 2016. Available online: https://support.google.com/glass/answer/3064128?hl=en (accessed on 2 September 2017).

53. Muensterer, O.J.; Lacher, M.; Zoeller, C.; Bronstein, M.; Kübler, J. Google Glass in pediatric surgery: An exploratory study. *Int. J. Surg.* **2014**, *12*, 281–289. [CrossRef] [PubMed]

54. Jack, R.E.; Schyns, P.G. The human face as a dynamic tool for social communication. *Curr. Biol.* **2015**, *25*, R621–R634. [CrossRef] [PubMed]

55. Klin, A.; Jones, W.; Schultz, R.; Volkmar, F.; Cohen, D. Visual fixation patterns during viewing of naturalistic social situations as predictors of social competence in individuals with autism. *Arch. Gen. Psychiatry* **2002**, *59*, 809–816. [CrossRef] [PubMed]

56. Kirchner, J.C.; Hatri, A.; Heekeren, H.R.; Dziobek, I. Autistic symptomatology, face processing abilities, and eye fixation patterns. *J. Autism Dev. Disord.* **2011**, *41*, 158–167. [CrossRef] [PubMed]

57. Tanaka, J.W.; Sung, A. The "Eye Avoidance" Hypothesis of Autism Face Processing. *J. Autism Dev. Disord.* **2016**, *46*, 1538–1552. [CrossRef] [PubMed]

58. Tang, J.; Falkmer, M.; Horlin, C.; Tan, T.; Vaz, S.; Falkmer, T. Face Recognition and Visual Search Strategies in Autism Spectrum Disorders: Amending and Extending a Recent Review by Weigelt et al. *PLoS ONE* **2015**, *10*, e0134439. [CrossRef] [PubMed]

59. Jones, W.; Carr, K.; Klin, A. Absence of preferential looking to the eyes of approaching adults predicts level of social disability in 2-year-old toddlers with autism spectrum disorder. *Arch. Gen. Psychiatry* **2008**, *65*, 946–954. [CrossRef] [PubMed]

60. Rutter, M.; Bailey, A.; Lord, C. *The Social Communication Questionnaire: Manual*; Western Psychological Services: Melton South, VIC, Australia, 2003.

61. Chandler, S.; Charman, T.; Baird, G.; Simonoff, E.; Loucas, T.; Meldrum, D.; Scott, M.; Pickles, A. Validation of the social communication questionnaire in a population cohort of children with autism spectrum disorders. *J. Am. Acad. Child Adolesc. Psychiatry* **2007**, *46*, 1324–1332. [CrossRef] [PubMed]

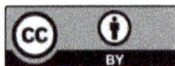

Journal of
Clinical Medicine

MDPI

Article

Development and Evaluation of Culturally and Linguistically Tailored Mobile App to Promote Breast Cancer Screening

Hee Yun Lee [1],*, Mi Hwa Lee [2], Zan Gao [3] and Karim Sadak [4]

[1]   School of Social Work, University of Alabama, Tuscaloosa, AL 35487, USA
[2]   College of Health and Human Performance, East Carolina University, Greenville, NC 27858, USA;
     leemih17@ecu.edu
[3]   School of Kinesiology, University of Minnesota, Minneapolis, MN 55455, USA; gaoz@umn.edu
[4]   Masonic Cancer Center, University of Minnesota Medical School, Minneapolis, MN 55455, USA;
     ktsadak@umn.edu
*   Correspondence: hlee94@ua.edu; Tel: +1-205-348-6553

Received: 26 June 2018; Accepted: 13 July 2018; Published: 24 July 2018

Abstract: Background: While a significant breast cancer burden exists for Korean American immigrant women, their cancer screening behavior is strikingly poor, and few interventions have focused on this population. To promote breast cancer screening behavior in Korean American immigrant women, a mobile phone multimedia messaging intervention (mMammogram) was developed. Objective: The current study explores the impact of mMammogram on changes to study participants' screening behavior and proposes suggestions for how the intervention can be improved for wide dissemination and implementation in the Korean American community. Material and Methods: Data were collected through qualitative research methods. Three focus groups were conducted with 14 Korean immigrant women who completed the mMammogram. Findings: Three themes emerged: (1) better understanding of breast cancer and screening through mMammogram (e.g., increased knowledge on breast cancer and screening methods, increased understanding of the importance of regular mammography, and reduced anxiety about mammography); (2) health navigators as a trigger to promote mammography (e.g., providing resources for free or low-cost mammograms and scheduling mammogram appointments); and (3) suggestions for mMammogram (e.g., technical issues and program period). Conclusions: Mobile app intervention that is culturally tailored, along with health navigation services, can be a feasible, effective, and acceptable tool to promote breast cancer screening behaviors in underserved immigrant women. A mobile app can cover a broad range of breast cancer health topics and the health navigator can further help women overcome barriers to screening. A health navigation service is critical in overcoming language, transportation, and health accessibility barriers and triggering a positive change in their health screening behavior, especially for newly arrived immigrant populations.

Keywords: breast cancer; mammogram; mobile phone-based health intervention; mHealth; app; health navigator; Korean American immigrant women

---

1. Introduction

Although the cancer mortality rate is decreasing in the United States (U.S.) among the general population, the rate remains on the rise for Asian Americans, specifically for the Korean American population [1]. Studies report that Korean Americans have one of the highest overall cancer mortality rates across Asian American subgroups [2]. For example, breast cancer has been cited as both the most frequently diagnosed cancer and the most common cause of cancer deaths for Korean American women [3]. Cancer screening has been shown to be an effective measure in reducing cancer morbidity, contributing to the decline in cancer mortality rates in the general U.S. population [2,4]. However, there is a lack of utilization of these screening tools among Korean Americans. Studies of Asian American subgroups found that Korean Americans have had the lowest overall cancer screening rate [5], and Korean American women reported the lowest breast cancer screening rates [4,6–8].

Korean American women experience a variety of barriers to breast cancer screening. Studies on the topic have identified several obstacles to screening, including low socioeconomic status, language barriers, difficulties accessing healthcare (e.g., inadequate health insurance and burdens of cost and time), lack of cultural awareness by healthcare providers, lack of knowledge about screening guidelines, culture-based health beliefs (e.g., the belief that screening is unnecessary in the absence of symptoms), cultural modesty or embarrassment in terms of physical examinations, a fatalistic view of cancer, and fear of screening results [8–12]. Alongside barriers, the literature has also cited a number of facilitators that have been found to promote increased mammogram use in Korean American women. The noted factors include perceived benefits of mammograms, perceived self-efficacy, and perceived susceptibility to breast cancer [13,14].

A handful of interventions specifically designed to address barriers and promote breast cancer screening in the Korean American community have been implemented. These community-based efforts include peer-led workshops, education sessions, a lay health worker intervention, and distribution of print material about screening guidelines [13,15–19]. These interventions have only been partially effective in promoting screening among this population. Key reasons cited in the research literature for such limited success include the fact that Korean American women are a hard-to-reach population due to geographical dispersion across the U.S. [17] and that past efforts have utilized a "one size fits all" approach rather than tailored interventions that target specific obstacles individuals face [18,19]. A more efficacious approach may be to develop a culturally appropriate, personalized intervention that promotes breast cancer screening among Korean American women and responds to the systemic sociocultural barriers present in this population.

An innovative and promising solution might be a mobile phone-based health intervention. It is likely to provide low-cost and effective methods of contacting hard-to-reach populations with tailored individual messages, covering broad content areas while also overcoming restrictions to place and time of delivery [20]. Mobile health, or mHealth—described as "the delivery of healthcare services and information via mobile communication devices" [21]—is emerging as a direct and effective medium to change health behavior. mHealth is an element or expansion of eHealth [22,23]: it is the broader trend that incorporates any health service information delivered through the Internet or related technology [24]. The growing mHealth field has already proven to be effective in the realm of health behavior change [25–27].

To promote breast cancer screening behavior of Korean American immigrant women, the intervention program called mobile Mammogram (mMammogram) was developed. The current study aims to explore the perspectives of Korean American immigrant women regarding their use of mMammogram, and how the program (1) promotes knowledge and positive attitude toward breast cancer screening; (2) motivates them to get breast cancer screening; and (3) may be improved for wide dissemination and implementation in the Korean American community. The current study provides critical information for developing a culturally relevant and personally tailored intervention to promote mammograms among underserved immigrant women and other disadvantaged minority groups which can effectively improve breast cancer health equity.

2. Materials and Methods

2.1. mMammogram

mMammogram was a 7-day mobile phone-based multimedia messaging program. mMammogram provided knowledge on breast cancer and screening methods along with guidelines, cultural barriers (e.g., fatalistic view and lack of preventive care concept), and information to access the healthcare system. This content was delivered in various formats of tailored messages using culture-specific emoticons, graphs, images, pictures, and videos in the Korean language. mMammogram also offered health navigation services, such as providing necessary resources (e.g., free or low-cost mammogram) and making an appointment for a mammogram. More detailed information about the mMammogram Randomized Clinical Trial (RCT) has been previously published [28].

2.2. Research Method and Data Collection

The research team utilized qualitative research methods to address the research aims. Three focus groups were conducted between June 2014 and February 2015 with a total of 14 Korean immigrant women who completed mMammogram prior to the focus groups. Six women participated in the first focus group, five in the second group, and three in the third group. Details of data collection (e.g., study participants' inclusion and exclusion criteria and detailed recruiting process on mMammogram) are described elsewhere [28]. University of Minnesota's Institutional Review Board approved this study.

The first author, along with two research staff members, facilitated and took notes during each focus group. The focus group interviews were semi-structured and included open-ended questions that asked participants about general feedback on (1) content, duration, and concerns of mMammogram; (2) changes in their knowledge, attitude, and motivation for screening receipt after participating in mMammogram; and (3) their screening experience if they had a mammogram after the intervention and their recommendation for dissemination in the Korean American community. Some examples of questions used in the focus group include: What are your perspective about the mMammogram intervention? What did you think of the content of the mMammogram program? Was it helpful to improve your knowledge in breast cancer screening? and What are your suggestions for wide dissemination of the mMammogram intervention in our community? All focus groups were conducted in Korean. Each focus group lasted approximately 1–1.5 h and was digitally recorded. Written consent was obtained from all 14 participants before starting the focus groups. Each participant received $20 for her time commitment.

3. Data Analysis

A thematic analysis [29] was used to analyze the data and to identify the essential themes discussed. The thematic analysis involves six steps: (1) being familiar with written transcription of verbal data; (2) generating initial codes; (3) searching and deciding on a set of codes, subcategories, and categories; (4) identifying themes and reviewing the themes; (5) defining and naming themes; and (6) producing the report. To follow the steps, first, all audio interview files were transcribed in Korean by three bilingual Korean research assistants and then reviewed by the research team. Second, two of three bilingual Korean research assistants coded all transcripts separately. Each person identified and highlighted every codable unit of text in the transcripts and compared their analyses (codes, subcategories, and categories). Based on the codes, the research team established and reviewed themes. Themes were cross-checked to ensure they were representative of the transcripts. Clear definitions and names for each theme were generated through the process. Finally, the most representative quotes were selected to present in this paper and translated into English. Final translations were examined by all authors who are bilingual and bicultural.

4. Findings

4.1. Study Participants

Table 1 indicates study participants' sociodemographic characteristics. The mean age of all participants was 50.57 years old (Standard Deviation (SD) = 6.64). On average, they lived in the U.S. for 14 years (SD = 9.71). The majority of the participants (92.9%) were married. With respect to educational background, half of the participants (50%) had completed university and around 42.9% finished high school. Approximately 64.3% were currently employed. More than two-thirds of the participants (71.4%) had health insurance and only 35.7% had a primary healthcare provider. Only 14.3% had regular check-ups. Around 28.6% of the participants reported that their most recent mammogram was before 2010 and 35.7% had never had a mammogram in their life.

Table 1. The sociodemographics of study participants.

	Age	Years in the U.S.	Marital Status	Highest Education Level	Employment Status	Health Insurance	Primary Health Care Provider	Regular Check-Up	Recent Mammogram
1	44	5	Married	High school	Employed	Yes	No	No	Never screened
2	60	3	Separated or divorced	High school	Employed	Yes	No	Yes	2012
3	57	5	Married	High school	Employed	Yes	Yes	No	2011
4	51	13	Married	University	Employed	Yes	Yes	Yes	2003
5	50	14	Married	High school	Employed	No	Yes	No	Never screened
6	45	6	Married	High school	Employed	No	No	No	2008
7	53	13	Married	High school	Unemployed	No	Yes	No	2012
8	52	28	Married	University	Employed	Yes	No	No	2009
9	48	20	Married	University	Unemployed	Yes	No	No	2009
10	46	4	Married	University	Employed	Yes	No	No	2010
11	58	14	Married	University	Unemployed	No	No	No	Never screened
12	40	12	Married	University	Unemployed	Yes	No	No	Never screened
13	61	35	Married	University	Unemployed	Yes	Yes	No	2011
14	43	24	Married	Graduate school	Employed	Yes	No	No	Never screened

4.2. Themes from Focus Groups

Overall, three themes were identified from the focus groups: (1) better understanding of breast cancer and screening; (2) health navigators as a trigger to promote mammography; and (3) suggestions for mMammogram. We indicated each participant's number when describing quotes to protect the confidentiality of each participant.

4.2.1. Theme 1. Better Understanding about Breast Cancer and Mammography

Study participants reported that mMammogram helped to (1) increase their awareness, positive attitude, and knowledge on breast cancer and breast cancer screening methods; (2) increase their understanding of the importance of regular mammography; and (3) reduce their anxiety about mammography, resulting in promoting their interests in screening participation.

(1) Increased awareness and knowledge on breast cancer and screening methods

Overall, almost all participants (n = 12) stated that mMammogram was helpful to learn basic knowledge of breast cancer, as well as the three breast cancer screening methods: breast self-exam, clinical breast exam, and mammogram. Several participants reported that they were unaware of how prevalent breast cancer is in the Korean American community, which naturally led to their limited awareness about breast cancer screening. Interestingly, after participating in the program, they started to pay attention to information related to breast cancer when they watched TV, listened to the radio, or had conversations with their friends. The participants reported that mMammogram makes them take breast cancer seriously and encourages them to consider getting a mammogram. For example, participant #1 decided to get a mammogram after completing the program:

"You know ... I was surprised by the fact that breast cancer is common in our community. I believed that it is a rare disease in our community. When people talk about breast cancer, I did not carefully listen to [them]. However, the statistical graph related to breast cancer incidence and mortality in Korean American women caught my attention. It makes me to consider it more serious, leading me to think about mammogram. Early detection is better, right?"

In addition, seven participants explained how their misperceptions about mammograms were corrected through mMammogram. The common misperceptions reported by the study participants included (1) people who are older do not need screening and (2) mammogram causes radiation exposure, which also may cause cancer. Four participants knew an older woman with breast cancer and they thought it was a very rare case, indicating that older women do not need to get screened. For example, one participant admitted that she made a joke about her 89-year old mother-in-law who got a mammogram. She could not understand why her old mother-in-law got a mammogram at that time, but she was able to understand after completing mMammogram. Now she knows that old age is a risk factor for breast cancer and that women should get a mammogram regardless of their age. Three other participants expressed their concern about radiation exposure; their concern even led them to not get a mammogram. For instance, participant #3 shared her story:

> "I used to get a mammogram every year or every other year . . . and my last mammogram was in 2011. I have several reasons to stop getting it. One of the reasons is possible harm from the radiation exposure during mammogram. I worried about cumulative radiation exposure for several years because radiation exposure could be a risk factor for breast cancer, you know. This program highlights the early detection of mammogram. Plus, a female doctor in the video said that mammogram only involves a tiny amount of radiation and the benefits of mammogram outweigh possible harm from the radiation exposure. I am fully aware of it now, which led me get a mammogram again. If I did not participate in this study, I would not get a mammogram for many years."

(2) Reminder of the importance of regular mammography

Some participants (*n* = 5) did not understand why women should get a mammogram on a regular basis. They had received a mammogram before, but they did not adhere to routine screening for several reasons, such as having no symptoms on their breasts, having a busy life, and having health insurance issues. For example, participant #6 did not follow her physician's recommendation. She was young and healthy, so she could not find reasons to get a mammogram again, even with her physician's continuous suggestion:

> "Whenever I saw a doctor, he recommended me to get a mammogram because my last mammogram was 7 years ago. However, I ignored his suggestion. You know, I am healthy enough. No symptoms on my breasts. Why should I get a mammogram? Plus, I have conducted breast self-exam and had clinical breast exam. I thought these two methods are enough to check my breast. However, my thoughts have changed after I completed this program. I realized that I needed to get a mammogram on a regular basis, regardless of my health status. I learned that the two methods are not sufficient to find cancer. I did not know that breast cancer is very common in Korean American women, which makes me feel anxious."

The participants reported that mMammogram was helpful in reminding them about their breast health and increasing their awareness of getting regular mammography. For instance, participant #2 said that she made a schedule to get a mammogram after completing the program. She used to get mammograms in Korea because of her breast symptoms, but she stopped receiving them after she came to the U.S. because her life was too busy and she did not feel the symptoms anymore. mMammogram reminded her that she should continue to care for her breasts.

(3) Reduced anxiety about mammography

Half of the participants (*n* = 7) reported that mMammogram—particularly, two videos about mammogram procedures—helped reduce their anxiety about breast cancer screening. The participants were highly satisfied with the videos that demonstrated the procedure of a mammogram. One video showed the mammogram procedure briefly. The other video showed a technician at a breast imaging center explaining the mammogram procedure in step-by-step detail, from the check-in process at the front desk to taking images of the breasts. The participants mentioned that they felt a bit more confident in getting a mammogram after watching the videos. They reported getting a sense of the whole procedure of mammography, which resulted in relieving their anxiety about going to a hospital to get a mammogram. For example, participant #14 said:

"I felt safe to get a mammogram after watching two videos about mammogram procedure. I learned that I don't need to take off all my clothes while imaging my breasts … just exposure one side of breast and then if it is done … move to the other side of breast. You know the video. A nurse showed the rooms where we can change our clothes and where the mammogram machine is. This all information was super helpful to relieve my anxiety about mammogram. Now I know what to expect when I go to hospital to get a mammogram"

More than half of the study participants (*n* = 8) showed passion for learning more about breast cancer, beyond what was covered in the program, such as breast density and its relationship with breast cancer incidence and various cases of breast cancer by stage and related treatment options. In addition, they were highly motivated to educate other women about the importance of breast cancer screening, including colleagues at work, friends, and family members. They wanted to share what they learned from the program with other women in the community who did not or were not able to participate in this study. Two participants said that, after completing mMammogram, they partly showed the program to their daughters to educate them on how to conduct a breast self-exam:

"I showed a part of the mMammogram application (app) program to my daughter, in particular the breast self-exam video. She is a college student and I think she needs to start self-examination." (Participant #3)

4.2.2. Theme 2. Health Navigators as a Trigger to Promote Mammography

As a part of mMammogram, health navigation services were offered to the study participants. The services included obtaining necessary resources (e.g., free or low-cost mammograms) for participants who did not have health insurance, scheduling mammogram appointments for participants, helping participants select a primary care physician, helping fill out forms at hospitals or clinics, transporting participants to receive a mammogram, and/or following up after receiving a mammogram for those who have abnormal results. The study participants had an option to contact bilingual health navigators to support them in getting a mammogram. The most common requests were checking whether their health insurance covered mammography and if they were eligible to get a mammogram for free or at low cost.

(1) Importance of Health Navigation Services

Some of the focus group participants (*n* = 9) reported difficulties accessing healthcare due to their limited English proficiency. They highlighted how bilingual health navigators were helpful in supporting their accessibility, resulting in increased screening uptake. Some participants (*n* = 5) mentioned the complexity of health insurance. For example, participant #4 reported that her company chooses different health plans every year, which presents more challenges to getting a mammogram:

"All the problem is rooted in health insurance. You know what? My health insurance plan is changed every year, which led me discourage to access health care. It used to change every two or three years. (…). The coverage is getting worse. I need to find a new family doctor again... and check my coverage which I do feel uncomfortable because of my English. I am getting tired of it. I sometimes think to visit Korea to get comprehensive health exam. That is going to be much easier and cheaper."

(2) Health Navigation Services and Regular Mammogram Receipt

The study participants reported how bilingual health navigators helped them overcome barriers to screening (e.g., health insurance and communication with healthcare providers). They also indicated intentions to continue getting mammograms if they are able to access a health navigation service. For instance, participant #1 shared her story:

"After participating in this program, I decided to get a mammogram. It was my first mammogram in my lifetime. I was nervous and worried about receiving mammogram because I am not familiar with U.S. health care system and my English is not enough to communicate with doctor or nurse. I believed that I was able to get a mammogram because of health navigator's support. She called my health insurance company to check my insurance coverage. And then, she scheduled a mammogram appointment for me and went to the clinic with me. Such a good service. I really appreciated all the things she did. You know, I would like to continue to get mammography every year if someone reminds me and assists me to get it."

4.2.3. Theme 3. Suggestions for Improvement and Dissemination of the mMammogram

Although study participants were highly satisfied with mMammogram, they suggested how the intervention could be improved for wider dissemination and implementation in the Korean American community. Their suggestions include larger subtitles on videos, addressing technical issues (e.g., Wi-Fi connection), extended schedule of message delivery, and adjusting the program period duration. For example, a total of eight videos were provided via mMammogram that included Korean or English subtitles. Some participants ($n = 8$) said that the subtitles on videos were too small to read via their phone, even though they were wearing glasses. They had to watch the videos several times to read the subtitles and understand the contents. Second, sometimes participants faced challenges to using their phone, such as issues with Wi-Fi connection. In addition, participants expressed a desire to receive messages later at night or at other times based on their schedules. In the current mMammogram system, study participants could select their preferred time to receive the messages between 8 a.m. and 8 p.m. They suggested they could control the starting time of the program, given that their schedules could change from day to day. Otherwise, they were unable to attend the program on time and missed it. Lastly, participants had different opinions regarding the program period. Some participants suggested a shorter period of 3–5 days, while others preferred a 7-day program.

5. Discussion

This study explored (1) how mMammogram helped Korean American immigrant women to increase their knowledge and positive attitude toward mammography; (2) how the program motivated them to complete breast cancer screening; and (3) how the program could be improved and disseminated in the Korean American community. Along with these findings, this study demonstrated that a mobile phone-based multimedia health intervention with health navigation services can be a feasible, effective, and acceptable tool to promote mammography uptake in underserved immigrant women.

We identified three themes: (1) better understanding of breast cancer and screening through mMammogram intervention; (2) importance of health navigator services to promote mammography, and (3) suggestions for mMammogram improvement and dissemination strategies. As noted in Theme 1, multimedia messages (e.g., images, pictures, and videos) through a mobile phone-based application have the advantage of being entertaining and individual-targeted to capture study participants' attention. For example, video content held great persuasive power in our intervention. Video messages were the most popular and well-accepted among the study participants, and they remembered the contents conveyed via videos much clearer and longer than other text messages. In particular, study participants liked two video clips that featured mammogram procedures and the importance of having a regular mammogram. Those who were unfamiliar with U.S. hospitals and who never had a mammogram previously got a sense of what would happen when they go to a clinic for mammography. This improved their confidence about mammography and promoted their interest in screening participation [30,31].

Another merit of a mobile phone-based health intervention is its easy dissemination, accessibility, and portability by having important health information at the user's fingertips. Plus, the study participants can keep the program if they want and open it anytime to remind themselves or inform other people. A few study participants who had a passionate interest in our program taught their daughters how to conduct a breast self-exam by showing them the videos from the program. This was an unintended impact of our intervention, which implies "ripple effects" in that they led to new effects beyond the intended primary target of the intervention [32]. The participants' daughters may now have increased awareness of breast cancer screening at an early age and may start their mammography in the right time frame.

As discussed in Theme 2, it is well-known that immigrants face various challenges in navigating the U.S. healthcare system due to lack of health insurance literacy and underutilization of healthcare services due to limited English proficiency. In particular, undocumented immigrants' barriers range from financial issues to fear of deportation [33]. Health navigation models of care have been employed as a strategy to support individuals with limited resources and multiple barriers, and health navigators have made significant differences to health equity in culturally and linguistically diverse communities [34–36]. Our study also indicated how health navigation services played critical roles in boosting the participants' accessibility to receiving breast cancer screenings. Study participants could contact trained health navigators while attending mMammogram. They felt assured that they could ask for help in their own language as their needs increased. With navigators' assistance, some participants had a mammogram for the first time in their lives. Plus, they showed their intention to continue getting a mammogram if a health navigation service offers. Given that the U.S. healthcare system is complicated, and the healthcare environment continues to change, health navigator services and educational programs could be employed as tools to reduce breast cancer disparities.

As seen in Theme 3, on the other hand, several challenges were reported while attending mMammogram intervention. One of the challenges of a mobile phone-base health intervention is the various sizes and types of smartphones. Some participants had the latest phones with big screens (5.5 inches or larger), while some had older versions of mobile phones. Those who had mini smartphones had difficulty reading the subtitles on the videos. Given that the size of participants' phones cannot be controlled, we may consider enlarging the subtitles or dubbing the video in participants' native language. We need to further consider developing an application that could be downloaded onto the iPad, where participants may read subtitles through a large window. Additionally, some participants faced challenges in using their phones due to weak Wi-Fi connections or a complicated process of downloading an app. They still felt challenged even after our research team taught them how to access to our app program and respond to it before the intervention. With only a short time for training, it might be hard to overcome all challenges faced by study participants. We may need to provide ongoing training via health navigation services or a handout on how to deal with common technical challenges. Another solution is to develop a web-based app which does not need to be downloaded and can be easily seen by smartphones and any other mobile devices.

6. Limitations

This study provides a valuable contribution to knowledge on how mHealth can be used to change health behavior, particularly for promoting breast cancer screening; however, some limitations may affect its applicability to other contexts. First, while a small sample size is not a limitation of qualitative research, the data were collected from one-time focus group meetings. However, the examination of the study participants' responses to open-ended questions regarding evaluation of the intervention after the completion of mMammogram facilitated further insights into the evaluation of and feedback on a mobile-phone text-messaging program. Lastly, the frequent interactions between study participants and research team members may impact participants' knowledge and motivation to receive a breast cancer screening, as well as their positive attitudes toward the intervention. Whenever study participants had questions related to the app (e.g., technical issue) or contents, they were allowed to contact us, which may positively impact intervention effectiveness and study results.

7. Implications for Health Practice and Policy

In conclusion, mobile apps can cover a broad range of breast cancer health topics, and the health navigator can further help women overcome barriers to screening. Specifically, for newly arrived immigrant populations, a health navigation service is critical in overcoming language, transportation, and health accessibility barriers and triggering a positive change in their health screening behavior. This study demonstrates the effectiveness of a culturally tailored mobile app intervention in increasing knowledge, attitude, and receipt of breast cancer screening in an immigrant group. Mobile app intervention should be combined with health navigation services, particularly when working with immigrant or refugee groups, to provide another layer of assistance which boosts confidence and comfort level in changing health behaviors. In addition, it was revealed that providing educational health information through visual images and videos is more effective than text messages. Overall, culturally and linguistically tailored multimedia messaging intervention combined with health navigation services is feasible and acceptable as an intervention tool to produce health behavior changes. The intervention can be easily translated into other types of cancer screening and cancer prevention behaviors, which will significantly reduce the current cancer burden vulnerability that immigrant and refugee communities currently face.

8. Conclusions

By applying the mobile phone-based multimedia messaging program, the most prominent findings include better understanding of breast cancer and screening through mMammogram intervention and the importance of health navigator to promote mammography, as well as suggestions for mMammogram improvements and dissemination strategies. Identifying these three themes provided important insights for mMammogram intervention to increase the breast cancer screening. The vital role of these three implies the mobile phone-based multimedia messaging program may be useful for reducing multiple challenges and barriers in navigating the healthcare system and increasing the level of health literacy implemented in the immigrant population.

In light of the present findings, to produce health behavior changes and mitigate challenges in the healthcare system, mobile apps must cover a wide range of health topics in different languages with health navigator services. Mobile apps should also be tailored to different cultures among the immigrant populations to trigger positive changes in increasing health literacy and receipt of cancer screening. Furthermore, the tailored multimedia messaging intervention also need to combine with visual images and videos. In sum, culturally and linguistically tailored multimedia messaging intervention combined with health navigation services is useful and effective to reduce the current cancer burden vulnerability faced by immigrant populations.

Author Contributions: All authors listed have contributed sufficiently to the project to be included as authors.

Funding: The study was supported by the fund from the Susan G. Komen for the Cure®Foundation (IIR12223971).

Acknowledgments: The research team appreciates the Foundation's generous funding to pilot this intervention study and the Korean American immigrant women who participated in this research.

Conflicts of Interest: The authors declare no conflict of interest.

References

1. Centers for Disease Control and Prevention. Breast Cancer. Available online: www.cdc.gov/cancer/breast/ (accessed on 18 August 2010).
2. Cannistra, S.A.; Niloff, J.M. Cancer of the uterine cervix. *N. Engl. J. Med.* **1996**, *334*, 1030–1037. [CrossRef] [PubMed]
3. Coughlin, S.S.; Uhler, R.J. Breast and cervical cancer screening practices among Asian and Pacific islander women in the United States, 1994–1997. *Cancer Epidemiol. Biomarkers Prev.* **2000**, *9*, 597. [PubMed]

4. McCracken, M.; Olsen, M.; Chen, M.S.; Jemal, A.; Thun, M.; Cokkinides, V.; Deapen, D.; Ward, E. Cancer incidence, mortality, and associated risk factors among Asian Americans of Chinese, Filipino, Vietnamese, Korean, and Japanese Ethnicities. *CA Cancer J. Clin.* **2007**, *57*, 190–205. [CrossRef] [PubMed]
5. Lee, H.Y.; Lundquist, M.; Ju, E.; Luo, X.; Townsend, A. Colorectal cancer screening disparities in Asian Americans and Pacific islanders: Which Groups are most Vulnerable? *Ethn. Health* **2011**, *16*, 501–518. [CrossRef] [PubMed]
6. Sadler, G.R.; Ryujin, L.; Nguyen, T.; Oh, G.; Paik, G.; Kustin, B. Heterogeneity within the Asian American community. *Int. J. Equity Health* **2003**, *2*, 12. [CrossRef] [PubMed]
7. Lee, H.Y.; Ju, E.; Vang, P.D.; Lundquist, M. Breast and cervical cancer screening disparity among Asian American women: Does race/ethnicity matter? *J. Women Health* **2010**, *19*, 1877–1884. [CrossRef] [PubMed]
8. Lee, E.E.; Fogg, L.; Menon, U. Knowledge and beliefs related to cervical cancer and screening among Korean american women. *West. J. Nurs. Res.* **2008**, *30*, 960–974. [CrossRef] [PubMed]
9. Gany, F.M.; Herrera, A.P.; Avallone, M.; Changrani, J. Attitudes, knowledge, and health-seeking behaviors of five immigrant minority communities in the prevention and screening of cancer: A focus group approach. *Ethn. Health* **2006**, *11*, 19–39. [CrossRef] [PubMed]
10. Kim, H.; Lee, K.-J.; Lee, S.-O.; Kim, S. Cervical cancer screening in Korean American women: Findings from focus group interviews. *J. Korean Acad. Nurs.* **2004**, *34*, 617–624. [CrossRef]
11. Lee, M.C. Knowledge, barriers, and motivators related to cervical cancer screening among Korean-American women: A focus group approach. *Cancer Nurs.* **2000**, *23*, 168–175. [CrossRef] [PubMed]
12. Im, E.-O.; Park, Y.S.; Lee, E.-O.; Yun, S.N. Korean Women's Attitudes toward breast cancer screening tests. *Int. J. Nurs. Stud.* **2004**, *41*, 583–589. [CrossRef] [PubMed]
13. Kim, J.H.; Menon, U.; Wang, E.; Szalacha, L. Assess the effects of culturally relevant intervention on breast cancer knowledge, beliefs, and mammography use among Korean American women. *J. Immigr. Minor. Health* **2010**, *12*, 586–597. [CrossRef] [PubMed]
14. Lee, H.; Kim, J.; Han, H.-R. Do cultural factors predict mammography behaviour among Korean immigrants in the USA? *J. Adv. Nurs.* **2009**, *65*, 2574–2584. [CrossRef] [PubMed]
15. Kim, J.H.; Menon, U. Pre- and postintervention differences in acculturation, knowledge, beliefs, and stages of readiness for mammograms among Korean American women. *Oncol. Nurs. Forum* **2009**, *36*, 80–92. [CrossRef] [PubMed]
16. Han, H.-R.; Lee, H.; Kim, M.T.; Kim, K.B. Tailored lay health worker intervention improves breast cancer screening outcomes in non-adherent Korean-American women. *Health Educ. Res.* **2009**, *24*, 318–329. [CrossRef] [PubMed]
17. Maxwell, A.E.; Jo, A.M.; Chin, S.-Y.; Lee, K.-S.; Bastani, R. Impact of a print intervention to increase annual mammography screening among Korean American women enrolled in the national breast and cervical cancer early detection program. *Cancer Detect. Prev.* **2008**, *32*, 229–235. [CrossRef] [PubMed]
18. Moskowitz, J.M.; Kazinets, G.; Wong, J.M.; Tager, I.B. "Health is strength": A community health education program to improve breast and cervical cancer screening among Korean American women in Alameda county, California. *Cancer Detect. Prev.* **2007**, *31*, 173. [CrossRef] [PubMed]
19. Juon, H.-S.; Choi, S.; Klassen, A.; Roter, D. Impact of breast cancer screening intervention on Korean-American women in Maryland. *Cancer Detect. Prev.* **2006**, *30*, 297–305. [CrossRef] [PubMed]
20. Griffiths, F.; Lindenmeyer, A.; Powell, J.; Lowe, P.; Thorogood, M. Why are health care interventions delivered over the internet? A systematic review of the published literature. *J. Med. Internet Res.* **2006**, *8*, e10. [CrossRef] [PubMed]
21. Torgan, C. The Mhealth Summit: Local & Global Converge. Kinetics—From Lab Bench to Park Bench. Available online: http://caroltorgan.com/mhealth-summit/ (accessed on 24 July 2018).
22. World Health Organization. *MHealth: New Horizons for Health through Mobile Technologies*; World Health Organization: Geneva, Switzerland, 2011; pp. 1–112.
23. Istepanian, R.S.H.; Laxminarayan, S.; Pattichis, C.S. *M-Health: Emerging Mobile Health Systems*; Springer: New York, NY, USA, 2006.
24. Eysenbach, G. What is e-health? *J. Med. Internet Res.* **2001**, *3*, E20. [CrossRef] [PubMed]
25. Fjeldsoe, B.S.; Marshall, A.L.; Miller, Y.D. Behavior change interventions delivered by mobile telephone short-message service. *Am. J. Prev. Med.* **2009**, *36*, 165–173. [CrossRef] [PubMed]

26. Cole-Lewis, H.; Trace, K. Text messaging as a tool for behavior change in disease prevention and management. *Epidemiol. Rev.* **2010**, *32*, 56–69. [CrossRef] [PubMed]
27. Wei, J.; Ilene, H.; Stan, K. A review of the use of mobile phone text messaging in clinical and healthy behaviour interventions. *J. Telemed. Telecare* **2011**, *17*, 41–48. [CrossRef] [PubMed]
28. Lee, H.; Ghebre, R.; Le, C.; Jang, Y.J.; Sharratt, M.; Yee, D. Mobile phone multilevel and multimedia messaging intervention for breast cancer screening: Pilot randomized controlled Trial. *JMIR Mhealth Uhealth* **2017**, *5*, e154. [CrossRef] [PubMed]
29. Braun, V.; Victoria, C. Using thematic analysis in psychology. *Qual. Res. Psychol.* **2006**, *3*, 77–101. [CrossRef]
30. Tuong, W.; Larsen, E.R.; Armstrong, A.W. Videos to influence: A systematic review of effectiveness of video-based education in modifying health behaviors. *J. Behav. Med.* **2014**, *37*, 218–233. [CrossRef] [PubMed]
31. Ruffinengo, C.; Elisabetta, V.; Giovanni, R. Effectiveness of an informative video on reducing anxiety levels in patients undergoing elective coronarography: An RCT. *Eur. J. Cardiovasc. Nurs.* **2009**, *8*, 57–61. [CrossRef] [PubMed]
32. Jagosh, J.; Bush, P.L.; Salsberg, J.; Macaulay, A.C.; Greenhalgh, T.; Wong, G.; Cargo, M.; Green, L.W.; Herbert, C.P.; Pluye, P. A Realist Evaluation of Community-Based Participatory Research: Partnership Synergy, Trust Building and Related Ripple Effects. *BMC Public Health* **2015**, *15*, 725. [CrossRef] [PubMed]
33. Hacker, K.; Anies, M.; Folb, B.L.; Zallman, L. Barriers to health care for undocumented immigrants: A literature review. *Risk Manag. Healthc. Policy* **2015**, *8*, 175–183. [CrossRef] [PubMed]
34. Lee, T.; Ko, I.; Lee, I.; Kim, E.; Shin, M.; Roh, S.; Yoon, D.; Choi, S.; Chang, H. Effects of nurse navigators on health outcomes of cancer patients. *Cancer Nurs.* **2011**, *34*, 376–384. [CrossRef] [PubMed]
35. Doolan-Noble, F.; Smith, D.; Gauld, R.; Waters, D.L.; Cooke, A.; Reriti, H. Evolution of a health navigator model of care within a primary care Setting: A case study. *Aust. Health Rev.* **2013**, *37*, 523–528. [CrossRef] [PubMed]
36. Dohan, D.; Schrag, D. Using navigators to improve care of underserved patients: Current practices and approaches. *Cancer* **2005**, *104*, 848–855. [CrossRef] [PubMed]

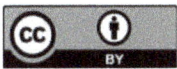

Journal of
Clinical Medicine

MDPI

Article

Technology-Enhanced Classroom Activity Breaks Impacting Children's Physical Activity and Fitness

Heidi Buchele Harris and Weiyun Chen *

School of Kinesiology, University of Michigan, Ann Arbor, MI 48109, USA; bucheleh@yahoo.com
* Correspondence: chenwy@umih.edu; Tel.: +1-734-615-0376

Received: 10 June 2018; Accepted: 28 June 2018; Published: 29 June 2018

Abstract: Background: This study examined the effects of a 4-week technology-enhanced physical activity (PA) interventions on students' real-time daily PA and aerobic fitness levels. Methods: 116 fifth-graders were assigned to one intervention group ($n = 31$) participating in daily physical activity engaging the brain with Fitbit Challenge (PAEB-C), another intervention group ($n = 29$) wearing Fitbits only (Fitbit-O) daily, five days per week, or the comparison group ($n = 56$). Four-week real-time PA data were collected from the intervention students via Fitbase. Three groups were pre- and post-tested aerobic fitness. Results: The PAEB-C students showed significantly higher steps and minutes of being very active and fairly active ($F = 7.999$, $p = 0.014$, $\eta = 0.121$; $F = 5.667$, $p = 0.021$, $\eta = 0.089$; $F = 10.572$, $p = 0.002$, $\eta = 0.154$) and lower minutes of being sedentary daily ($F = 4.639$, $p = 0.035$, $\eta = 0.074$) than the Fitbit-O group. Both Fitbit groups exhibited significantly greater increases in aerobic fitness scores than the comparison group over time ($F = 21.946$, $p = 0.001$, $\eta = 0.303$). Boys were more physically active and fit than girls. Conclusions: Technology-enhanced PA intervention was effective for improving real-time PA and aerobic fitness.

Keywords: real-time physical activity; wearable technology; fitness; Fitbits

1. Introduction

To obtain physical and mental health benefits, children are recommended to participate in 60 or more minutes of moderate-to-vigorous physical activity (MVPA) per day, and to demonstrate a healthy level of aerobic fitness [1–3]. However, one in three children did not meet the recommended daily MVPA minutes, and failed to meet aerobic fitness standards [4–6]. To address the critical concerns, health professionals have advocated that schools provide realistic settings for PA intervention [1–7]. More than 95% of youth are enrolled in schools and spend about half of their waking hours in schools [1–6]. Therefore, introducing physical activity (PA) to each school day may be beneficial in helping children to meet daily physical activity guidelines and improve aerobic fitness [1–6].

Integrating PA into daily classroom breaks is an important strategy for increasing daily PA levels of children during school [8–13]. A growing number of classroom-based PA intervention studies have shown that students who participated in daily 10-min classroom physical activity (i.e., TAKE 10!) or 15 min of physically active academic lessons (i.e., Physical Activity Across the Curriculum (PAAC)), on a regular basis, achieved significantly greater levels of daily MVPA compared to control students [10–13]. Further, Carlson et al. [12] found that ten-minute classroom PA breaks, in addition to physical education and recess, significantly increased the likelihood of obtaining 30 min of PA per day during school. Ma et al. [13] found that daily 4-min high intensity classroom PA breaks increased PA levels during school. However, most of studies did not examine the effects of the classroom PA breaks on improving children's fitness levels [8–13]. Empirical studies show that physical fitness is one of the enabling factors that provide the physical foundations necessary for enjoyable and successful PA engagement in youth [14–17]. Physically fit children are willing to engage in PA and to maintain their PA behaviors, whereas physically unfit children tend to be physically inactive [14–17]. Importantly, these links are reciprocal, as children's participation in PA provides opportunities for improving physical fitness as well [14–17].

Wearable technology has been used as a self-monitoring tool for promoting physical activity participation [18–21]. In the Futurestep study by Mikkola et al. [20], the results indicated that students' use of Polar heart rate monitors increased an awareness of their own fitness level and physical activity level and improved their motivation for PA participation. In a systematic review of activity monitors and PA, Lubans et al. [21] found that twelve out of fourteen studies using activity monitors significantly increased PA levels in terms of steps, distances, durations, and intensities. Fitbit is specifically designed to work at the individual level by providing detailed personalized data, such as minute-by-minute data, and composite data on steps, distance traveled, MVPA, heart rate, and intensity [18–20]. Fitbit has been evidenced to be a reliable and valid self-monitor, self-evaluation, and motivational tool to facilitate an individual's engagement in PA [18–21]. Lubans [21] notes that although technologies may not be a solution to our global health epidemic, they could be a way to facilitate behavioral change at an individual level.

To the best of our knowledge, Fitbit has not been integrated into the classroom PA break intervention studies, nor has Fitbit been used as a daily intervention strategy to promote real-time PA levels and aerobic fitness levels in school-aged children. To fill the gaps, this study aimed to investigate the impact of the technology-enhanced classroom-based PA intervention on daily real-time PA levels and aerobic fitness levels. Our research hypotheses are (1) students in the two intervention groups: Physical Activity Engaging the Brain + Fitbit Challenge (PAEB-C) group, and Fitbit Only (Fitbit-O) group, will meet the recommended daily MVPA minutes; and (2) students in the two intervention groups will show a greater increase in aerobic fitness levels compared to the control group over time. The significance of this study lies in integration of Fitbits into daily classroom-based activity breaks and assessing students' daily real-time PA levels over the course of the interventions.

2. Methods

2.1. Participants and Research Design

Participants were fifth-grade students recruited from five classes in two elementary schools, matched by minority status and percentage of students receiving free and reduced lunch. A quasi-experimental design was used to assign one school to the experimental school and another school to the control school. In the experimental school, one fifth-grade class was assigned to the Physical Activities Engaging the Brain + Fitbit Challenge (PAEB-C) condition, and another was assigned to the Fitbit Only (Fitbit-O) condition. This study was conducted over the course of seven weeks. The first week was used for recruitment. The second (pre-test) and last weeks (post-test) were used to administer aerobic fitness tests to the students, and the four weeks in the middle were for the intervention.

Prior to the data collection, approvals from the Institutional Review Board and the school district were granted (HUM00102732). A copy of the study guidelines and a consent form were sent to the students' parents/guardians. Then, a second letter was sent to home if no consent was returned by the end of the week. Parents' signed consents were secured for the study prior to asking assent of the children. Children were given the written assent form just prior to the study. The classroom teacher read, out loud, the assent form, which described the purpose of the study and the student's involvement in this study. A total of 96.9% of the students from the PAEB-C group (N = 31), 87.5% of the students from the Fitbit-O group (N = 29), and 87.7% in the control group (N = 56) consented to participate in this study. As a result, this included 116 fifth-grade students aged 10–11 years (57 girls vs. 59 boys). In the intervention school, 60% of the participants self-identified as a race other than white, with 30% African American. At the comparison school, 48% self-identified as a race other than white, with 19% African American.

2.2. Treatment

2.2.1. Fitbit-O Group

The Fitbit Charger + Heart Rate[TM] tracker was used as a self-monitoring and self-motivating tool for students to participate in PA daily. The Fitbit Charger + Heart Rate[TM] tracker is the device that uses a non-invasive wireless sensor on the wrist to measure heart rate. The Fitbit Charger + Heart Rate[TM] device relies on an accelerometer to offer direct and immediate feedback in terms of steps, distance, floors climbed, and heart rate. Thus, the students in the Fitbit-O group wore their Fitbit Charger + Heart Rate[TM] device daily, five school days per week for four weeks. They received immediate as well as weekly feedback, to monitor their own progress and the progress of their classmates.

2.2.2. PAEB-C Group

The PAEB-C was designed to deliberately use both sides of the body, in unison and apart from each other, to coordinate both sides of the body and activate both hemispheres of brain. While the teacher showed a six-minute PAEB activity video once a day after the students had been sitting for 20 min, the students followed the video to immediately perform the PAEB activity for five days per week over the four-week intervention. The QuickTime videos were labeled Day 1 through Day 20. During the first week of the intervention, the PAEB were done very slowly, while in weeks 2 and 3, the activities were slightly faster. Finally, during the week 4, the speed was further increased. First, fine motor movements were rhythmically repeated eight, then four time, and last two, first in unison, and then opposite each other. Next, patterned hand movements focused on changing direction, going forward, sideways, up and down, also in the same rhythmic format. Then, gross motor movements included making figure eights, by simultaneously pairing arm movements in the same direction, by changing the direction and having the arms go in opposite directions. Lastly, gross motor skills utilized the entire body movement. For example, children went from a split to a squat stance, first in unison, then in opposite directions, so when the video instructor jumped sideways, the participants were encouraged to squat. These series of PAEB sequences were done throughout the intervention. The teacher reported missing the PAEB for 3 days (85% of the time).

In addition, the students wore their Fitbit Charger + Heart Rate[TM] device daily, five school days per week for four weeks, following the same procedures used in the Fitbit-O group, except for use of Fitbit Challenge. Regarding the Fitbit Challenge, the PAEB-C students were encouraged to set their own individual goals each week. For example, during the first week of the intervention, the students were encouraged to increase their steps each day by 2000, with the goal of reaching at least 10,000 steps a day. Also, the PAEB-C students were informed of the daily and weekly challenges. The Fitbit Challenges came in the form of a log sheet, on which students were encouraged to record their PA to see if they meet their weekly challenges. The challenges included counting steps and setting a goal, estimating how many steps the whole classroom would take, setting a goal based on distance (miles), and a climbing challenge (floors). Each Monday, the classroom totals were sent to the teacher, highlighting the previous week's goals. On each Monday, the classroom teachers were given reports that showed weekly averages for steps and distance traveled and floors climbed for their classes.

2.2.3. Control Group

The students in the control group neither wore the Fitbit and nor participated in any PA-related classroom breaks. Instead, they had regular classroom breaks based on the school schedule.

2.3. Data Collection

2.3.1. Fitbits

Prior to giving the Fitbit Charger + Heart Rate™ devices to the students, the investigator taught the students (1) where to put their Fitbits on the battery charger on Fridays; (2) how to check the battery; (3) if their Fitbit's battery was low they need to charge it; and (4) how to immediately see their real-time steps, distance, calories burned, and the heart rate on the Fitbits they are wearing. Also, the investigator explained the wearing protocols: wear the Fitbit Charger Heart Rate™ device from Monday through Friday at all times, but students were allowed to take the device off when bathing and during other water activities. In addition, they were told that they would not get in trouble if they took them off, but they were encouraged to wear them as often as possible. Students in the Fitbit-O group and in the PAEB-C group wore their Fitbits day and night from Monday morning (as they arrived at the classroom), until Friday afternoon, whereupon they put the Fitbits in the charging station before they left for home on the weekend during the four weeks of the intervention.

On each Friday during the four weeks of the intervention, after students had left the school, the researcher went to the school and uploaded the information from the Fitbits onto a secure Fitbit Software database, Fitabase. This is a password protected site which is accessible only by the researcher and the data management team from Fitabase. The researcher recorded which Fitbits had been placed on the charging station, and which Fitbits were missing. The teachers were asked to remind their students to bring the Fitbits in on Fridays so that the data could be recorded. Teachers were also given printouts of the classroom's average number of steps and minutes, as well as the classrooms total number of steps and distance traveled. Fitbits were collected after students had spent twenty days in the schools wearing them.

2.3.2. Fitness Assessment

Physical education teachers in both schools provided the study team with the results from an aerobic fitness assessment. The intervention school and the control school pre- and post-tested students' aerobic fitness using the FitnessGram® test (i.e., Progressive Aerobic Cardiovascular Endurance Run (PACER), one-mile run) during weeks 2 and 7 of the study. The FitnessGram test is a validated and reliable health-related fitness assessment toolkit designed by Cooper Institute [22]. The PACER and one-mile run were used to assess levels of cardiovascular endurance [22]. The PACER test and/or one-mile run test were used by PE teachers in each school for the fifth-grade students' report cards. All of the students in both schools participated in the fitness assessments.

2.4. Data Analysis

This study used average daily steps of the 20 days collected from the Fitbit Charger + Heart Rate™ trackers. Then, the data was translated into composite measures of sedentary, light active (LA), fairly active (FA), very active (VA) minutes, and steps via the Fitabase software. These were determined based upon metabolic equivalents (METs). METS are organized by the World Health Organization (WHO, 2015) into working versus resting metabolic rates. A unit of 1 MET is equivalent to sitting (sedentary), 2–3 METs are considered light activity, 4–6 METs is fairly active, and greater than 6 METs is considered very active. Daily data from the Fitbits was excluded from analysis if the student took fewer than 1000 steps or if they had fewer than 840 min of wearing the Fitbit. This resulted in losing an average of one day per person during the four-week study, or an average of 3.97 ($\pm$4.83) steps and 0.72 ($\pm$1.19) minutes for the Fitbit-O group and 1.87 ($\pm$2.21) steps and 0.90 ($\pm$1.56) minutes for the PAEB-C group. Neither group lost individual students ($N = 60$). Daytime sedentary minutes were calculated by subtracting the age-based average of 9 hours of sleep per night (WebMD, 2016). Therefore, 540 sedentary minutes were subtracted before sedentary averages were calculated. A ratio of fairly and very active minutes/total activity minutes was created. Descriptive statistics of each variable was computed for the two Fitbit groups. The Multivariate Analysis of Variance (MANOVA) was used to analyze if there is an overall significant difference in the five PA variables and sedentary variable between the two Fitbit groups controlling for gender and race. Subsequently, the Analysis of Variance (ANOVA) was conducted separately for the steps, very active (VA) minutes, fairly active (FA) minutes, and light active (LA) minutes, sedentary, and fairly and very active (FVA) minutes between the two groups. Additionally, an interaction effect was performed to see if gender and race moderated physical activity levels. Partial eta squared was calculated to determine the effect size of the intervention effect on each Fitbit variable.

Students' aerobic testing scores used to group into high fit (HF), healthy fitness zone (HFZ), and low fit (LF) based on the FitnessGram standards for healthy fitness zone for boys and girls [22]. Then, each fitness zone was coded as: 3 = HF, 2 = HFZ, and 1 = LF. Descriptive statistics of the coded fitness scores for the three groups were computed. A composite of HFZ and HF was used to determine the percentages of students who were at or above the healthy fitness zones (HFZs). The percentages of students meeting the HFZs by each group at the pre- and the post-test were calculated. A 2 (pre-test vs. post-test) × 3 (PAEB-C, Fitbit-O, and the control) ANOVA was conducted while controlling for gender and race. Subsequently, post hoc comparison method was analyzed to determine if there were any significant increases in HFZs between the two groups at a time. All statistical analyses were conducted with IBM SPSS statistics 24 and a significant level of $p < 0.05$ was set.

3. Results

3.1. Daily Real-Time Physical Activity Levels between the Two Intervention Groups

Table 1 presents the descriptive statistics of each Fitbit variable between the two groups.

Table 1. Mean steps and minutes of physical activity between the two intervention groups. Fitbit-O, Fitbit Only; PAEB-C, Physical Activity Engaging the Brain + Fitbit Challenge.

	Fitbit-O	PAEB-C
	$M \pm SD$	$M \pm SD$
Steps	8954.54 ± 2518.59	11151.78 ± 3421.68
Very Active (VA)	4.09 ± 5.00	7.96 ± 7.32
Fairly Active (FA)	11.28 ± 8.00	22.98 ± 17.75
Light Active (LA)	230.57 ± 82.23	247.78 ± 76.33
Sedentary	454.34 ± 203.23	347.75± 179.51
Fairly and Very Active (FVA)/Total Activity	1.3 ± 1	2.9 ± 2.3

The PAEB-C group showed higher numbers of average daily real-time steps and higher average daily real-time minutes in very active (VA), fairly active (FA), and light active (LA) variables compared to the students in Fitbit-O group. Further, the PAEB-C group were fairly and very active (FVA) for about 31 min, while the Fitbit-O group were FVA for 15 min daily. By contrast, the PAEB-C group had lower average daily sedentary minutes compared to the Fitbit-O group.

The results of the MANOVA revealed an overall significant difference in average daily steps, VA minutes, FA minutes, LA minutes, and sedentary minutes when controlling for gender and race between the two groups ($F = 2.418$, $p = 0.039$, $\eta = 0.215$). Subsequently, the ANOVA revealed that the PAEB-C group took significant more daily steps than the Fitbit-O group ($F = 7.999$, $p = 0.014$, $\eta = 0.121$). Likewise, the PAEB-C group spent significant more minutes being VA ($F = 5.667$, $p = 0.021$, $\eta = 0.089$), FA ($F = 10.572$, $p = 0.002$, $\eta = 0.154$), and FVA ($F = 11.701$, $p = 0.001$, $\eta = 0.168$) daily than did the Fitbit-O group. No significant difference in LA minutes between the two groups was found ($F = 0.707$, $p = 0.404$, $\eta = 0.012$). By contrast, the Fitbit-O group spent significant more minutes being sedentary per day than the PAEB-C group ($F = 4.639$, $p = 0.035$, $\eta = 0.074$). Table 2 presents descriptive statistics of five Fitbit variables by groups and gender.

Table 2. Descriptive statistics of five Fitbit variables by groups and gender.

		Fitbit-O	PAEB-C
		$M \pm SD$	$M \pm SD$
Steps			
	Boys	9139.64 ± 1872.23	12,221.84 ± 4161.87
	Girls	8814.95 ± 2839.23	10,270.55 ± 2460.06
Very Active (VA)			
	Boys	5.47 ± 5.77	10.83 ± 7.05
	Girls	3.36 ± 4.54	5.61 ± 6.84
Fairly Active (FA)			
	Boys	14.35 ± 10.16	29.97 ± 17.22
	Girls	9.67 ± 6.33	17.22 + 10.90
Light Active (LA)			
	Boys	249.41 ± 49.17	223.42 ± 73.07
	Girls	220.66 ± 94.92	267.84± 75.10
Sedentary			
	Boys	380.64 ± 167.19	385.78 ± 195.47
	Girls	491.43 ± 214.01	318.30 ± 164.90

No significant interaction of group by gender in each PA variable and sedentary minutes was found. However, regardless of intervention type, boys were significantly more likely to participate in VA minutes ($F = 6.383$, $p = 0.014$, $\eta = 0.099$), FA minutes ($F = 7.408$, $p = 0.009$, $\eta = 0.113$), and FVA minutes ($F = 7.167$, $p = 0.010$, $\eta = 0.110$). By contrast, no gender difference was found in light minutes ($F = 0.172$, $p = 0.680$, $\eta = 0.003$) and sedentary minutes ($F = 0.252$, $p = 0.617$, $\eta = 0.003$).

3.2. Intervention Effects on Aerobic Fitness Levels

Table 3 shows the descriptive statistics of average aerobic fitness scores and percentages of meeting the HFZs among the three groups at the pre- and the post-test.

Table 3. Average aerobic fitness scores and percentage of healthy fitness zones (HFZs) at the pre- and post-test by groups.

	Pre-Test		Post-Test	
	$M \pm SD$	% HFZs	$M \pm SD$	% HFZs
PAEB-C	1.26 ± 0.45	26%	1.61 ± 0.50	61%
Fitbit-O	1.26 ± 0.45	26%	1.56 ± 0.51	56%
Control	1.52 ± 0.71	39%	1.38 ± 0.71	26%

At the pre-test, only 26% of the PAEB-C and Fitbit-O students were in HFZs, while 39% of the control students were in the HFZs. The two Fitbit groups' mean aerobic fitness score was 1.26, while the control group was 1.52. By contrast, at the post-test, 61% of the PAEB-C students and 56% of the Fitbit-O students were in HFZs, while 26% the control students were in HFZs. The PAEB-C's average aerobic fitness score was 1.61 and the Fitbit-O's was 1.56, whereas the control group's was 1.32.

The results of the repeated measure ANOVA revealed significant main effect of time in aerobic fitness score ($F = 19.273$, $p = 0.000$, $\eta = 0.160$), indicating the three groups showed significant improvement in the aerobic fitness testing score from pre- to post-test. Further, the repeated measure ANOVA revealed a significant interaction between time × treatment ($F = 21.946$, $p = 0.000$, $\eta = 0.303$). Subsequently, the post hoc analysis revealed significant comparisons in the mean fitness scores from pre- to post-test between the PAEB-C and the control group ($F = 29.327$, $p = 0.000$), and between the

Fitbit-O and the control group ($F = 25.007$, $p = 0.000$), but no significant difference between the two Fitbit groups (see Figure 1).

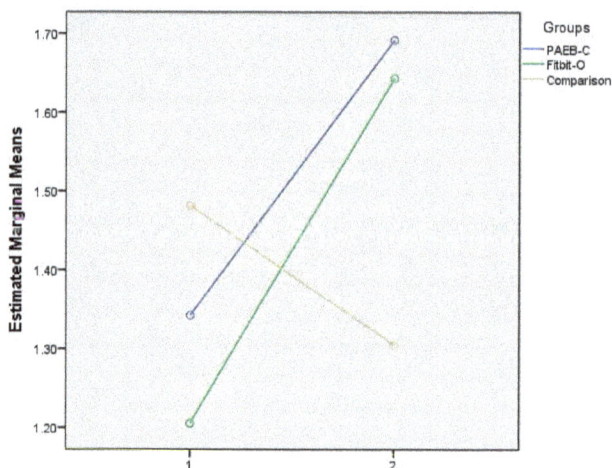

Figure 1. Mean scores of aerobic fitness among the three groups from pre- to post-test.

4. Discussion

This study was central to examining the effects of the technology-enhanced physical activity interventions on real-time daily PA and aerobic fitness levels in school-aged children. The students in the PAEB-C group, who engaged in daily classroom-based activity breaks in conjunction with the Fitbit Challenge program, exceeded 10,000 steps daily, on average, and took, on average, 2206 more steps/day than the Fitbit-O group. Consistent with the results, a systematic review by Dobbins, Husson, DeCorby, and LaRocca [23] concluded that school-based physical activity interventions were more likely to improve MVPA minutes by as little as five and up to forty-five minutes. Similarly, classroom-based activity break studies have shown improved PA levels [10–13,24].

Another promising result was that the PAEB-C group had 107 fewer sedentary minutes/day than the Fitbit-O group. Supporting the previous studies, the results indicated that engaging the students in daily classroom-based activity breaks may be a feasible way to reduce their sedentary time during school day [10–13]. Reducing prolonged sedentary behaviors have a significant impact on a child's overall health, as well as cognitive functions (i.e., attention, concentration, and information processing) [10–13]. However, the PAEB activities alone could not account for these differences. Since the PAEB activities are mostly fine and small gross motor skills, they predominantly fell into the light and fairly active categories. This suggests that the Fitbit Challenge may have played an important role in increasing steps and reducing sedentary minutes. Children engaging in both PAEB activities and the Fitbit Challenges were motivated by them to be more active than the Fitbit-O group.

It is important to note that the PAEB-C group, on average, spent 30.94 min, and the Fitbit-C group spent 15.47 min engaging in very active (vigorous) and fairly active (moderate) PA daily over the course of four weeks. Their daily real-time physical activity minutes are far lower than the recommended daily 60 min or more of MVPA by the 2008 Physical Activity Guidelines [4]. However, the PAEB-C group engaged 248 min, and the Fitbit-O group engaged 231 min, in being light active, daily. This is consistent with the findings by Van der Niet et al. [24] who found that students' time was spent mostly in PA that consisted of light PA.

In addition, this study showed the gender discrepancy in daily MVPA. Though the PAEB-C group took more very active and fairly active minutes than the Fitbit-O group, most of these differences can be attributed to time spent in very active and fairly active PA by boys. Boys were more likely to participate in very active and fairly active PA than girls throughout the study. In a study of 1111 fourth- and fifth-grade students' daily PA in year 1, and 1012 fourth- and fifth-grade students' daily PA in year 2 of the Healthy Kids and Smart Kids project, Chen et al. [14] found that boys self-reported they were more physically active than girls in daily PA during school and outside of school in both years. Similarly, Ridgers, Salmon, Parrish, Stanley, and Okely [25] found the boys were more likely to participate in a higher amount of MVPA minutes than girls.

As expected, the two Fitbits groups showed greater increases in aerobic fitness compared to the control group from pre- to the post-test. After the four-week interventions, 61% of the PAEB-C and 56% of the Fitbit-O students were in the HFZs. Similarly, Chen et al. [14] reported 59% of 265 fifth-grade students met the HFZ standards in PACER test at the end of participating in one-school year Healthy Kids and Smart Kids project. By contrast, the percentages of meeting the HFZs dropped from 39% to 26% for the comparison school. These changes occurred during a time when seasonal changes sometimes act to reduce fitness levels [9]. Fedewa et al. [9] found that though students participate in daily classroom-based PA breaks, their daily average steps decreased during winter season. However, this study showed that the seasonal factor seemed not to negatively influence the two Fitbits groups' aerobic fitness scores at the post-test. Rather, the two Fitbit groups showed significant increases in aerobic fitness scores. The results suggest that the students' wearing the Fitbit daily, checking their real-time daily steps taken, and self-monitoring their progress toward meeting the weekly-based goal, are effective intervention strategies for improving their aerobic fitness levels, in addition to merely engaging in classroom activity breaks. The results might be attributed to the reciprocal relationship between regular PA participation and physical fitness [15]. Supporting this point, Chen et al. [14] found that children's total weekly PA minutes in and outside school were significantly associated with healthy level of aerobic fitness. Similarly, previous studies found a significant association between amount of PA and aerobic fitness in school-aged children [14–17]. Another possible reason for the two Fitbits groups' significant increases in aerobic fitness would be that Fitbits do allow for students to immediately monitor their real-time heart rates. The study suggests that Fitbits can be used to encourage students to spend a greater amount of time in their target heart rate zones. In addition, the overall excitement of wearing a Fitbit for four weeks, the wearable device effect, might also play a role in increasing students' aerobic fitness levels.

The limitation of the study was that fitness testing data were based upon one-mile run and the PACER tests. Originally, both schools planned to do the one-mile test, but the Fitbit school underwent construction during the study, which did not allow them to take the one-mile run at the post-test. However, both tests were typically used to assess aerobic fitness levels based on the gender- and age-specific standards for low fit, healthy fitness zone, and high fit in the FitnessGram® [22]. Another limitation of this study was not using the Fitbit Charger + Heart Rate™ device to collect the students' average daily heart rate data. The future study could use this essential data to examine the participants' daily heart rates patterns over the course of the intervention, and how their average daily heart rates are associated with increased physical activity participation and aerobic fitness levels. Also, this study was not focused on examining how the students' wearing the Fitbit device daily motivated their participation in physical activities and improved their aerobic fitness. A future study may examine how wearing the Fitbits daily will influence participants' intrinsic and extrinsic motivations for physical activity, which in turn, is conducive to developing habitual physical activity behaviors.

5. Conclusions

The students' daily real-time MVPA minutes did not meet the recommended 60 min of MVPA daily. However, the integration of Fitbits into daily classroom activity breaks were effective intervention strategies for engaging students in more minutes of MVPA and reducing their sedentary minutes compared to the intervention strategy that merely integrated Fitbits into their daily life. Boys were more likely to be physically active than girls, when wearing the Fitbits. Use of Fitbits as a daily and real-time intervention strategy along with daily classroom-based activity breaks for four weeks significantly increased proportions of students meeting HFZs.

Author Contributions: Conceptualization, W.C.; Methodology, W.C.; Validation, W.C. and H.B.H.; Formal Analysis, H.B.H.; Investigation, H.B.H.; Resources, W.C. and H.B.H.; Data Curation, H.B.H. and W.C.; Writing—Original Draft Preparation, H.B.H. and W.C.; Writing—Review & Editing, W.C.; Supervision, W.C.; Project Administration, W.C.; Funding Acquisition, W.C.

Funding: This research was funded by Hartwig Endowment Fund of School of Kinesiology, University.

Acknowledgments: The authors would like to thank the teachers, children and the district for participating in this project.

Conflicts of Interest: The authors declare no conflicts of interest.

References

1. Institute of Medicine of the National Academies. *Educating the Student Body: Taking Physical Activity and Physical Education to School*; IOM: Washington, DC, USA, 2013.
2. US Department of Health and Human Services. *Physical Activity Guidelines for Americans, 2008*; US Department of Health and Human Services: Washington, DC, USA, 2008.
3. Centers for Disease Control and Prevention. School health guidelines to promote healthy eating and physical activity. *MMWR Recomm. Rep.* **2011**, *60*, 1–76.
4. Bassett, D.R.; Fitzhugh, E.C.; Heath, G.W.; Erwin, P.C.; Frederick, G.M.; Wolff, D.L.; Welch, W.A.; Stout, A.B. Estimated energy expenditures for school-based policies and active living. *Am. J. Prev. Med.* **2013**, *44*, 108–113. [CrossRef] [PubMed]
5. Ogden, C.L.; Carroll, M.D.; Kit, B.K.; Flegal, K.M. Prevalence of childhood and adult obesity in the United States, 2011–2012. *JAMA* **2014**, *311*, 806–814. [CrossRef] [PubMed]
6. Pate, R.R.; Freedson, P.S.; Sallis, J.F.; Taylor, W.C.; Sirard, J.; Trost, S.G.; Dowda, M. Compliance with physical activity guidelines: Prevalence in a population of children and youth. *Ann. Epidemiol.* **2002**, *12*, 303–308. [CrossRef]
7. World Health Organization. Physical Activity and Young People: Recommended Levels of Physical Activity for Children Aged 5–17 Years. 2015. Available online: http://www.who.int/dietphysicalactivity/factsheet_young_people/en/ (accessed on 25 February 2016).
8. Rasberry, C.N.; Lee, S.M.; Robin, L.; Laris, B.A.; Russell, L.A. The association between school-based physical activity, including physical education, and academic performance: A systematic review of the literature. *Prev. Med.* **2011**, *52*, S10–S20. [CrossRef] [PubMed]
9. Fedewa, A.L.; Ahn, S.; Erwin, H.; Davis, M.C. A randomized controlled design investigating the effects of classroom-based physical activity on children's fluid intelligence and achievement. *Sch. Psychol. Int.* **2015**, *36*, 135–153. [CrossRef]
10. Donnelly, J.E.; Greene, J.L.; Gibson, C.A.; Smith, B.K.; Washburn, R.A.; Sullivan, D.K.; DuBose, K.; Mayo, M.S.; Schmelzle, K.H.; Ryan, J.J.; et al. Physical activity across the curriculum (PAAC): A randomized controlled trail to promote physical activity and diminish overweight and obesity in elementary school children. *Prev. Med.* **2009**, *49*, 336–341. [CrossRef] [PubMed]
11. Stewart, J.A.; Dennison, D.A.; Kohl, H.W.; Doyle, A. Exercise level and energy expenditure in the TAKE 10!® in class physical activity program. *J. Sch. Health* **2004**, *74*, 397–400. [CrossRef] [PubMed]
12. Carlson, J.A.; Engelberg, J.K.; Cain, K.L.; Sallis, J.F. Implementing classroom physical activity breaks: Associations with student physical activity and classroom behavior. *Prev. Med.* **2015**, *81*, 67–72. [CrossRef] [PubMed]
13. Ma, J.K.; Le Mare, L.; Gurd, B.J. Classroom-based high-intensity interval activity improves off-task behaviour in primary school students. *Appl. Physiol. Nutr. Metab.* **2014**, *39*, 1332–1337. [CrossRef] [PubMed]
14. Chen, W.; Hammond-Bennett, A.; Hypnar, A.; Mason, S. Health-related physical fitness and physical activity in elementary school students. *BMC Public Health* **2018**, *18*, 195. [CrossRef] [PubMed]
15. Stodden, D.F.; Goodway, J.D.; Langendorfer, S.J.; Rpberton, M.A.; Rudisill, M.E.; Garcia, C.; Garcia, L.E. A developmental perspective on the role of motor skill competence in physical activity: An emergent relationship. *Quest* **2008**, *60*, 290–306. [CrossRef]

16. Okely, A.D.; Booth, M.L.; Patterson, W. Relationship of cardiorespiratory endurance of fundamental movement skill proficiency among adolescents. *Pediatr. Exerc. Sci.* **2001**, *13*, 380–391. [CrossRef]

17. Chen, W.; Hypnar, A.; Mason, S.; Hammond-Bennett, A.; Zalmout, S. Elementary school students' daily physical activity behaviors: A contributing role of quality physical education teaching in comprehensive school-based physical activity program. *J. Teach. Phys. Educ.* **2014**, *33*, 592–610. [CrossRef]

18. Lewis, Z.H.; Lyons, E.J.; Jarvis, J.M.; Baillargeon, J. Using an electronic activity monitor system as an intervention modality: A systematic review. *BMC Public Health* **2015**, *5*, 585. [CrossRef] [PubMed]

19. Preuschl, E.; Baca, A.; Novatchkov, H.; Kornfeind, P.; Bichler, S.; Boecskoer, M. Mobile motion advisor— A feedback system for physical exercise in schools. *Procedia Eng.* **2010**, *2*, 2741–2747. [CrossRef]

20. Mikkola, H.; Kumpulainen, K.; Rahikkala, A.; Pitkanen, M.; Korkeamaki, R.L.; Hytonen, M. Futurestep— Enhancing children's wellbeing by using activity monitors in formal and informal contexts. In Proceedings of the 4th International Technology, Education and Development Conference (Inted 2010), Valencia, Spain, 8–10 March 2010; pp. 5687–5694.

21. Lubans, D.R.; Morgan, P.J.; Tudor-Locke, C. A systematic review of studies using pedometers to promote physical activity among youth. *Prev. Med.* **2009**, *48*, 307–315. [CrossRef] [PubMed]

22. Meredith, M.D.; Welk, G.J. *FitnessGram and Activitygram Test Administration Manual*, 4th ed.; Human Kinetics: Champain, IL, USA, 2007.

23. Dobbins, M.; Husson, H.; DeCorby, K.; LaRocca, R.L. School-based physical activity programs for promoting physical activity and fitness in children and adolescents aged 6 to 18. *Cochrane Database Syst. Rev.* **2013**, *2*, CD007651. [CrossRef] [PubMed]

24. Van der Niet, A.G.; Hartman, E.; Smith, J.; Visscher, C. Modeling relationships between physical fitness, executive functioning, and academic achievement in primary school children. *Psychol. Sport Exerc.* **2014**, *15*, 319–325. [CrossRef]

25. Ridgers, N.D.; Salmon, J.; Parrish, A.; Stanley, R.M.; Okely, A.D. Physical activity during school recess: A systematic review. *Am. J. Prev. Med.* **2012**, *43*, 320–328. [CrossRef] [PubMed]

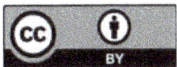

Journal of
Clinical Medicine

MDPI

Article

Effectiveness of Combined Smartwatch and Social Media Intervention on Breast Cancer Survivor Health Outcomes: A 10-Week Pilot Randomized Trial

Zachary C. Pope [1], Nan Zeng [1], Rui Zhang [1,2], Hee Yun Lee [3] and Zan Gao [1,*]

[1]   School of Kinesiology, University of Minnesota, 1900 University Ave. SE, Minneapolis, MN 55455, USA;
       popex157@umn.edu (Z.C.P.); zengx185@umn.edu (N.Z.); zhan1386@umn.edu (R.Z.)
[2]   College of Pharmacy, and Institute for Health Informatics, University of Minnesota,
       8-116 Phillips-Wangensteen Building, 516 Delaware Street SE, Minneapolis, MN 55455, USA
[3]   School of Social Work, The University of Alabama, 1022 Little Hall, Box 870314, Tuscaloosa, AL 35487, USA;
       hlee94@ua.edu
*   Correspondence: gaoz@umn.edu; Tel.: +1-(612)-626-4639; Fax: +1-(612)-626-7700

Received: 16 May 2018; Accepted: 5 June 2018; Published: 7 June 2018

Abstract: Physical activity (PA) among breast cancer survivors (BCS) can improve this population's health and quality of life (QoL). This study evaluated the effectiveness of a combined smartwatch- and social media-based health education intervention on BCS's health outcomes. Thirty BCS ($\overline{X}_{age}$ = 52.6 ± 9.3 years; $\overline{X}_{Wt}$ = 80.2 ± 19.6 kg) participated in this 10-week, 2-arm randomized trial, with BCS randomized into: (1) experimental group (n = 16): received Polar M400 smartwatches for daily PA tracking and joined a Facebook group wherein Social Cognitive Theory-related PA tips were provided twice weekly; and (2) comparison group (n = 14): only joined separate, but content-identical Facebook group. Outcomes included PA, physiological, psychosocial, and QoL variables. Specifically, PA and energy expenditure (EE) was assessed by ActiGraph GT3X+ accelerometers while physiological, psychosocial, and QoL were examined via validated instruments at baseline and post-intervention. No baseline group differences were observed for any variable. Ten BCS dropped out of the study (experimental: 4; comparison: 6). Compared to completers, dropouts differed significantly on several outcomes. Thus, a per-protocol analysis was performed, revealing significant group differences for changes in social support (t = −2.1, p = 0.05) and barriers (t = −2.2, p = 0.04). Interestingly, the comparison group demonstrated improvements for both variables while the intervention group demonstrated slightly decreased social support and no change in barriers. Notably, both groups demonstrated similarly increased daily light PA, moderate-to-vigorous PA, EE, and steps of 7.7 min, 5.1 min, 25.1 kcals, and 339 steps, respectively, over time. Despite extensive user training, several experimental BCS found the Polar M400 use difficult—possibly decreasing intervention adherence. Future interventions should utilize simpler smartwatches to promote PA among middle-aged clinical/non-clinical populations.

Keywords: physical activity; quality of life; social cognitive theory; wearable technology

---

1. Introduction

Invasive or in situ forms of breast cancer were diagnosed among approximately 330,000 women in 2017 [1]. Improved treatment options have led to increased breast cancer survival rates, with 3.1 million breast cancer survivors residing in the U.S. [1,2]. It is noteworthy, however, that studies comparing women never previously diagnosed with breast cancer to breast cancer survivors have observed lower quality of life (e.g., poorer physical functioning; increased depression/anxiety rates; greater fatigue) and poorer physical health among breast cancer survivors [3,4]. While medicinal

J. Clin. Med. **2018**, *7*, 140; doi:10.3390/jcm7060140

www.mdpi.com/journal/jcm

treatments (e.g., Tamoxifen use) may be prescribed following breast cancer treatment and the beginning of remission, health behavior changes are now more commonly being recommended to breast cancer survivors—the most frequent being increased physical activity participation [3,5–10]. Given the ubiquitous nature of modern-day technology, researchers are seeking to leverage several technologies (e.g., smartphone applications, wearable technology, social media) to improve health among various populations through increased physical activity and reduced sedentary behavior [11,12]. Currently, smartwatches are among the most popular technologies being used to assist individuals in living more active and healthier lifestyles.

As a popular form of wearable technology, smartwatches are projected to comprise an approximately $10 billion USD market by 2019 [13]. Smartwatches from companies like Polar, Apple, and Fitbit are most popular within this market due to: (1) attractive price points ($100–250 USD); and (2) the ability to track health metrics like step counts, heart rate, energy expenditure, stairs climbed, and sleep, among other metrics—data which can be sent via Bluetooth to an associated smartphone application for easy interpretation and facilitation of the self-regulation (i.e., tracking and modification) of health behaviors [14,15]. Yet, while some studies [16] have observed smartphone application-based physical activity interventions to be effective in promoting improved physical activity and quality of life among breast cancer survivors, little to no research has been conducted on the effectiveness of smartwatches in the promotion of this population's health. This is noteworthy as qualitative research has found breast cancer survivors to be interested and open to the use of smartwatches in the self-regulation of physical activity and sedentary behaviors [17].

Of the paucity of high-quality randomized trials which evaluated the effectiveness of smartwatches in the promotion of physical activity, populations investigated have included: overweight and obese individuals [18–20], older adults [21], adults [22], and college students [23–25]. Findings from these studies have been mixed. For example, Cadmus-Bertram et al. [18,19] observed significantly increased moderate-to-vigorous physical activity and steps/day over 16 weeks among overweight and obese postmenopausal women using the Fitbit to track health behaviors when compared to a control group receiving standard care (e.g., exercise counseling), with marginally positive findings also observed in another study by Thorndike et al. [22] among medical residents and Rote [24] among college students. Yet, other literature among overweight and obese men and women [20], older adults [21], and college students [23,25] has not observed provision of a smartwatch to result in greater improvements in physical activity versus control.

The mixed findings of the preceding studies may be attributable to: (1) little provision of health education despite the need for health literacy in long-term health behavior engagement [26,27]; and (2) lack of an established theoretical framework to guide study design/implementation notwithstanding the importance of health behavior theory in promoting increased intervention effectiveness [28]. This suggests that future randomized trials might be more effective if a theoretically-based health education piece is included. A theory which might be particularly effective in future randomized trials given its concentration on personal-level factors (i.e., self-efficacy, enjoyment, barriers, and outcome expectancy) and micro-environmental factors (i.e., social support) is the Social Cognitive Theory [29,30]. Briefly, this theory posits reciprocal determinism between an individual's characteristics, environmental factors, and behavior [30]. For example, if an intervention can increase an individual's self-efficacy for physical activity (i.e., an individual characteristic) and promote greater social support for physical activity (i.e., an environmental factor), this individual is more likely to participate in physically active behavior(s). One manner by which a Social Cognitive Theory-based health education intervention might be delivered is through social media as this technological medium could be used to promote: (1) improvements in individual characteristics via health education; and (2) social support given the inclusion of all intervention participants on intervention-related social media pages upon which the participants can interact and support one another's health-related endeavors. Data has indicated females to comprise the majority of U.S. Facebook users, with women ≥25 years old representing 40% of all U.S. Facebook users [31]. As the use of theory to frame an intervention's development/implementation may increase intervention effectiveness [32,33], providing breast cancer survivors with Social Cognitive Theory-based health education tips via Facebook might assist this population in living healthier, more active lifestyles in addition to improving quality of life—a strategy which has, in fact, been suggested by breast cancer survivors in recent research [17].

Therefore, the purpose of this 10-week pilot randomized trial was to evaluate the effectiveness of a combined smartwatch and theoretically-based, social media-delivered health education intervention in promoting improved physical activity participation, physiological/psychosocial health, and quality of life as well as reduced sedentary behavior among breast cancer survivors. By providing experimental group participants a Polar M400 smartwatch and a Social Cognitive Theory-based [29,30], Facebook-delivered health education intervention, it was hypothesized that: (1) experimental group participants would have larger increases in physical activity, energy expenditure, and steps/day in addition to greater decreases in sedentary behavior than comparison group participants receiving only the Facebook-delivered health education intervention given the experimental group's additional ability to monitor Polar M400 health metrics like steps per day and daily activity duration; (2) experimental group participants would experience greater improvements in weight, body composition, and cardiorespiratory fitness versus comparison. This was hypothesized as it was believed the experimental group might modify caloric consumption and increase physical activity participation based upon the Polar M400's energy expenditure and steps per day/daily activity time readings, respectively—behaviors which would be supplemented by the health education being delivered via this group's respective Facebook group; and (3) more favorable changes in Social Cognitive Theory-related psychosocial constructs and quality of life would be observed in the experimental group versus comparison partially resulting from the greater hypothesized changes for physical activity and physiological outcomes among the experimental group. Observations may assist health professionals in developing large-scale, low-burden, and well-integrated physical activity interventions among breast cancer survivors and other clinical populations which can effectively improve health outcomes during or following treatment.

2. Materials and Methods

This manuscript's construction was guided by the CONSORT guidelines [34] for the reporting of randomized trials.

2.1. Study Design

A 10-week two-arm parallel randomized pilot trial study design was implemented, with data collected from November 2016 to April 2017. Baseline and 10-week assessments of 7-day habitual physical activity and sedentary behavior as well as evaluations of physiological, psychosocial, and quality of life outcomes were performed. Given the pilot nature of the trial, use/acceptability of the intervention was also assessed. Notably, the current investigation built upon the researchers' previous smartphone- and social media-based health education intervention study [16], with three distinct differences. First, the current study used the Polar M400 smartwatch as opposed to a smartphone application because most breast cancer survivors in the previous study stated the need to open their smartphone to track/document physical activity was burdensome and that the "always on" physical activity tracking capabilities of smartwatches would be preferable during future interventions. Second, the Facebook-delivered health education intervention used in the current study, while similar to the previous study, included the addition of a workout program (see Procedures) designed around the unique limitations of breast cancer survivors (e.g., functional limitations imposed by mastectomies and/or comorbidities). Finally, the previous study was a single group pre-post intervention design, not a randomized trial as implemented in the present investigation. All procedures performed with participants were in accordance with the standards of the Institution and/or national research committee and with the 1964 Helsinki declaration and its later amendments or comparable ethical standards [35]. Testing was not performed until University institutional review board approval and participant informed consent were obtained.

2.2. Recruitment and Inclusion/Exclusion Criteria

Posted flyers in the University's Masonic Cancer Center and surrounding medical buildings, University-wide emails, online postings, and word-of-mouth were all used to recruit eligible breast cancer survivors. Breast cancer survivors interested in study participation contacted one of the researchers (ZCP) and were screened against the following criteria: (1) females of any race/ethnicity; (2) ≥21-years-old; (3) prior stage 0–III breast cancer diagnosis; (4) breast cancer treatment finished 3 months to 10 years earlier with no recurrence; (5) possessed an active Facebook account; and (6) willingness to complete the Physical Activity Readiness Questionnaire [36] and be randomized into an experimental or comparison group. Exclusion criteria were: (1) any ongoing breast cancer treatment; and (2) contraindication(s) to physical activity participation (e.g., pacemaker implant, medical condition) as indicated by the Physical Activity Readiness Questionnaire which could potentially limit study participation.

2.3. Measures

Demographic/clinical variables. Breast cancer survivors self-reported age, race/ethnicity, birthplace, education/annual income level, marital/employment status, breast cancer diagnosis stage, treatment type, months since diagnosis, remission duration, and Tamoxifen use.

2.3.1. Primary Outcome

Physical activity levels/energy expenditure. ActiGraph GT3X+ accelerometers were employed at baseline and 10 weeks to evaluate: mean daily duration of sedentary behavior, light physical activity, and moderate-to-vigorous physical activity as well as energy expenditure in kcalories and steps/day. Previous research [37] has observed the ActiGraph GT3X+ to be valid in physical activity measurement among adults in free-living conditions. Per recommendations made in previous literature [38], breast cancer survivors wore the accelerometer for 7 days to ensure collection of physical activity data on at least 2 weekdays and 1 weekend day. Data was analyzed using the following empirically-based cut points in counts/minute: sedentary behavior: 0–99; light physical activity: 100–2019; moderate-to-vigorous physical activity: ≥2020 [39]. Any day with less than 10 h of valid wear time for any participant was excluded from the analysis [38].

2.3.2. Secondary Outcomes

Anthropometry, body composition, and cardiorespiratory fitness. To measure height to the nearest half-centimeter and weight/body fat percentage, trained research assistants used a Seca stadiometer (Seca, Hamburg, Germany) and a Tanita BC-558 IRONMAN® Segmental Body Composition Monitor (Tanita, Tokyo, Japan), respectively. Validity of bioelectrical impedance for field measurements of body fat percentage has been observed in other adult populations [40]. Finally, the YMCA 3-min Step Test was used to evaluate cardiorespiratory fitness, with palpation of the radial artery for 1 min following the test to acquire a post-test heart rate in beats/minute [41]. These measurements were taken at baseline and 10 weeks.

Psychosocial variables. Psychometrically validated questionnaires were used to assess social support, barriers, self-efficacy, enjoyment, and outcome expectancy. In detail, a 5-item social support measure adapted from the Patient-Centered Assessment and Counseling for Exercise questionnaire [42] queried breast cancer survivors regarding how often significant others encouraged them to be physically active using a 5-point Likert-type scale (1: almost never to 5: almost always). For physical activity barriers, breast cancer survivors rated the degree of agreement between personal barriers and hypothetical barriers on a 14-item measure which employed a 4-point Likert-type scale (1: strongly disagree to 4: strongly agree) [43]. A 9-item measure developed by Rodgers et al. [44] examined breast cancer survivors' self-efficacy as they rated how confident they felt in specific exercise situations (e.g., " … exercise when you feel discomfort" or " … exercise when you lack energy") using a percentage scale (0%: not confident at all to 100%: extremely confident in 10% increments). A modified 5-item measure constructed by Harter [45] evaluated physical activity enjoyment as breast cancer survivors rated their agreement with statements like "Engaging in physical activity is the thing I like to do best" using a 5-point Likert-type scale (1: strongly disagree to 5: strongly agree). Finally, a 9-item measure developed by Trost et al. [46] assessed breast cancer survivors' outcome expectancy as they rated agreement with responses originating from the stem "If I was to exercise on most days it would … ", with sample responses like "give me more energy" and "help to control my weight". This questionnaire employed a 5-point Likert-type scale (1: strongly disagree to 5: strongly agree). These questionnaires were administered at baseline and 10 weeks.

Quality of life. Evaluation of physical functioning, anxiety, depression, fatigue, sleep, ability to participate in social roles/activities, and pain occurred via the Patient Reported Outcome Measurement Information System [47], with all outcomes assessed via 5-point Likert-type scales aside from that of pain intensity. Specifically, to assess physical functioning, breast cancer survivors rated how current physical abilities (e.g., "Are you able to get in and out of bed?") were made more difficult due to current health (1: without any difficulty to 5: unable to do). A 7-day recall of symptom frequency (1: never to 5: always) was used to assess anxiety, depression, and ability to participate in social roles/activities. Symptom frequency was also reported for fatigue, sleep, and pain, with responses ranging from 1: not at all to 5: very much. Finally, sleep quality was evaluated using a 5-point Likert-type scale (1: very poor to 5: very good), with pain intensity assessed on a 0 to 10 scale (0: no pain to 10: worst pain imaginable). Prior research has indicated the validity of the Patient Reported Outcome Measurement Information System in clinical populations [48]—including cancer populations [49]. This questionnaire was administered at baseline and 10 weeks.

Use/acceptability. A post-intervention self-reported survey among experimental participants evaluated: weekly frequency of Polar M400 wear, weekly frequency/mean duration of Polar M400 use during exercise, and Polar M400 enjoyment (dichotomous "yes" or "no" response). Experimental participants were also asked to list any negative features of the smartwatch. Moreover, both groups were surveyed at post-intervention regarding: implementation frequency of Facebook-delivered health education tips and whether they perceived the health education tips as helpful (dichotomous "yes" or "no" response).

2.4. Procedures

Breast cancer survivors interested in participating contacted a study researcher (ZCP), with potential participants screened against inclusion criteria. Baseline testing was then scheduled for eligible breast cancer survivors. Baseline testing began with a battery of questionnaires evaluating demographic/clinical characteristics, psychosocial constructs, and quality of life indices. Next, breast cancers survivors' height, weight, body composition, and cardiorespiratory fitness were measured. Participants were then given an ActiGraph GT3X with instructions on how and when the accelerometer needed to be worn over the following 7 days. During the 7 days the breast cancer survivors wore the accelerometer during baseline testing, a random numbers table was used to randomize participants into the experimental or comparison group, with a 1:1 allocation ratio. Upon returning the accelerometer, each participant met with the researcher (ZCP) to learn their group allocation and discuss use of the Polar M400 and/or the Facebook group components of their respective intervention.

Experimental group participants were instructed first on the use of the Polar M400—a powerful no-frills smartwatch capable of tracking health metrics such as energy expenditure, steps/days, and daily physical activity duration, among other metrics. Notably, while the Polar M400 is equipped with a triaxial accelerometer, the smartwatch also possesses global positioning system capabilities and Bluetooth compatibility—the latter allowing the smartwatch to sync to an associated smartphone application and/or internet-based portal [50]. Given the Polar M400's numerous functions, the researcher spent approximately 15 min with each experimental participant providing a tutorial of the smartwatch's functions, subsequently providing the Polar M400 manual to experimental group participants as well. Next, experimental group participants were given a tutorial of the Facebook page used throughout the intervention to provide twice-weekly Social Cognitive Theory-related health education tips (see Supplementary Materials). These tips were developed to assist participants' integration of physical activity into their daily routine by improving participants' physical activity-related self-efficacy, outcome expectancy, social support, and enjoyment while reducing barriers. These tips have been used with success in a previous intervention among breast cancer survivors [16]. For example, health education tips written to increase participants' outcome expectancy, enjoyment, and social support used empirically-based facts to remind participants of the improved mood/quality of life and physiological outcomes which may occur due to increased physical activity participation while also providing some ideas by which to make physical activity more fun and social. Experimental group participants were also told that they could post physical activity-related statistics to the Facebook group from their Polar M400 and/or comment within the Facebook group at their discretion to support one another toward physical activity goals.

Comparison group participants received identical instructions to those listed above regarding accessing and using a separate, content-identical Facebook group, with each participant asked to discontinue smartwatch use throughout the duration of the study. Finally, both groups also received a periodized strength and aerobic training program (see Supplementary Materials) via the Facebook group developed by the first author (an ACSM Certified Exercise Physiologist) with the physical limitations of breast cancer survivors—particularly those of the upper body—accounted for. This workout program was not mandatory to implement, however. Notably, both Facebook groups were completely private (i.e., closed) and unsearchable via Facebook. To ensure intervention fidelity, both groups were contacted every other week throughout the study and encouraged to continue using the Polar M400 (experimental group) and/or reading and attempting to implement the Facebook-delivered health education tips (both groups). Successful study completion resulted in receipt of a $100 gift card compensation. Experimental group participants were not allowed to keep the Polar M400 following study completion.

2.5. Statistical Analysis

First, intervention use/acceptability was evaluated descriptively—providing context for subsequent results. Second, descriptive statistics for all other outcomes at each time point were calculated, with an outlier analysis and Shapiro–Wilks tests of normality also performed. To evaluate baseline group differences in each categorical and continuous variable, chi-square and independent *t*-tests were then conducted, respectively. Third, mean change for each outcome variable was calculated by subtracting the value measured at baseline from the measurements taken at 10 weeks. Finally, Mann–Whitney U tests and independent *t*-tests were used to investigate group differences over time in the mean change of primary (i.e., moderate-to-vigorous physical activity, light physical activity, steps/day, and energy expenditure) and secondary (i.e., weight, body fat percentage, cardiorespiratory fitness, psychosocial constructs, and quality of life) outcomes. Notably, non-normal data distributions were observed for all physical activity outcomes and quality of life outcomes and, therefore, Mann–Whitney U tests were employed to evaluate differences in mean change between groups over time. Normally distributed data distributions were observed for physiological and psychosocial variables; thus, independent *t*-tests assessed differences in mean change over time in these outcomes, with Levene's Test for Equality of Variance used to examine homogeneity and determine the correct p-value(s) to report. Given the exploratory nature of the pilot trial, alpha was not adjusted, remaining at a p-value of 0.05 for all analyses.

3. Results

3.1. Baseline Comparisons and Participant Flow

Participant flow through the study is outlined within the CONSORT Diagram (see Figure 1). Forty-two breast cancer survivors expressed interest in the study, with 30 breast cancer survivors subsequently found eligible for baseline testing and randomization. Baseline values for these breast cancer survivors' demographic and clinical outcomes are presented in Table 1, with baseline comparisons of physical activity, physiological, psychosocial, and quality of life outcomes included in Table 2. No baseline group differences were observed for any variable suggesting efficacy of the randomization procedures.

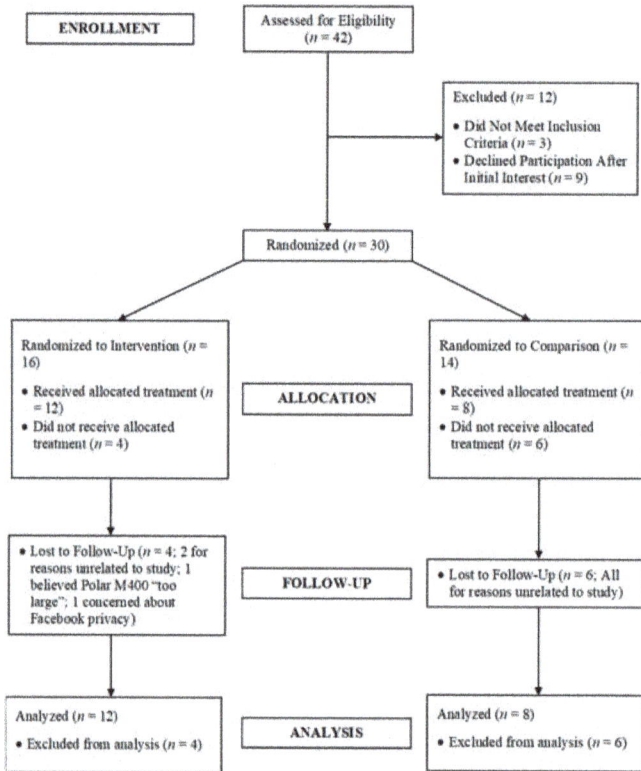

Figure 1. CONSORT study participant flow diagram.

Table 1. Participant baseline comparisons for clinical and demographic characteristics *.

	Demographic Characteristics ($n = 30$)				
	Experimental ($n = 16$)		Comparison ($n = 14$)		
	Avg. ($M \pm SD$)	Freq. (Counts)	Avg. ($M \pm SD$)	Freq. (Counts)	*p*-Value
Age (years)	50.6 ± 7.4		54.9 ± 11.0		0.23
Race/ethnicity					
• Caucasian		16		13	0.28
• Hispanic		0		1	

Table 1. *Cont.*

	Demographic Characteristics (*n* = 30)				
	Experimental (*n* = 16)		Comparison (*n* = 14)		
	Avg. (*M* ± SD)	Freq. (Counts)	Avg. (*M* ± SD)	Freq. (Counts)	*p*-Value
Educational status					
● Some college/technical school		2		2	
● College graduate		5		4	0.98
● Graduate school		9		8	
Health insurance					
● Private		16		12	0.12
● Medicaid		0		2	
Employment status					
● Full time		9		7	
● Part time		5		4	0.46
● Retired		0		2	
● Housewife		2		1	
Marital status					
● Married		14		10	
● Separated/divorced		1		2	0.60
● Widowed		0		1	
● Living with unmarried partner		1		1	
Annual income (USD)					
● $10,001–20,000		1		1	
● $30,001–40,000		1		2	
● $40,001–50,000		0		1	0.65
● $50,000–74,999		0		1	
● $75,000–99,999		4		3	
● ≥$100,000		10		6	
	Clinical Characteristics (*n* = 30)				
Time in remission	60.7 ± 39.7		48.7 ± 31.7		0.37
Months since diagnosis					
● ≤12 months		0		1	
● 13 to 24 months		5		1	
● 25 to 36 months		2		3	0.12
● 49 to 60 months		0		3	
● ≥61 months		9		6	
Diagnosed breast cancer stage					
● Stage 0		3		1	
● Stage 1		4		5	0.68
● Stage 2		7		5	
● Stage 3		2		3	
Treatment type					
● Surgery only		2		4	
● Surgery + radiation		2		1	0.64
● Surgery + chemo		5		5	
● Surgery + radiation + chemo		7		4	
Tamoxifen use					
● Yes		10		9	0.92
● No		6		5	
Follow-up care in past 12 months					
● Yes		16		14	1.00
● No		0		0	
Clinical breast exam frequency					
● Never		1		0	
● Every 3–6 months		2		2	
● Every 6–12 months		5		5	0.57
● Once yearly		6		7	
● Other		2		0	
Comorbidities					
● None		13		14	
● 1		1		0	0.23
● ≥2		2		0	

* Intent-to-treat analysis presented. Avg. = average; *M* = Mean; SD = Standard Deviation; Freq. = Frequency.

Table 2. Baseline comparisons for participants' primary and secondary outcomes [*,a].

	Experimental (*n* = 16)	Comparison (*n* = 14)	*p*-Value
	Primary Outcomes		
Daily MVPA	26.7 ± 18.4	20.9 ± 17.6	0.40
Daily LPA	72.9 ± 44.1	77.3 ± 48.2	0.80
Daily SB	378.0 ± 192.5	361.7 ± 201.0	0.82
Daily EE	272.5 ± 166.6	303.1 ± 240.9	0.69
Daily steps	4099.8 ± 2651.6	3092.7 ± 2214.0	0.27
	Secondary Outcomes		
	Physiological variables		
Weight (kg)	76.0 ± 13.0	85.0 ± 24.9	0.24
Body fat (%)	39.4 ± 5.5	38.6 ± 9.8	0.81
Cardiorespiratory fitness	113.2 ± 20.7	106.1 ± 23.4	0.39
	Psychosocial variables		
Self-efficacy [#]	73.3 ± 22.1	80.3 ± 14.5	0.33
Social support [$]	2.8 ± 1.1	2.1 ± 1.0	0.06
Enjoyment [$]	3.2 ± 0.5	3.3 ± 0.5	0.55
Barriers [@]	2.0 ± 0.5	1.9 ± 0.4	0.57
Outcome expectancy [$]	3.9 ± 0.5	4.1 ± 0.5	0.55
	Quality of life variables		
Physical functioning [**]	1.2 ± 0.4	1.3 ± 0.3	0.64
Anxiety [**]	1.8 ± 0.8	1.5 ± 0.7	0.34
Depression [**]	1.3 ± 0.3	1.1 ± 0.3	0.21
Fatigue [**]	2.5 ± 1.1	2.3 ± 0.6	0.51
Sleep quality [**]	3.1 ± 1.0	3.4 ± 0.9	0.39
Sleep disturbances [**]	2.9 ± 0.6	2.6 ± 0.5	0.17
Social roles/activities limitations [**]	2.2 ± 1.1	2.1 ± 0.8	0.76
Pain limitations [**]	1.7 ± 0.8	1.5 ± 0.6	0.51
Pain intensity [&]	2.0 ± 1.3	2.2 ± 1.9	0.72

[*] All values Mean ± Standard Deviation; [a] Intent-to-treat analysis presented; [#] Evaluated on a percentage confidence scale from 0% (Not confident at all) to 100% (Extremely confident); [$] Evaluated on 5-point Likert-type scale; [@] Evaluated on 4-point Likert-type scale; [**] Evaluated on a 5-point Likert-type scale; [&] Evaluated on a scale from 0 (no pain) to 10 (worst pain imaginable).

Ten breast cancer survivors dropped out of the study (66.6% retention rate; experimental group: 4; comparison group: 6). Eight breast cancer survivors dropped out due to reasons unrelated to the study. Regarding the other two dropouts, one participant dropped out due to the perception that the Polar M400 was "too large" and inhibiting her daily work, with the other dropping out due to concerns about Facebook privacy (despite the Facebook groups being entirely private and unsearchable). Compared to completers, dropouts had less private insurance coverage, longer duration since diagnosis, and lower annual income, daily light physical activity, moderate-to-vigorous physical activity, EE, and steps. Given these differences, a per-protocol analysis was completed when evaluating changes in health outcomes from baseline to 10 weeks.

3.2. Intervention Use/Acceptability

All experimental group participants reported wearing the Polar M400 6–7 days/week. The weekly mean frequency and duration per session for the use of this device during exercise was 4.55 ± 1.74 sessions/week and 53.9 ± 16.7 min/session, respectively. Only 7 of the 12 experimental participants reported enjoying Polar M400 use, however, with these participants stating the following as negative device features: was difficult to sync to phone/computer; had trouble tracking activities like biking and swimming; the size of the smartwatch was "too big", with most breast cancer survivors stating the device's buttons would get inadvertently pressed when dressing and undressing given the thickness of the smartwatch; and the smartwatch use was not as "straightforward" to use as other smartwatches as the device used buttons on the side of the device to toggle through black-and-white screens and did not possess a color touchscreen with easily accessible tabs akin to other smartwatches like the Fitbit. Regarding the Facebook health education intervention, participants across both groups reported implementing the tips provided 1.2 ± 1.0 times/weekly, with 16 out of 20 participants enjoying these health education tips.

3.2.1. Primary Outcomes

Table 3 contains descriptive statistics for breast cancer survivors' mean daily moderate-to-vigorous physical activity, light physical activity, sedentary behavior, energy expenditure, and steps/day at baseline and 10 weeks. No statistically significant group differences were observed for change over time for any variable. However, both the experimental and comparison groups demonstrated increased mean daily moderate-to-vigorous physical activity (+3.5 and +7.5 min, respectively), light physical activity (+7.5 and +8.1 min, respectively), energy expenditure (+26.7 and +22.6 calories, respectively), and steps/day (+342.7 and +334.4 steps/day, respectively) from baseline to 10 weeks. Notably, mean daily sedentary behavior remained stable over time, but slight increases were observed within the experimental (+2.4 min) and comparison (+0.4 min) groups.

Table 3. Descriptive statistics for physical activity-related outcomes by group at baseline and 10 weeks [*,a].

	Experimental (*n* = 12)		Comparison (*n* = 8)		*p*-Value [b]
	Baseline	10 Weeks	Baseline	10 Weeks	
Daily MVPA	30.7 ± 13.2	34.2 ± 18.7	30.2 ± 16.2	37.8 ± 20.4	0.49
Daily LPA	91.4 ± 28.8	98.9 ± 29.5	100.4 ± 31.6	108.5 ± 47.9	0.76
Daily SB	464.4 ± 50.7	466.8 ± 34.7	449.2 ± 54.9	449.6 ± 53.2	0.82
Daily EE	333.1 ± 113.3	359.9 ± 147.4	395.5 ± 229.9	418.0 ± 188.9	0.44
Daily steps	4832.4 ± 1816.4	5175.1 ± 2308.2	4411.6 ± 1624.7	4746.0 ± 2044.9	0.76

[*] All values Mean ± Standard Deviation; [a] Per-protocol analysis presented; [b] *p*-value represents group difference in change from baseline to 10 weeks for a given outcome as assessed via Mann–Whitney U tests.

3.2.2. Secondary Outcomes

Table 4 provides descriptive statistics for all physiological and psychosocial outcomes at baseline and 10 weeks while Table 5 provides descriptive statistics for all quality of life outcomes at the same time points.

Table 4. Descriptive statistics for physiological and psychosocial variables by group at baseline and 10 weeks [*,a].

	Experimental (*n* = 12)		Comparison (*n* = 8)		*p*-Value [b]
	Baseline	10 Weeks	Baseline	10 Weeks	
	Physiological variables				
Weight (kg)	76.6 ± 13.3	76.9 ± 12.2	78.0 ± 22.6	78.0 ± 23.0	0.62
Body fat (%)	39.8 ± 6.0	40.2 ± 5.4	36.0 ± 10.6	35.0 ± 10.8	0.12
Cardiorespiratory fitness	110.4 ± 18.5	105.7 ± 21.7	104.8 ± 29.3	100.3 ± 21.6	0.97
	Psychosocial variables				
Self-efficacy [#]	75.6 ± 25.1	67.9 ± 26.5	78.2 ± 12.1	71.8 ± 14.8	0.98
Social support [$]	3.0 ± 1.1	2.7 ± 1.3	2.4 ± 1.1	3.0 ± 1.1	0.05
Enjoyment [$]	3.3 ± 0.5	3.2 ± 0.5	3.2 ± 0.6	3.3 ± 0.6	0.53
Barriers [@]	2.0 ± 0.5	2.0 ± 0.5	2.1 ± 0.2	1.8 ± 0.4	0.04
Outcome expectancy [$]	4.1 ± 0.5	3.9 ± 0.5	4.0 ± 0.6	4.0 ± 0.6	0.34

[*] All values Mean ± Standard Deviation; [a] Per-protocol analysis presented; [b] *p*-value represents group difference in change from baseline to 10 weeks for a given outcome as assessed via independent *t*-tests; [#] Evaluated on a percentage confidence scale from 0% (Not confident at all) to 100% (Extremely confident); [$] Evaluated on 5-point Likert-type scale; [@] Evaluated on 4-point Likert-type scale.

Table 5. Descriptive statistics for quality of life outcomes by group at baseline and 10 weeks *,a.

	Experimental (*n* = 12)		Comparison (*n* = 8)		*p*-Value b
	Baseline	**10 Weeks**	**Baseline**	**10 Weeks**	
Physical functioning **	1.1 ± 0.2	1.1 ± 0.2	1.2 ± 0.2	1.1 ± 0.2	0.78
Anxiety **	1.8 ± 0.8	2.0 ± 0.8	1.7 ± 0.7	1.5 ± 0.7	0.19
Depression **	1.2 ± 0.3	1.4 ± 0.4	1.1 ± 0.3	1.1 ± 0.1	0.41
Fatigue **	2.3 ± 1.0	2.3 ± 0.8	2.4 ± 0.6	2.2 ± 0.9	0.31
Sleep quality **	3.1 ± 0.9	3.3 ± 0.6	3.6 ± 0.9	3.5 ± 0.9	0.62
Sleep disturbances **	2.8 ± 0.6	2.5 ± 0.4	2.5 ± 0.5	2.5 ± 0.4	0.64
Social roles/activities limitations **	2.0 ± 0.9	1.8 ± 0.7	1.9 ± 0.7	1.9 ± 0.5	0.64
Pain limitations **	1.5 ± 0.5	1.5 ± 0.6	1.4 ± 0.5	1.4 ± 0.4	1.0
Pain intensity &	1.8 ± 1.0	1.8 ± 1.8	2.0 ± 1.9	1.8 ± 1.4	0.97

* All values Mean ± Standard Deviation; a Per-protocol analysis presented; b *p*-value represents group difference in change from baseline to 10 weeks for a given outcome as assessed via Mann–Whitney U tests; ** Evaluated on a 5-point Likert-type scale; & Evaluated on a scale from 0 (no pain) to 10 (worst pain imaginable).

3.3. Physiological Changes over Time

Breast cancer survivors' weight was observed to be largely unchanged within both groups from baseline to 10 weeks, but the comparison group did demonstrate a larger, albeit non-significant ($p > 0.05$), decrease in body fat percentage (−1.0%) compared to the experimental group (+0.5%) during the intervention. Additionally, while improvements in cardiorespiratory fitness over time were not significantly different between groups, both groups demonstrated reduced heart rate following the YMCA 3-min Step Test at 10 weeks (experimental: −4.8 beats/minute; comparison: −4.5 beats/minute).

3.4. Psychosocial Construct Changes over Time

Significant group differences for changes in social support ($t = -2.1$, $p = 0.05$) and barriers ($t = -2.2$, $p = 0.04$) were observed. Interestingly, from baseline to 10 weeks, the comparison group demonstrated improved physical activity-related social support and decreased barriers while the experimental group demonstrated slightly decreased social support and no change in barriers.

3.5. Quality of Life Changes over Time

No significant group differences over time were observed for any quality of life outcome. It is noteworthy, however, that the experimental group demonstrated decreased social role limitations and reductions in sleep disturbances, with a subsequent increase in sleep quality, from baseline to 10 weeks.

4. Discussion

Breast cancer survivors are at risk of greater physical inactivity, poorer physiological/psychological health, and reduced quality of life due to past breast cancer treatment [3,4]. Given physical activity's demonstrated effects on breast cancers survivors' health outcomes, health behavior change interventions have become common recommendations among this population [5–10]. As breast cancer survivors have found acceptable and expressed interest in the use of smartwatches to self-regulate physical activity and sedentary behavior [17], this pilot randomized trial examined the effectiveness of a combined smartwatch- and social media-based health education intervention in the promotion of improved physical activity and health indices among breast cancer survivors. Observations suggested this type of intervention might promote improvements in physical activity and certain health outcomes, but that smartwatch complexity needs to be considered as the experimental group did not demonstrate significantly different improvements over time versus the comparison group.

The current investigation's first hypothesis was that greater increased physical activity, energy expenditure, and steps/day in addition to reduced sedentary behavior would be observed among the experimental group versus the comparison group. Observations were not congruent with this hypothesis as both groups demonstrated similarly increased moderate-to-vigorous physical activity, light physical activity, energy expenditure, and steps/day during the intervention period with mean increases of approximately 5 min, 8 min, 25 kcalories, and 340 steps/day, respectively. Despite no statistically significant group differences, these findings may have some clinical/practical significance. Specifically, research has indicated sedentary behavior to increase breast cancer recurrence risk by up to 34% among breast cancer survivors [51]. Reasons for the increased recurrence risk are many, not the least of which has to do with adiposity and its effects on cancer-related hormones. Briefly, increased adiposity among breast cancer survivors has been positively correlated with insulin resistance as well as poorer regulation of insulin growth factor-1 (IGF-1) and estrogen—two hormones frequently implicated in breast cancer development and recurrence [52]. Fortunately, physical activity has been shown to promote appropriate regulation of insulin, IGF-1, and estrogen [53]. Thus, the combined ~13 min/day increase in moderate-to-vigorous physical activity and light physical activity from baseline to 10 weeks is noteworthy as this increase contributed to ~1.5 h/week more of physical activity among the current sample. Nonetheless, it is necessary to question why the experimental group did not experience greater increases in the preceding primary outcomes than the comparison group.

Examination of the experimental groups' opinion of the Polar M400 smartwatch may provide some answers. Explicitly, five out of the 12 breast cancer survivors in the experimental group expressed frustration with the smartwatch, with participants finding the smartwatch too complex, hard to connect to the associated smartphone application, and too big. These remarks are congruent with recent literature among breast cancer survivors during which it was found breast cancer survivors prefer simple, easy-to-use smartwatches with larger screens when using these devices to self-regulate physical activity and sedentary behavior [17]. Indeed, while powerful, the Polar M400 is not as intuitive as other smartwatches available on the market (e.g., Apple Watch 3, Fitbit Ionic) given the fact that Polar has long marketed their products to the sport performance industry and has only recently begun to develop and market smartwatches. Therefore, future studies among breast cancer survivors may utilize smartwatches which are more mainstream and easier-to-use—keeping in mind that breast cancer survivors are often middle-aged females and that research does suggest a negative relationship between age and technological literacy, adoption, and use [54,55].

The preceding observations regarding the usability of the Polar M400 might have also influenced the conclusions made regarding the study's second hypothesis wherein it was stated that the experimental participants would have greater improvements in physiological outcomes versus comparison participants. Indeed, no difference in mean body weight changes were observed between groups, with the lower heart rate observed following the step test nearly identical for both groups (approximately 5 beats/minute; indicative of improved cardiorespiratory fitness). Interestingly, decreased body fat percentage was observed among comparison participants while slightly increased body fat percentage was seen among experimental participants during the intervention. Yet, it is difficult to know whether these changes represent actual changes in body fat percentage due to the intervention as the magnitude of these changes is within the margin of error commonly reported for bioelectrical impedance testing on individuals of higher body fat percentage akin to that observed in the current investigation [56]. While the lower heart rate following step testing is promising given the fact improved cardiorespiratory fitness has been observed to negatively correlate with breast cancer survivors' risk of breast cancer recurrence [57], decreased body weight and body fat percentage is still highly desired given the aforementioned influence of adiposity on key cancer hormones [52,53].

The final hypothesis of this study was that the experimental participants would experience greater beneficial changes in social cognitive theory-related psychosocial constructs and quality of life indices versus the comparison group. Observations, again, were not congruent with this hypothesis. Interestingly, significantly greater increases in social support were observed among comparison participants versus experimental participants who demonstrated slightly decreased social support over time. It is noteworthy, however, that experimental participants had marginally significantly higher social support at baseline versus comparison participants ($p = 0.06$), with both groups completing the intervention with approximately the same social support scores. Therefore, these paradoxical findings might be attributed more to regression towards the mean than the effects of the intervention. Notably, experimental participants did demonstrate greater reductions in social role limitations and sleep disturbances in addition to a slight increase in sleep quality versus comparison participants during the intervention. These observations are positive as social role limitations and fatigue (among other factors) have been observed to be a major determinants of quality of life among breast cancer survivors [58]. Moreover, sleep disturbances have been shown to moderate the effect of vasomotor symptoms associated with the onset of breast cancer treatment-induced menopause (e.g., hot flashes) on depressive symptoms among breast cancer survivors approximately the same age as women in the current study [59]. This suggests the less frequent sleep disturbances (and improved sleep quality) indicated among experimental participants might confer health benefits in the long term. Nonetheless, more research with larger and more diverse samples is needed to investigate how to effectively promote improved psychosocial and quality of life health outcomes among breast cancer survivors.

Strengths of the current study include: (1) investigation of breast cancer survivors—a population not often targeted for physical activity interventions; (2) use of a combined smartwatch and social media-delivered health education intervention; (3) utilization of Social Cognitive Theory to develop and implement the intervention; and (4) evaluations of physiological, psychosocial, and quality of life indices in addition to a full spectrum of objectively-assessed physical activity analyses (i.e., durations of sedentary behavior, light physical activity, and moderate-to-vigorous physical activity). Despite these strengths, limitations are present and should be accounted for when interpreting the study's findings. To begin, the study was not blinded. Although group allocation was concealed as best as possible from participants, several breast cancer survivors in the present study knew one another from various breast cancer survivors support groups raising the concern of contamination between groups. Second, while the request was made to comparison participants to discontinue smartwatch use throughout the duration of the intervention, it might be possible that some participants did not follow these directives or utilized other means of health behavior tracking in place of a smartwatch (e.g., a smartphone-based health application). Third, the study concentrated exclusively on promoting physical activity and reducing sedentary behavior, with no dietary component included. Diet has been cited as an important consideration when seeking to promote improved health among breast cancer survivors given the dietary effects which can be present on hormones related to breast cancer development/metastasis such as estrogen, insulin, and IGF-1 [53]. As interventions targeting both dietary and physical activity behaviors have been shown to be more effective than interventions targeting dietary or physical activity behaviors exclusively [60], including both emphases in future interventions is advised. Further, measurements of biomarkers in future studies might also be advised to increase the generalizability of the effects an intervention of this type might have in a clinical setting. Indeed, not only have biomarkers like estrogen, insulin, and IGF-1 been implicated in breast cancer development/recurrence [52,53] but, more recently, myokines have been observed important to breast cancer development [61]. Specifically, this latter research has indicated that muscular contraction can increase myokine secretion which may have a therapeutic effect on organ metabolism and potentially reduce the likelihood of breast cancer recurrence among breast cancer survivors. Myokine measurements might also be correlated with lean mass measurements made by body composition assessment techniques with demonstrated high accuracy like hydrodensiometry and dual x-ray absorptiometry [62]. Nonetheless, the current study's methodology was sufficient to investigate whether a combined smartwatch- and theoretically-based, social media-delivered health education intervention was feasible among breast cancer survivors. Although ActiGraph GT3X+ accelerometer has demonstrated acceptable validity and reliability in assessing sedentary and physical activity behavior among adults, more accurate motion sensor in measuring sedentary and light physical activity (e.g., activPAL) may be used in future studies with this population [63]. Additionally, the small sample size limited statistical power, with the fact the sample was well-educated and of high socioeconomic status limiting study generalizability. Larger and more diverse samples are suggested for future investigations. Finally, given the increasing popularity of the Social Ecological Model and the important role the neighborhood environment plays in enhancing physical activity and quality of life, researchers might include neighborhood environment in the research design in the future [64].

5. Conclusions

The current study suggests that a theoretically based health education intervention delivered using social media may be able to promote increased physical activity and select improved health indices among breast cancer survivors. However, observations do not suggest smartwatch use confers any additional benefit to an intervention of this type. Indeed, despite extensive user training, most experimental participants found the Polar M400 difficult to use—possibly decreasing intervention adherence. Future interventions should utilize simpler smartwatches to promote PA among middle-aged clinical/non-clinical populations as technology-based interventions of this type still show promise in providing low-burden, well-integrated health promotion options for these populations.

Supplementary Materials: The following are available online at http://www.mdpi.com/2077-0383/7/6/140/s1.

Author Contributions: While conducting this study, Z.C.P. played a role in developing the idea as well as a large role in collecting and analyzing these data while also writing the manuscript. N.Z. played a role in data collection/sorting and a large role in editing the manuscript. R.Z. played a role in developing the idea and editing the manuscript. H.Y.L. played a role in interpreting the data analysis and editing the manuscript. Z.G. played a large role in developing the idea, overseeing data collection/analysis, and editing the manuscript.

Funding: This study was funded by a research grant from the Grant-in-Aid Program at the University of Minnesota-Twin Cities (Grant #: 111179).

Acknowledgments: The University of Minnesota played no part in the development, implementation, analysis, or writing of the study/manuscript. The results of this study are presented clearly, honestly, and without fabrication, falsification, or inappropriate data manipulation.

Conflicts of Interest: The authors declare no conflict of interest.

References

1. Amercian Cancer Society. How Common Is Breast Cancer? Available online: https://www.cancer.org/cancer/breast-cancer/about/how-common-is-breast-cancer.html (accessed on 16 May 2018).
2. Howlader, N.; Noone, A.; Krapcho, M.; Miller, D.; Bishop, K.; Altekruse, S.; Kosary, C.; Yu, M.; Ruhl, J.; Tatalovich, Z.; et al. *Seer Cancer Statistics Review*; National Cancer Institute: Bethesda, MD, USA, 2016.
3. Phillips, S.; McAuley, E. Physical activity, quality of life, and survivorship in breast cancer survivors: A brief review. *CML Breast Cancer* **2012**, *24*, 77–84.
4. Jadoon, N.; Munir, W.; Shahzad, M.; Choudhry, Z. Assessment of depression and anxiety in adult cancer outpatients: A cross-sectional study. *BMC Cancer* **2010**, *10*, 594. [CrossRef] [PubMed]
5. Phillips, S.; McAuley, E. Physical activity and fatigue in breast cancer survivors: A panel model examining the role of self-efficacy and depression. *Cancer Epidemiol. Prev. Biomark.* **2013**, *22*, 773–781. [CrossRef] [PubMed]
6. Phillips, S.; McAuley, E. Physical activity and quality of life in breast cancer survivors: The role of self-efficacy and health status. *Psychol. Oncol.* **2014**, *23*, 27–34. [CrossRef] [PubMed]
7. Harrison, S.; Hayes, S.; Newman, B. Age-related differences in exercise and quality of life among breast cancer survivors. *Med. Sci. Sports Exerc.* **2010**, *42*, 67–74. [CrossRef] [PubMed]
8. Mack, D.; Meldrum, L.; Wilson, P.; Sabiston, C. Physical activity and psychological health in breast cancer survivors: An application of basic psychological needs theory. *Appl. Psychol. Health Well Being* **2013**, *5*, 369–388. [CrossRef] [PubMed]

9.   Smith, A.; Alfano, C.; Reeve, B.; Irwin, M.; Bernstein, L.; Baumgartner, K.; Bowen, D.; McTiernan, A.; Ballard-Barbash, R. Race/ethnicity, physical activity, and quality of life in breast cancer survivors. *Cancer Epidemiol. Prev. Biomark.* **2009**, *18*, 656–663. [CrossRef] [PubMed]

10. Taylor, D.; Nichols, J.; Pakiz, B.; Bardwell, W.; Flatt, S.; Rock, C. Relationships between cardiorespiratory fitness, physical activity, and psychosocial variables in overweight and obese breast cancer survivors. *Int. J. Behav. Med.* **2010**, *17*, 264–270. [CrossRef] [PubMed]

11. Lewis, B.; Napolitano, M.; Buman, M.; Williams, D.; Nigg, C. Future directions in physical activity intervention research: Expanding our focus to sedentary behaviors, technology, and dissemination. *J. Behav. Med.* **2017**, *40*, 112–126. [CrossRef] [PubMed]

12. Brandt, C.; Clemensen, J.; Nielsen, J.; Sondergaard, J. Drivers of successful long-term lifestyle change, the role of e-health: A qualitative study. *BMJ Open* **2018**, *8*, e017466. [CrossRef] [PubMed]

13. Statista. Consumer Wearables Revenues in the United States from 2014 to 2019 (in Billion U.S. Dollars). Available online: https://www.statista.com/statistics/503455/consumer-wearables-revenues-in-the-us (accessed on 16 May 2018).

14. Almalki, M.; Gray, K.; Sanchez, F. The use of self-quantification systems for personal health information: Big data management activities and prospects. *Health Inf. Sci. Syst.* **2015**, *3*, S1. [CrossRef] [PubMed]

15. Lyons, E.; Lewis, Z.; Mayrsohn, B.; Rowland, J. Behavior change techniques implemented in electronic lifestyle activity monitors: A systematic content analysis. *J. Med. Internet Res.* **2014**, *16*, e192. [CrossRef] [PubMed]

16. Pope, Z.; Lee, J.; Zeng, N.; Lee, H.; Gao, Z. Feasibility of smartphone application and social media intervention on breast cancer survivors' health outcomes. *Transl. Behav. Med.* **2018**. [CrossRef] [PubMed]

17. Nguyen, N.; Hadgraft, N.; Moore, M.; Rosenberg, D.; Lynch, C.; Reeves, M.; Lynch, B. A qualitative evaluation of breast cancer survivors' acceptance of and preferences for consumer wearable technology activity trackers. *Support. Care Cancer* **2017**, *25*, 3375–3384. [CrossRef] [PubMed]

18. Cadmus-Bertram, L.; Marcus, B.; Patterson, R.; Parker, B.; Morey, B. Randomized trial of a fitbit-based physical activity intervention for women. *Am. J. Prev. Med.* **2015**, *49*, 414–418. [CrossRef] [PubMed]

19. Cadmus-Bertram, L.; Marcus, B.; Patterson, R.; Parker, B.; Morey, B. Use of the fitbit to measure adherence to a physical activity intervention among overweight or obese, postmenopausal women: Self-monitoring trajectory during 16 weeks. *J. Med. Internet Res.* **2015**, *3*, e96. [CrossRef] [PubMed]

20. Wang, J.; Cadmus-Bertram, L.; Natarajan, L.; White, M.; Madanat, H.; Nichols, J.; Ayala, G.; Pierce, J. Wearable sensor/device (fitbit one) and sms text-messaging prompts to increase physical activity in overweight and obese adults: A randomized controlled trial. *Telemed. E-Health* **2015**, *21*, 782–792. [CrossRef] [PubMed]

21. Thompson, W.; Kuhle, C.; Koepp, G.; McCrady-Spitzer, S.; Levine, J. "Go4life" exercise counseling, accelerometer feedback, and activity levels in older people. *Arch. Gerontol. Geriatr.* **2014**, *58*, 314–319. [CrossRef] [PubMed]

22. Thorndike, A.; Mills, S.; Sonnenberg, L.; Palakshappa, D.; Gao, T.; Pau, C.; Regan, S. Activity monitor intervention to promote physical activity of physicians-in-training: Randomized controlled trial. *PLoS ONE* **2014**, *9*, e100251. [CrossRef] [PubMed]

23. Kim, Y.; Lumpkin, A.; Lochbaum, M.; Stegemeier, S.; Kitten, K. Promoting physical activity using wearable activity tracker in college students: A cluster randomized trial. *J. Sports Sci.* **2018**, 1–8. [CrossRef] [PubMed]

24. Rote, A. Physical activity intervention using fitbits in an introductory college health course. *Health Educ. J.* **2017**, *76*, 337–348. [CrossRef]

25. Melton, B.; Buman, M.; Vogel, R.; Harris, B.; Bigham, L. Wearable devices to improve physical activity and sleep: A randomized controlled trial of college-aged african american women. *J. Black Stud.* **2016**, *47*, 610–625. [CrossRef]

26. Nielsen-Bohlman, L.; Panzer, A.; Kindig, D. *Health Literacy: A Prescription to End Confusion*; The National Academies Press: Washington, DC, USA, 2004.

27. Rikard, R.; Thompson, M.; McKinney, J.; Beauchamp, A. Examining health literacy disparities in the United States: A third look at the national assessment of adult literacy (NAAL). *BMC Public Health* **2016**, *16*, 975. [CrossRef] [PubMed]

28. Patten, M. The role of theory in research. In *Understanding Research Methods: An Overview of the Essentials*, 9th ed.; Patten, M., Ed.; Pyrczak Publishing: Glendale, CA, USA, 2014; pp. 27–29.

29. Statista. Distribution of Facebook Users in the United States as of January 2017, by Age Group and Gender. Available online: https://www.statista.com/statistics/187041/us-user-age-distribution-on-facebook/ (accessed on 16 May 2018).

30. Brug, J.; Oenema, A.; Ferreira, I. Theory, evidence, and intervention mapping to improve behavior, nutrition, and physical activity interventions. *Int. J. Behav. Nutr. Phys. Act.* **2005**, *2*, 2. [CrossRef] [PubMed]

31. Thomas, J.; Nelson, J.; Silverman, S. Developing the problem and using the literature. In *Research Methods in Physical Activity*, 6th ed.; Thomas, J., Nelson, J., Silverman, S., Eds.; Human Kinetics: Champaign, IL, USA, 2011; pp. 25–50.

32. Bandura, A. Self-efficacy: Toward a unifying theory of behavioral change. *Psychol. Rev.* **1977**, *84*, 191–215. [CrossRef] [PubMed]

33. Bandura, A. *Social Foundations of thought and Action: A Social Cognitive Theory*; Prentice Hall: Englewood Cliffs, NJ, USA, 1986.

34. Schulz, K.; Altman, D.; Moher, D.; Group, C. Consort 2010 statement: Updated guidelines for reporting parallel group randomised trials. *BMC Med.* **2010**, *8*, 18. [CrossRef] [PubMed]

35. World Medical Association. *World Medical Association Declaration of Helsinki: Ethical Principles for Medical Research Involving Human Subjects*; World Medical Association: Washington, DC, USA, 2008; pp. 1–5.

36. Canadian Society for Exercise Physiology. Par-Q Forms. Available online: http://www.csep.ca/view.asp?ccid=517 (accessed on 16 May 2018).

37. Kaminsky, L.; Ozemek, C. A comparison of the actigraph gt1m and gt3x accelerometers under standardized and free-living conditions. *Physiol. Meas.* **2012**, *33*, 1869–1876. [CrossRef] [PubMed]

38. Trost, S.; McIver, K.; Pate, R. Conducting accelerometer-based activity assessments in field-based research. *Med. Sci. Sports Exerc.* **2005**, *37*, S531–S543. [CrossRef] [PubMed]

39. Troiano, R.; Berrigan, D.; Dodd, K.; Masse, L.; Tilert, T.; McDowell, M. Physical activity in the united states measured by accelerometer. *Med. Sci. Sports Exerc.* **2008**, *40*, 181–188. [CrossRef] [PubMed]

40. Aandstad, A.; Holtberget, K.; Hageberg, R.; Holme, I.; Anderssen, S. Validity and reliability of bioelectrical impedance analysis and skinfold thickness in predicting body fat in military personnel. *Mil. Med.* **2014**, *179*, 208–217. [CrossRef] [PubMed]

41. Golding, L.; Meyers, C.; Sinning, W. *Y's Way to Physical Fitness: The Complete Guide to Fitness Testing and Instruction*, 4th ed.; Human Kinetics: Champaign, IL, USA, 1998.

42. Carlson, J.; Sallis, J.; Wagner, N.; Calfas, K.; Patrick, K.; Groesz, L.; Norman, G. Brief physical activity-related psychosocial measures: Reliability and construct validity. *J. Phys. Act. Health* **2012**, *9*, 1178–1186. [CrossRef] [PubMed]

43. Sechrist, K.; Walker, S.; Pender, N. Development and psychometric evaluation of the exercise benefits/barriers scale. *Res. Nurs. Health* **1987**, *10*, 357–365. [CrossRef] [PubMed]

44. Rodgers, W.; Wilson, P.; Hall, C.; Fraser, S.; Murray, T. Evidence for a multidimensional self-efficacy for exercise scale. *Res. Q. Exerc. Sport* **2008**, *79*, 222–234. [CrossRef] [PubMed]

45. Harter, S. Effectance motivation reconsidered: Toward a developmental model. *Hum. Dev.* **1978**, *21*, 34–64. [CrossRef]

46. Trost, S.; Pate, R.; Saunders, R.; Ward, D.; Dowda, M.; Felton, G. A prospective study of the determinants of physical activity in rural fifth-grade children. *Prev. Med.* **1997**, *26*, 257–263. [CrossRef] [PubMed]

47. National Institutes of Health. Patient Reported Outcome Measurement Information System: Instrument Details. Available online: http://www.nihpromis.org/measures/instrumentdetails (accessed on 16 May 2018).

48. Lin, F.-J.; Pickard, A.; Krishnan, J.; Joo, M.; Au, D.; Carson, S.; Gillespie, S.; Henderson, A.; Lindenauer, P.; McBurnie, M.; et al. Measuring health-related quality of life in chronic obstructive pulmonary disease: Properties of the eq 5d 5l and promis 43 short form. *BMC Med. Res. Methodol.* **2014**, *14*, 78. [CrossRef] [PubMed]

49. Yost, K.; Eton, D.; Garcia, S.; Cella, D. Minimally important differences were estimated for six promis-cancer scales in advanced-stage cancer patients. *J. Clin. Epidemiol.* **2011**, *64*, 507–516. [CrossRef] [PubMed]

50. Polar. Polar M400 Gps Running Watch. Available online: https://www.polar.com/us-en/products/sport/M400 (accessed on 16 May 2018).

51. Arnold, M.; Leitzmann, M.; Freisling, H.; Bray, F.; Romieu, I.; Renehan, A.; Soerjomataram, I. Obesity and cancer: An update of the global impact. *Cancer Epidemiol.* **2016**, *41*, 8–15. [CrossRef] [PubMed]

52. Belardi, V.; Gallagher, E.; Novosyadlyy, R.; LeRoith, D. Insulin and IGFs in obesity-related breast cancer. *J. Mammary Gland Biol. Neoplasia* **2013**, *18*, 277–289. [CrossRef] [PubMed]
53. Dieli-Conwright, C.; Lee, K.; Kiwata, J. Reducing the risk of breast cancer recurrence: An evaluation of the effects and mechanisms of diet and exercise. *Curr. Breast Cancer Rep.* **2016**, *8*, 139–150. [CrossRef] [PubMed]
54. Pew Research Center. Older Adults and Technology Use. Available online: http://www.pewinternet.org/2014/04/03/older-adults-and-technology-use/ (accessed on 16 May 2018).
55. Van Volkom, M.; Stapley, J.; Amaturo, V. Revisiting the digital divide: Generational differences in technology use in everyday life. *N. Am. J. Psychol.* **2014**, *16*, 557–574.
56. Faria, S.; Faria, O.; Cardeal, M.; Ito, M. Validation study of multi-frequency bioelectrical impedance with dual-energy X-ray absorptiometry among obese patients. *Obes. Surg.* **2014**, *24*, 1476–1480. [CrossRef] [PubMed]
57. Loprinzi, P.; Cardinal, B.; Winters-Stone, K.; Smit, E.; Loprinzi, C. Physical activity and the risk of breast cancer recurrence: A literature review. *Oncol. Nurs. Forum* **2012**, *39*, 269–274. [CrossRef] [PubMed]
58. Fallowfield, L.; Jenkins, V. Psychosocial/survivorship issues in breast cancer: Are we doing better. *JNCI J. Natl. Cancer Inst.* **2015**, *107*. [CrossRef] [PubMed]
59. Accortt, E.; Bower, J.; Stanton, A.; Ganz, P. Depression and vasomotor symptoms in young breast cancer survivors: The mediating role of sleep disturbance. *Arch. Women Ment. Health* **2015**, *18*, 565–568. [CrossRef] [PubMed]
60. Kohl, H., III; Murray, T. (Eds.) Overweight and obesity. In *Foundations of Physical Activity and Public Health*; Human Kinetics: Champaign, IL, USA, 2012; pp. 95–117.
61. Dethlefsen, C.; Pedersen, K.S.; Hojman, P. Every exercise bout matters: Linking systemic exercise responses to breast cancer control. *Breast Cancer Res. Treat.* **2017**, *162*, 399–408. [CrossRef] [PubMed]
62. Kenney, W.; Wilmore, J.; Costill, D. (Eds.) Body composition and nutrition for sport. In *Physiology of Sport and Exercise*; Human Kinetics: Champaign, IL, USA, 2015; pp. 371–405.
63. Alberto, F.; Nathanael, M.; Mathew, B.; Ainsworth, B.E. Wearable monitors criterion validity for energy expenditure in sedentary and light activities. *J. Sport Health Sci.* **2017**, *6*, 103–110. [CrossRef]
64. Theodoropoulou, E.; Stavrou, N.; Karteroliotis, K. Neighborhood environment, physical activity, and quality of life in adults: Intermediary effects of personal and psychosocial factors. *J. Sport Health Sci.* **2017**, *6*, 96–102. [CrossRef]

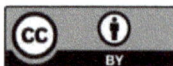

Journal of
Clinical Medicine

MDPI

Article

Preschoolers' Technology-Assessed Physical Activity and Cognitive Function: A Cross-Sectional Study

Minghui Quan [1] [ORCID], Hanbin Zhang [1], Jiayi Zhang [2], Tang Zhou [1], Jinming Zhang [3], Guanggao Zhao [4], Hui Fang [1], Shunli Sun [1], Ru Wang [1,*] and Peijie Chen [1,*]

[1]   School of Kinesiology, Shanghai University of Sport, Shanghai 200438, China;
      quanminghui@163.com (M.Q.); zhb20092009@163.com (H.Z.); tzhou_1023@foxmail.com (T.Z.);
      ffanghui@163.com (H.F.); sunsl087@outlook.com (S.S.)
[2]   Editorial Department of Medicine and Health, China Science Publishing and Media Ltd.,
      Shanghai 200032, China; jiayi_0827@126.com
[3]   Department of Kinesiology, College of Sport Medicine and Rehabilitation, Taishan Medical University,
      Taian 271016, China; jmzhang@tsmc.edu.cn
[4]   Department of Physical Education, Nanchang University, Nanchang 330031, China; zhaogg2002@163.com
*   Correspondence: wangru0612@163.com (R.W.); chenpeijie@sus.edu.cn (P.C.);
      Tel.: +86-21-5125-3240 (R.W.); +86-21-5125-3003 (P.C.)

Received: 19 April 2018; Accepted: 7 May 2018; Published: 8 May 2018

Abstract: Early childhood is a critical period for development of cognitive function, but research on the association between physical activity and cognitive function in preschool children is limited and inconclusive. This study aimed to examine the association between technology-assessed physical activity and cognitive function in preschool children. A cross-sectional analysis of baseline data from the Physical Activity and Cognitive Development Study was conducted in Shanghai, China. Physical activity was measured with accelerometers for 7 consecutive days, and cognitive functions were assessed using the Chinese version of Wechsler Young Children Scale of Intelligence (C-WYCSI). Linear regression analyses were used to assess the association between physical activity and cognitive function. A total of 260 preschool children (boys, 144; girls, 116; mean age: 57.2 ± 5.4 months) were included in analyses for this study. After adjusting for confounding factors, we found that Verbal Intelligence Quotient, Performance Intelligence Quotient, and Full Intelligence Quotient were significantly correlated with light physical activity, not moderate to vigorous physical activity, in boys. Standardized coefficients were 0.211, 0.218, and 0.242 (all $p < 0.05$) in three different models, respectively. However, the correlation between physical activity and cognitive functions were not significant in girls ($p > 0.05$). These findings suggest that cognitive function is apparently associated with light physical activity in boys. Further studies are required to clarify the sex-specific effect on physical activity and cognitive functions.

Keywords: motor activity; intelligence quotient; young children

---

1. Introduction

Cognitive function is the ability to process information acquired from individual surroundings by the brain and includes the ability to learn and remember information, organize, plan and problem-solve, focus, maintain and shift attention, and understand and use language [1]. The stage of childhood is a critical period to develop cognitive function, as cognitive function in childhood may be an important indicator for future physical health, mental health, wealth, and public safety [2]. Therefore, identifying related factors in the development of cognitive function in childhood has drawn researchers' attention due to its substantial benefits extending into adulthood.

Physical activity (PA), a component of lifestyle, is considered to be a potentially important factor in altering our brain health and mental function [3]. In recent years, many studies have examined the effects of PA on cognitive function. There is an increasing body of evidence suggesting that in children and adolescents, PA, particularly moderate to vigorous physical activity (MVPA), is closely associated with cognitive functions [4,5]. Furthermore, a systematic review concluded that there is a positive association between PA and cognitive function in children [6]. Animal evidence suggests that aerobic exercise can enhance human brain structure, prevent age-related brain tissue loss, and improve cognitive performance [7], so increased PA can enhance brain function. Previous human studies also indicated that PA in schools may enhance academic attainment, and higher levels of physical fitness in children may be associated with improved neurocognitive processing [8]. Increased physical activity may therefore provide cognitive and educational benefits across childhood and adolescence. So, moderate and vigorous PA was recommended for children and adolescents, and the importance of establishing healthy and appropriate behaviors in children is crucial for long-term effects. However, different types, amounts, and frequencies of PA were adopted in these studies. Moreover, in preschool stage, a key period for personality development, to the best of our knowledge, studies assessing the association between PA and cognitive functions is limited. Furthermore, previous trials were individually underpowered or primarily of weak quality to address this issue, and the few observational studies addressing it have mixed results [9].

Therefore, in the current study, the aim is to examine the PA conditions in preschool children and the association between the technology-assessed PA and cognitive functions, while adjusting for confounding factors that associated with cognitive function on the basis of previous studies, such as children's cardiorespiratory fitness, daily behavior, and mother's education [6,10,11].

2. Methods

2.1. Participants

This cross-sectional study is a baseline data analysis from The Physical Activity and Cognitive Function Study (Trial Registration: ChiCTR-OOC-15007439) [12]. A total of 346 (boys, 201; girls, 145) preschool children were recruited from seven urban kindergartens in Shanghai, China. All the parents/guardians of potential participants have been fully informed of the protocol and aims of the study by parents' meeting held in the kindergarten. Signed informed consent forms were obtained from parents/guardians of the participants before this study began. The protocol was also approved by The Ethics Advisory Committee of Shanghai University of Sport.

2.2. Measures and Procedures

Participants' cognitive functions were evaluated using a short form of the Chinese version of Wechsler Young Children Scale of Intelligence (C-WYCSI) [13], due to constraints in assessment time. The short form consisted of four subtests, taking approximately 30 min to complete, and was also widely adopted in previous studies investigating cognitive function [14,15]. Furthermore, the short form of C-WYCSI was validated and the association of its scores and estimated Full Intelligence Quotient (FIQ) was also confirmed in our pilot study for preschool children ($n = 31$, $r = 0.90$, $p < 0.01$). The short-form items consisted of two tests: the Verbal Intelligence Quotient (VIQ: Information and Vocabulary) test and the Performance Intelligence Quotient (PIQ: Picture Completion and Block Design) test. The Information subtest involved asking participants to answer questions about everyday knowledge; participants received a 1 or 0 score for each correct or incorrect answer (total, 0–23 scores). For the Vocabulary subtest, children were asked to identify the true answer from four pictures corresponding to the word instructed by the tester; children scored 1 or 0 for each correct or incorrect response (total, 0–44 scores). The Picture Completion subtest required children to identify and point out the missing part of the picture; children received a 1 or 0 score for each correct or incorrect answer (total, 0–25 scores). Finally, the Block Design subtest included a design either from the tester or the test booklet; children scored from 0 to 4 depending on how quickly they completed each design (total, 0–29 scores). After assessment, raw scores were converted to standard scores based on the instruction manual. Standardized scores of VIQ and PIQ were equal to the sum of two Verbal and Performance subtest scores, respectively. FIQ was estimated using weighted scores of each subtest according to the instruction manual (normal mean = 100, SD = 15.0). Children were divided into five groups based on their FIQ scores: significantly below normal, slightly below normal, normal, slightly above normal, and significantly above normal were defined as <70, 70–<90, 90–110, >110–130, and >130 scores, respectively.

Physical activity was measured over 7 consecutive days during waking hours with ActiGraph accelerometers (GT3X+, ActiGraph, Pensacola, FL, USA) on the right hip. The activity was captured by a 1 s sampling interval and categorized as either light or moderate to vigorous PA (LPA, MVPA) based on cutoff counts developed by Pate and colleagues for preschool children [16]. LPA corresponded with 101–1679 counts per minute (CPMs) and MVPA was equal or greater than 1680 CPMs. Individual data were validated into analyses when participating in at least 3 days (including 1 weekend day) of monitored PA, with a minimum of 8 h each day [17].

Children characteristics included sex, ages (months), heights, body weights, mother's education, family structures, and household income. Body mass index (BMI) was calculated using the formula weight/height^2 (kg/m^2) and BMI status was classified as normal, overweight, and obese using the cut points developed by International Obesity Task Force (IOTF) [18]. Mother's education was considered as a critical influence on children's cognitive function [11], and the education level was divided into six groups: less than high school, high school, some college/associate's degree, bachelor degree, master's degree, and doctor degree. "Living with both parents" and "living only with mother or father, or other situation" was used to evaluate family support. Household income was divided into six groups according to median household incomes in China: None, <4000 RMB/month, 4000–8000 RMB/month, 8001–15,000 RMB/month, 15,001–30,000 RMB/month, and >30,000 RMB/month (1 RMB ≈ 0.16 US dollars).

Children's daily behavior was an important indicator of physical activity [19] and was associated with cognitive functions [10]. Therefore, it was included as a covariate in the regression models. In this study, the past 2 months of children's daily behavior were measured using four items from the Chinese Child Behavior Checklist for Preschool Children. The items, completed by their teacher, were as follows: (1) whether the child shows lack of concentration or non-persistent attention; (2) whether the child is introverted and unwilling to talk; (3) whether the child is over-fatigued; and (4) whether the child has slow actions or anenergia. Items were rated by a 3-point scale (0 = not true, 1 = sometimes true, or 2 = often true). Finally, children's behavior scores were divided into three groups based on the total scores: low (4–6 scores), median (7–9 scores), and high (10–12 scores).

Cardiorespiratory fitness was assessed by the multistage 20 m shuttle run test, which measured cardiorespiratory fitness by running back and forth for 20 m with a starting speed of 8.5 km/h and increasing by 0.5 km/h with each level thereafter (1 min). Maximal performance was determined when the participant failed to follow the pace for two consecutive attempts or stopped due to exhaustion. Results were expressed as laps; one lap corresponded to 20 m. The multistage 20 m shuttle run test is widely used for assessing cardiorespiratory fitness in preschool children and has shown to have a high reliability [20]. Due to the young age of participants, each child had an adult running with them during the process to make sure the test was successfully completed.

2.3. Statistical Analyses

Analyses were performed using SPSS version 22.0 (SPSS Inc., Chicago, IL, USA). The normal distribution test was conducted using Kolmogorov–Smirnov test, and variables were described as mean ± SD for the normally distributed variables or median (interquartile ratio, IQR) for non-normally distributed variables. Independent *t* tests, Mann–Whitney *U* tests, or chi-square tests were used to assess sex differences for normally distributed, non-normally distributed, or categorical variables, respectively.

Linear regression analyses were used to explore the association between different intensities of PA and cognitive functions. Variables were transformed to normal distribution using the log or square root method before linear regression, if necessary. To understand total variance explained by different factors, cognitive function regressed in three models: Model 1 LPA and MVPA entered the model and was unadjusted for confounding factors; Model 2 was adjusted for sociodemographic and children's daily behavior (including age, BMI status, mother's education, family structure, household income, and child behavior scores); Model 3 was further adjusted for cardiorespiratory fitness. Because PA and physical fitness have been suggested to be strongly linked with sex, our linear regression analyses were stratified for sex. Furthermore, to test the robustness and avoid high correlation between LPA and MVPA causing confusion of our results, LPA, MVPA, and total time engaged in physical activity (TPA, equal to sum of LPA and MVPA) were separately entered into the regression model again following the three steps described above. A two-sided p value ≤ 0.05 was considered as statistically significant.

3. Results

A total of 325 of 346 participants completed the C-WYCSI test. Among them, 11 preschool children were excluded from analyses because of noncooperation during the test ($n = 6$) or intellectual disability ($n = 5$, FIQ: 54.2–73.8). Characteristics of 260 participants (144 boys; 116 girls) who have complete data of cognitive functions, PA, and confounding factors are shown in Table 1. On average, the age of participants was 57.2 months (55.4% boys), the majority (79.2%) of preschool children were considered as healthy weight according to IOTF, and the percentage of overweight/obesity, LPA, and MVPA in boys were significantly higher than girls. However, the correlation between physical activity and cognitive functions were not significant in girls ($p > 0.05$).

Table 1. Characteristics of the analyzed sample.

	Total ($n = 260$)	Boys ($n = 144$)	Girls ($n = 116$)	p for Sex
Age (month)	57.2 ± 5.4	57.6 ± 5.4	56.7 ± 5.3	0.200
BMI (kg/m^2)	16.2 ± 1.9	16.5 ± 1.9	15.9 ± 1.8	**0.001**
Normal	206	106	100	**0.013**
Overweight/Obesity	54	38	16	
Mother's education				0.236
Less than high school	10	3	7	
High school	44	28	16	
College/associate degree	82	42	40	
Bachelor's degree	94	57	37	
Master's degree	19	8	11	
Doctor degree	11	6	5	
Family structure				0.502
Living with both parents	251	140	111	
Others	9	4	5	
Household income (RMB/month)				0.866
<4000	5	3	2	
4000–8000	42	22	20	
8001–15,000	115	65	50	
15,001–30,000	80	46	34	
>30,000	18	8	10	
Child behavior scores (count)				<0.001
Low (4–6 scores)	165	77	88	
Median (7–9 scores)	88	60	28	
High (10–12 scores)	7	7	0	
Cardiorespiratory Fitness (lap)	11.0 (10–14)	11 (9.25–14.0)	12 (10.0–14.75)	0.328

Table 1. *Cont.*

	Total (*n* = 260)	Boys (*n* = 144)	Girls (*n* = 116)	*p* for Sex
Physical activity (min/day)				
LPA	98.4 ± 17.1	100.6 ± 17.9	95.6 ± 15.7	**0.021**
MVPA	71.8 ± 17.3	74.1 ± 18.7	69.0 ± 15.0	**0.021**
Cognitive function				
VIQ	23 (19.0–26.0)	22 (19.0–26.0)	23 (19.0–26.0)	0.558
FIQ	25 (22.0–27.0)	25 (21.0–27.0)	25 (23.0–27.75)	0.255
FIQ	110.5 ± 12.4	110.0 ± 13.0	111.3 ± 11.6	0.370

Note: BMI, body mass index; LPA, light physical activity; MVPA, moderate to vigorous physical activity; VIQ, Verbal Intelligence Quotient; PIQ, Performance Intelligence Quotient; FIQ, Full Intelligence Quotient. The mean ± SD or median (interquartile ratio, IQR) was reported for normal or non-normal distribution variables.

The results showed that LPA, but not MVPA, is significantly correlated with VIQ, PIQ, and FIQ, even when adjusting for several potential confounding factors in the final model in boys. Corresponding standardized coefficients were 0.211, 0.218, and 0.242 (all *p* < 0.05), respectively (Table 2). However, the association between LPA and different categories of IQ were not found in girls in this study. Furthermore, the results were similar with those described above when LPA and MVPA were separately entered into the model; only LPA positively correlated with FIQ, solely in boys (β = 0.208, *p* < 0.05). In addition, when TPA replaced LPA and MVPA into the model, the results also suggested TPA positively associated with VIQ, and FIQ, solely in boys (β = 0.236 and 0.179, all *p* < 0.05).

Table 2. Linear regression analyses between cognitive function and physical activity.

Predictor Variables	VIQ		PIQ		FIQ	
	β	95% CI	β	95% CI	β	95% CI
Boys						
Model 1 *						
LPA	0.203	−0.009, 0.407	0.191	−0.031, 0.416	**0.224**	**0.008, 0.441**
MVPA	0.162	−0.048, 0.356	−0.001	−0.218, 0.217	0.082	−0.130, 0.290
R^2		0.099		0.022		0.069
Model 2 †						
LPA	**0.197**	**0.009, 0.377**	0.188	−0.019, 0.398	**0.218**	**0.029, 0.408**
MVPA	0.064	−0.120, 0.242	−0.076	−0.280, 0.131	−0.016	−0.202, 0.171
R^2		0.300		0.152		0.291
Model 3 ‡						
LPA	**0.211**	**0.018, 0.395**	**0.218**	**0.007, 0.433**	**0.242**	**0.048, 0.435**
MVPA	0.043	−0.150, 0.232	−0.122	−0.335, 0.096	−0.051	−0.245, 0.146
R^2		0.297		0.157		0.293
Girls						
Model 1 *						
LPA	0.028	0.271, 0.212	0.064	−0.161, 0.289	0.007	−0.225, 0.240
MVPA	−0.009	−0.265, 0.245	0.108	−0.124, 0.353	0.037	−0.206, 0.286
R^2		−0.017		0.006		−0.016
Model 2 †						
LPA	−0.073	−0.311, 0.156	0.025	−0.205, 0.255	−0.038	−0.268, 0.191
MVPA	−0.025	−0.276, 0.220	0.103	−0.134, 0.353	0.029	−0.212, 0.274
R^2		0.090		0.011		0.060
Model 3 ‡						
LPA	−0.023	−0.252, 0.203	0.027	−0.206, 0.261	−0.003	−0.232, 0.226
MVPA	−0.143	−0.414, 0.092	0.097	−0.157, 0.363	−0.053	−0.312, 0.196
R^2		0.157		0.002		0.087

Note: β, standardized coefficients; R^2, adjusted R square; LPA, light physical activity; MVPA, moderate to vigorous physical activity; VIQ, Verbal Intelligence Quotient; PIQ, Performance Intelligence Quotient; FIQ, Full Intelligence Quotient; the *p* values less than 0.05 are bolded; * Model 1: unadjusted; † Model 2: adjusted for age, BMI status, mother's education, family structure, household income, and child behavior scores; ‡ Model 3: further adjusted for cardiorespiratory fitness, which was log-transformed before being entered into the model.

4. Discussion

In this cross-sectional study, the major finding was that LPA was significantly and positively associated with intelligence quotient in boys, but not in girls. Based on the evidence available, the most recent systematic review concluded that there is a positive association between PA and cognitive function in children, although more studies are needed to identify the effects of different types, amounts, and frequencies of PA on cognitive function [6]. Moreover, in general, MVPA was recommended for children and adolescents because of the "intensity threshold" of PA benefit [21]. However, findings from this study are not in agreement with the results of previous studies, which found only LPA was evidently correlated with cognitive function, as measured by standardized IQ testing, in preschool children. A potential reason has been suggested to explain why different intensities of PA may play a different role among different age groups. One of the hypotheses of PA's effect on cognitive function was mediated by cardiorespiratory fitness [22], which increased responding to LPA in preschool children but may need higher intensity stimulation in children and adolescents. Nevertheless, it is not suggested that we can ignore the importance of MVPA, although only LPA is shown to be correlated with cognition in this study. Further, total minutes of PA (TPA, sum of LPA and MVPA) also presented a notable association with VIQ and FIQ when TPA took the place of LPA and MVPA in the model. Moreover, the current guidelines of PA recommend accumulating at least 180 min of PA daily at any intensity, and especially highlight the importance of TPA for preschool children [23]. Engaging in both LPA and MVPA lead to increases in the amount of TPA and, therefore, neither of them can be ignored.

The positive association between PA and cognitive functions solely found in boys in this study is also contrary to a recent review article, which showed the sex-dependent effect was more significant in girls [1]. A possible explanation for the findings was the lower level of cardiorespiratory fitness in girls at baseline which could result in more apparent physiological effect in the analysis [24]. Considering the possible influencing factors in this study, there were several explanations for our current results. First, boys engaged in more PA than girls, possibly having a dose–response effect, allowing boys to accrue greater cognitive function benefits. Especially, accumulating evidence from animal to human studies demonstrated that engaging in more physical activity can increase expression and concentration of brain-derived neurotrophic factor in hippocampus [25], which has been to play a crucial role in brain plasticity and functions [26]. Second, contrary to adolescents, preschool children, especially boys, were found to have lower levels of cardiorespiratory fitness in this study. This may have been a physiological effect derived from boys' PA stimulation. Furthermore, hypothalamic–pituitary–adrenal (HPA) axis response to PA is sex-dependent, possibly causing the sex-dependent effect [27]. For example, higher activation of HPA axis to PA in boys initiates a number of physiological changes, such as stimulating protein synthesis, which serves as the basis for a number of hormones, including adrenocorticotropic hormone (ACTH) and bendorphin that improve cognition, behavior response, and homeostatic challenges [28]. Additionally, sex difference is also a result of genetic variation, parental and familial factors, and one's acquired behaviors and perceptions, with the latter often shaped by unique experiences at the individual, parental, and familial levels [29].

Our study has several strengths. First, PA was measured using an accelerometer, which avoided the recall bias of proxy report by parents or teachers. Second, several potential confounding factors were adjusted in the statistical analyses. Third, our results were strengthened by combining and separating LPA and MVPA into linear regression models. However, our study also has several limitations. First, for feasibility, we used a convenience sample in this observational study. Second, our cross-sectional study design has limited ability to draw a causal relation of our findings. We cannot illustrate whether PA improves cognitive functions in boys or whether preschool aged boys with high levels of cognitive function simply tend to participant in more PA. Last, the accelerometer was worn over the hip, which limited the ability to capture activities with little displacement of the body, such as cycling. However, the hip was probably the best placement to capture whole-body movements and was also the site most often used by various studies [30].

J. Clin. Med. **2018**, *7*, 108

5. Conclusions

In conclusion, our findings suggest PA has a significant and positive association with cognitive functions in boys, especially LPA. On the basis of this study, we indicated the benefit of cognitive function derived from LPA and recommend sex-dependent responses should be considered in future studies. Moreover, more prospective and intervention studies are needed to clarify the causal relation and mechanisms of our observed sex-specific effect.

Author Contributions: M.Q. conceived and designed the study, analyzed the data and drafted the manuscript. H.Z., J.Z., T.Z., J.Z., G.Z., H.F. and S.S. conducted the experiments and collected the data. M.Q. and G.Z. performed the literature search. R.W. and P.C. advised on analysis and interpretation of the data, and critically revised the manuscript.

Acknowledgments: This work was supported by the Science and Technology Commission of Shanghai Municipality, China (12XD1404500); the National Natural Science Foundation of China (81703252); the Humanity and Social Science Youth foundation of Ministry of Education of China (15YJC890029); and a grant from the Shanghai Municipal Education Committee (HJTY-2014-A10).

Conflicts of Interest: The authors declare no conflicts of interest.

References

1. Esteban-Cornejo, I.; Tejero-Gonzalez, C.M.; Sallis, J.F.; Veiga, O.L. Physical activity and cognition in adolescents: A systematic review. *J. Sci. Med. Sport* **2015**, *18*, 534–539. [CrossRef] [PubMed]
2. Moffitt, T.E.; Arseneault, L.; Belsky, D.; Dickson, N.; Hancox, R.J.; Harrington, H.L.; Houts, R.; Poulton, R.; Roberts, B.W.; Ross, S. A gradient of childhood self-control predicts health, wealth, and public safety. *Proc. Natl. Acad. Sci. USA* **2011**, *108*, 2693–2698. [CrossRef] [PubMed]
3. Carvalho, A.; Rea, I.M.; Parimon, T.; Cusack, B.J. Physical activity and cognitive function in individuals over 60 years of age: A systematic review. *Clin. Interv. Aging* **2014**, *9*, 661–682. [PubMed]
4. Moreau, D.; Kirk, I.J.; Waldie, K.E. High-intensity training enhances executive function in children in a randomized, placebo-controlled trial. *eLife* **2017**, *6*, e25062. [CrossRef] [PubMed]
5. Benzing, V.; Heinks, T.; Eggenberger, N.; Schmidt, M. Acute cognitively engaging exergame-based physical activity enhances executive functions in adolescents. *PLoS ONE* **2016**, *11*, e0167501. [CrossRef] [PubMed]
6. Donnelly, J.E.; Hillman, C.H.; Castelli, D.; Etnier, J.L.; Lee, S.; Tomporowski, P.; Lambourne, K.; Szabo-Reed, A.N. This summary was written for the American College of Sports Medicine, b. Physical activity, fitness, cognitive function, and academic achievement in children: A systematic review. *Med. Sci. Sports Exerc.* **2016**, *48*, 1223–1224. [CrossRef] [PubMed]
7. Dishman, R.K.; Berthoud, H.R.; Booth, F.W.; Cotman, C.W.; Edgerton, V.R.; Fleshner, M.R.; Gandevia, S.C.; Gomez-Pinilla, F.; Greenwood, B.N.; Hillman, C.H. Neurobiology of exercise. *Obesity* **2006**, *14*, 345–356. [CrossRef] [PubMed]
8. Davis, C.L.; Tomporowski, P.D.; Mcdowell, J.E.; Austin, B.P.; Miller, P.H.; Yanasak, N.E.; Allison, J.D.; Naglieri, J.A. Exercise improves executive function and achievement and alters brain activation in overweight children: A randomized controlled trial. *Health Psychol. Off. J. Div. Health Psychol. Am. Psychol. Assoc.* **2011**, *30*, 91–98. [CrossRef] [PubMed]
9. Carson, V.; Hunter, S.; Kuzik, N.; Wiebe, S.A.; Spence, J.C.; Friedman, A.; Tremblay, M.S.; Slater, L.; Hinkley, T. Systematic review of physical activity and cognitive development in early childhood. *J. Sci. Med. Sport* **2016**, *19*, 573–578. [CrossRef] [PubMed]
10. Liu, J.; Zhou, G.; Wang, Y.; Ai, Y.; Pinto-Martin, J.; Liu, X. Sleep problems, fatigue, and cognitive performance in chinese kindergarten children. *J. Pediatr.* **2012**, *161*, 520–525.e2. [CrossRef] [PubMed]
11. Santos, D.N.; Assis, A.M.; Bastos, A.C.; Santos, L.M.; Santos, C.A.; Strina, A.; Prado, M.S.; Almeida-Filho, N.M.; Rodrigues, L.C.; Barreto, M.L. Determinants of cognitive function in childhood: A cohort study in a middle income context. *BMC Public Health* **2008**, *8*, 202. [CrossRef] [PubMed]
12. Zhao, G.; Quan, M.; Su, L.; Zhang, H.; Zhang, J.; Zhang, J.; Fang, H.; Cao, Z.; Zhu, Z.; Niu, Z. Effect of physical activity on cognitive development: Protocol for a 15-year longitudinal follow-up study. *Biomed. Res. Int.* **2017**, *2017*, 8568459. [CrossRef] [PubMed]

13. Gong, Y.-X.; Dai, X.-Y. China-wechsler younger children scale of intelligence (c-wycsi). *Psychol. Sci.* **1986**, *2*, 23–30.

14. Kramer, M.S.; Aboud, F.; Mironova, E.; Vanilovich, I.; Platt, R.W.; Matush, L.; Igumnov, S.; Fombonne, E.; Bogdanovich, N.; Ducruet, T.; et al. Breastfeeding and child cognitive development: New evidence from a large randomized trial. *Arch. Gen. Psychiatry* **2008**, *65*, 578–584. [CrossRef] [PubMed]

15. Li, X.; Atkins, M.S. Early childhood computer experience and cognitive and motor development. *Pediatrics* **2004**, *113*, 1715–1722. [CrossRef] [PubMed]

16. Pate, R.R.; Almeida, M.J.; McIver, K.L.; Pfeiffer, K.A.; Dowda, M. Validation and calibration of an accelerometer in preschool children. *Obesity* **2006**, *14*, 2000–2006. [CrossRef] [PubMed]

17. Cain, K.L.; Sallis, J.F.; Conway, T.L.; Van Dyck, D.; Calhoon, L. Using accelerometers in youth physical activity studies: A review of methods. *J. Phys. Act. Health* **2013**, *10*, 437–450. [CrossRef] [PubMed]

18. Cole, T.J.; Bellizzi, M.C.; Flegal, K.M.; Dietz, W.H. Establishing a standard definition for child overweight and obesity worldwide: International survey. *BMJ* **2000**, *320*, 1240–1243. [CrossRef] [PubMed]

19. Ek, A.; Sorjonen, K.; Nyman, J.; Marcus, C.; Nowicka, P. Child behaviors associated with childhood obesity and parents' self-efficacy to handle them: Confirmatory factor analysis of the lifestyle behavior checklist. *Int. J. Behav. Nutr. Phys. Act.* **2015**, *12*, 36. [CrossRef] [PubMed]

20. Ortega, F.B.; Cadenas-Sánchez, C.; Sánchez-Delgado, G.; Mora-González, J.; Martínez-Téllez, B.; Artero, E.G.; Castro-Piñero, J.; Labayen, I.; Chillón, P.; Löf, M. Systematic review and proposal of a field-based physical fitness-test battery in preschool children: The prefit battery. *Sports Med.* **2015**, *45*, 533–555. [CrossRef] [PubMed]

21. Kwak, L.; Kremers, S.P.; Bergman, P.; Ruiz, J.R.; Rizzo, N.S.; Sjöström, M. Associations between physical activity, fitness, and academic achievement. *J. Pediatr.* **2009**, *155*, 914–918.e1. [CrossRef] [PubMed]

22. Suwabe, K.; Hyodo, K.; Byun, K.; Ochi, G.; Fukuie, T.; Shimizu, T.; Kato, M.; Yassa, M.A.; Soya, H. Aerobic fitness associates with mnemonic discrimination as a mediator of physical activity effects: Evidence for memory flexibility in young adults. *Sci. Rep.* **2017**, *7*, 5140. [CrossRef] [PubMed]

23. Tremblay, M.S.; Chaput, J.P.; Adamo, K.B.; Aubert, S.; Barnes, J.D.; Choquette, L.; Duggan, M.; Faulkner, G.; Goldfield, G.S.; Gray, C.E. Canadian 24-h movement guidelines for the early years (0–4 years): An integration of physical activity, sedentary behaviour, and sleep. *BMC Public Health* **2017**, *17*, 874. [CrossRef] [PubMed]

24. Carlson, S.A.; Fulton, J.E.; Lee, S.M.; Maynard, L.M.; Brown, D.R.; Kohl, H.W., 3rd.; Dietz, W.H. Physical education and academic achievement in elementary school: Data from the early childhood longitudinal study. *Am. J. Public Health* **2008**, *98*, 721–727. [CrossRef] [PubMed]

25. Zoladz, J.A.; Pilc, A. The effect of physical activity on the brain derived neurotrophic factor: From animal to human studies. *J. Physiol. Pharmacol.* **2010**, *61*, 533–541. [PubMed]

26. Park, H.; Poo, M.M. Neurotrophin regulation of neural circuit development and function. *Nat. Rev. Neurosci.* **2013**, *14*, 7–23. [CrossRef] [PubMed]

27. Baker, L.D.; Frank, L.L.; Foster-Schubert, K.; Green, P.S.; Wilkinson, C.W.; McTiernan, A.; Plymate, S.R.; Fishel, M.A.; Watson, G.S.; Cholerton, B.A. Effects of aerobic exercise on mild cognitive impairment: A controlled trial. *Arch. Neurol.* **2010**, *67*, 71–79. [CrossRef] [PubMed]

28. Lee, R.S.; Sawa, A. Environmental stressors and epigenetic control of the hypothalamic-pituitary-adrenal axis. *Neuroendocrinology* **2014**, *100*, 278–287. [CrossRef] [PubMed]

29. Ogilvie, K.M.; Rivier, C. Gender difference in hypothalamic-pituitary-adrenal axis response to alcohol in the rat: Activational role of gonadal steroids. *Brain Res.* **1997**, *766*, 19–28. [CrossRef]

30. Cliff, D.P.; Reilly, J.J.; Okely, A.D. Methodological considerations in using accelerometers to assess habitual physical activity in children aged 0–5 years. *J. Sci. Med. Sport* **2009**, *12*, 557–567. [CrossRef] [PubMed]

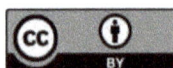

Journal of
Clinical Medicine

MDPI

Article

Reliability of Using Motion Sensors to Measure Children's Physical Activity Levels in Exergaming

Nan Zeng [1], Xingyuan Gao [2], Yuanlong Liu [3], Jung Eun Lee [4] and Zan Gao [1,*]

1   School of Kinesiology, University of Minnesota Twin Cities, Minneapolis, MN 55455, USA;
     zengx185@umn.edu
2   Department of Education, East China Normal University, Shanghai 200062, China; xygao@dedu.ecnu.edu.cn
3   Department of Health, Physical Education and Recreation, Western Michigan University,
     Kalamazoo, MI 49008, USA; yuanlong.liu@wmich.edu
4   Department of Applied Human Sciences, University of Minnesota Duluth, Duluth, MN 55812, USA;
     junelee@d.umn.edu
*   Correspondence: gaoz@umn.edu; Tel.: +1-612-626-4639

Received: 2 April 2018; Accepted: 30 April 2018; Published: 2 May 2018

Abstract: Objectives: This study examined the reliability of two objective measurement tools in assessing children's physical activity (PA) levels in an exergaming setting. Methods: A total of 377 children (190 girls, M_{age} = 8.39, SD = 1.55) attended the 30-min exergaming class every other day for 18 weeks. Children's PA levels were concurrently measured by NL-1000 pedometer and ActiGraph GT3X accelerometer, while children's steps per min and time engaged in sedentary, light, and moderate-to-vigorous PA were estimated, respectively. Results: The results of intraclass correlation coefficient (ICC) indicated a low degree of reliability (single measures ICC = 0.03) in accelerometers. ANOVA did detect a possible learning effect for 27 classes ($p < 0.01$), and the single measures ICC was 0.20 for pedometers. Moreover, there was no significant positive relationship between steps per min and time spent in moderate-to-vigorous physical activity (MVPA). Finally, only 1.3% variance was explained by pedometer as a predictor using Hierarchical Linear Modeling to further explore the relationship between pedometer and accelerometer data. Conclusions: The NL-1000 pedometers and ActiGraph GT3X accelerometers have low reliability in assessing elementary school children's PA levels during exergaming. More research is warranted in determining the reliable and accurate measurement information regarding the use of modern devices in exergaming setting.

Keywords: pedometers; accelerometers; measurement; physical activity levels; active video games

---

1. Introduction

Prevalence of insufficient physical activity (PA) among children and adolescents serves as a major contributor to non-communicable diseases such as obesity, depression, Type II diabetes, and cardiovascular diseases [1]. As such, a call has been made to gather effective methods of promoting more PA among children in the hopes of maintaining PA participation into adolescence and adulthood. One such method to promote PA levels among children is exergaming (also known as active video games). Exergaming is an emerging technology that requires the players to be physically active while providing performers with the opportunity for health enhancement, thereby thwarting the perception of videogame playing is always sedentary [2]. Compared with traditional PA, exergaming is often perceived as motivating and fun among children because it makes an attractive option in the quest to promote an active and healthy lifestyle within the school settings [3]. Previous studies have found exergaming is a feasible means for children to engage in higher amounts of PA [4,5], and thus exergaming has been integrated into school-based programs to promote children's PA [6–10].

J. Clin. Med. **2018**, *7*, 100

In addition, exergaming has been utilized for clinical purposes such as pediatric weight management, and improvement on executive functions of children with autism spectrum disorder and with attention deficit hyperactivity disorder (ADHD) [11–14]. Evidence has shown that exergaming has the potential to serve as an important addition to therapies for children with such conditions. As exergaming is becoming more popular in pediatric clinical setting, valid methods of assessing PA levels in children are critical to understanding the relationship between PA intervention and health promotion.

Nowadays, numerous techniques exist for measuring PA. These techniques can be grouped as observation, self-reported instruments, and motion sensors. Although direct observation is considered a gold standard in measuring PA [15], this may not be feasible in many situations because of expectancy bias, observation effect, and even privacy issues on participants [16]. In addition, self-reported instruments such as questionnaire is recommended not to be used in children below the age of 10 or 11 years, because these children do not have the required cognitive skills which may lead them to over-report their PA levels [17]. Consequently, objective assessment tools such as motion sensors are increasingly being used to assess PA levels in children.

More recently, pedometers and accelerometers have been widely used in assessing children's PA levels in exergaming settings. For instance, Gao and colleagues [8] used NL-1000 pedometers to monitor children's step counts and moderate-to-vigorous PA (MVPA) in Dance Dance Revolution (DDR). In addition, a number of studies measured children's energy expenditure (EE) and time spent in sedentary, light PA, and MVPA utilizing Actigraph GT1M and ActiGraph GT3X accelerometers during exergaming [2,18,19]. These devices are more advantageous because they are not dependent upon individual's memory, whereas self-reported instruments rely heavily on personal memory to judge the intensity, duration, and frequency of PA. More specifically, pedometers and accelerometers are capable of providing explicit information on the total accumulated quantity of EE and pattern of PA performed throughout the course of the day. As a result, pedometers and accelerometers are perceived more accurate and less subjective as compared to traditional self-reported instruments such as questionnaires and PA logs [20].

In fact, motion sensors have been proven to be reliable in some PA settings. For example, Steeves and colleagues [21] indicated that Omron HJ-303 Pedometer was trustworthy during treadmill running and walking, while the evidence of reliability on GT3X accelerometer was found in assessing activities of daily living [22]. Although many studies have attempted to assess children's PA levels utilizing pedometers and accelerometers, comparatively little attention is paid to the reliability of using such motion sensors in exergaming settings. To the best of our knowledge, there has been no work on proving reliability of using these motion sensors to measure children's PA levels during exergaming. Without the evidence of fidelity on these measures, it is difficult to draw conclusions regarding the effectiveness of exergames-based PA interventions. We believe objectively and accurately quantifying the amount of PA in exergaming is important because it will help us better understand the effectiveness of exergames on children's behavior and health outcomes. Therefore, the purpose of this study was to examine the reliability of using two popular PA monitors (NL-1000 pedometer and ActiGraph GT3X accelerometer) in assessing healthy elementary school children's PA levels during exergaming.

2. Materials and Methods

2.1. Participants and Research Setting

A total of 377 (190 girls, 187 boys) first through fourth grade children (aged 6–11 years, $M_{age} = 8.39$, $SD = 1.55$) enrolled in a suburban Title I elementary school in West region of the United States. Participants attended two structured PA programs for 150 min every week (30 min × 5 school days). The two PA programs consisted of three 30-min physical education (PE) and two 30-min exergaming classes in the first week (i.e., children went to PE classes on Monday, Wednesday, Friday, and attended exergaming classes on Tuesday and Thursday). In the second week, students played 30-min exergames on Monday, Wednesday, and Friday, and participated in 30-min PE classes on Tuesday and Thursday.

The third and fourth week repeated the process of the first two weeks. That is, students were offered equal numbers of PE and exergaming classes every month. This PA pattern was employed throughout the duration of the 18 weeks at school. Children from 20 classes attended the programs with class as the unit. The class size ranged from 17 to 22. The specific inclusion criteria for this study were (1) children were first through fourth grade and aged 6–11 years, (2) without a diagnosed physical or mental disability according to school records, and (3) with parental consent and child assent. Participants in this population were selected because this age range is a critical period for children to develop and maintain a physically active lifestyle.

In this study, children's PA behaviors only during exergaming were included to determine the reliability of motion sensors in assessing PA. Twelve exergaming stations were set up in a classroom, each station was equipped with eight different Wii exergames including, but not limited to: Wii Fit, Wii Cardio Workout, Just Dance, and Wii Sports. The children were instructed to learn how to play these games prior to the testing (e.g., imitate the movement projected by on-screen avatars). The selected exergames are school-age appropriate that require a variety of body movements such as jumping, kicking, punching, and ducking. A trained teacher supervised the children during exergaming. Each station accommodated up to two children to play, and children rotated from one station to another station and every 8–10 min allowing for a short duration transition. As such, all children in one class had the opportunity to play exergaming simultaneously, and were also able to play different exergames during the program. Prior to initiating data collection, The University Institutional Review Board approved the study protocol and informed consent forms were obtained from guardians and children.

2.2. Instruments

The NL-1000 pedometer. The NL-1000 (New Lifestyles Inc., Lee's Summit, MO, USA) is an advanced waist-worn pedometer that uses a piezoelectric sensor to quantify daily step counts, track the intensity of each step and displaying intensity as MVPA time accumulation [19]. The data of steps and MVPA time can be read directly from the screen, meaning that no downloading or cleaning of data is required. The NL-1000 has been shown to accurately detect steps taken in both laboratory and free-living settings for children [23,24]. In this study, the pedometer data were captured during monitoring period, and steps per min (step counts/30 min) were calculated as the outcome variable.

ActiGraph GT3X accelerometer. The ActiGraph GT3X (ActiGraph Co., Pensacola, FL, USA) is a compact (3.8 × 3.7 × 1.8 cm), lightweight (27 g) and rechargeable accelerometer, which uses a solid-state tri-axial accelerometer to collect motion data on three axes for the highest levels of analytic capabilities available [25]. The ActiGraph GT3X measures and records time-varying accelerations ranging in magnitude from 0.05 to 2.5 G's. The output is digitized by a 12-bit analog to digital convertor (ADC) at a rate of 30 Hz [25]. The signal passes through a digital filter that band-limits the accelerometer to the frequency range of 0.25–2.5 Hz once digitized [21]. Most recently, researchers have demonstrated acceptable validity and reliability of ActiGraph GT3X when using with children in school and free-living conditions [26,27]. Given a short-duration PA (30 min) of each class and the aims of this study, activity count was set at 1 s epoch length. That is, in-class PA levels were quantified as average activity counts per second (30 Hertz) for the intensities of the activities. PA levels were classified into sedentary, light, moderate, and vigorous categories according to the cut-points set by Evenson and colleagues [28]. The following cut points were applied to define different PA levels (sedentary: 0 to 100; light PA: 101 to 2295, and MVPA: 2296 and above). In the present study, children's time spent in sedentary, light PA, and MVPA were used as the outcome variables to classify PA intensities.

2.3. Procedures

Graduate research assistants were recruited from the University and were trained to assist the program supervisor of the study. Prior to data collection, the research assistants explained the purpose of the study to the participants, including activity sequence and instruction on how to appropriately wear motion sensors. At the start of practice, all children were assigned an identification number that matched up with the number on their pedometers and accelerometers. Each child then was asked to equip a pedometer and an accelerometer that were tied around the waist by an elastic belt and worn on the right side of hip. Although all children in this study had previous experience wearing pedometers and accelerometers in the exergaming program, the research team still assisted the students to make sure all the motion sensors were attached correctly. As such, the reactivity effect was minimized. For each participant, the time was recorded for placement and removal of the pedometers and accelerometers by the program supervisor. The pedometers and accelerometers were collected at the end of the class. Specifically, upon completion of the exergaming session, children took off the belts and reported their step counts pedometer data to the program supervisor and research assistants. In the meantime, accelerometers were retrieved and data were downloaded into ActiLife 6.0 (Actigraph Corps., Pensacola, FL, USA) for data sorting and processing. Data from accelerometers were truncated and matched to the initial time frames when PA occurred for each participant. Finally, all the data were imported into a SPSS data file for descriptive statistical analyses.

2.4. Data Reduction and Analyses

A total of 377 participants took part in the 18-week exergaming program. Due to holidays and other cancellations of class, children actually completed 27 days exergaming session. Among these sessions, day 7, day 11, day 15, day 16, day 22, and day 23 were excluded since they had less than 300 trails. In addition, 188 trails were excluded due to default listwise deletion function of intraclass correlation coefficient (ICC). As a consequence, each participant received 21 repeated assessments. Data were analyzed as follows: First, descriptive statistics for the outcome variables (i.e., standard deviations and means of steps/min, time spent in sedentary, light PA, and MVPA) were performed to describe the data characteristics. Second, the test-retest reliability for outcome variable was estimated using ICC with 95% confidence interval. A two-way mixed effects model was chosen for type of model. Consistency type was selected for the type of index, and single measures were reported. Reliability coefficients were categorized with values less than 0.4 considered poor; 0.41 to 0.6, moderate; 0.61 to 0.8, substantial; and greater than 0.8, excellent reliability [29]. Third, Pearson correlation was computed to estimate the linear relationship between accelerometer (i.e., time engaged in MVPA) and pedometer measurements (i.e., steps per min). Finally, given the present study involved a hierarchically structured data set where the measurements were nested within individual, data were analyzed using Hierarchical Linear Modeling (HLM) [30]. HLM is a flexible approach that can be applied to evaluate inter-individual differences in intra-individual changes over time [31]. That is, HLM separates inter-individual variance from intra-individual so that each participant has his/her own curve. In addition, HLM accounts for the shared variance by multiple observations within the same participant and extends multiple regression to nested or repeated-measures data [32]. Since there were several observations of each person, waves of data were nested within a person. In this study, measurements were nested within students and students were further nested within classes, so three levels were applied to the final analysis. The Level 3 experimental unit was class; the level 2 was student; and the Level 1 was measurement with time spent in MVPA and steps per min as the outcome variables. The ICC and Pearson correlation analyses were performed via the SPSS 20.0 version, and the HLM was conducted using HLM 7.0 software (Scientific Software International Inc., Lincolnwood, IL, USA) for the statistical modeling of thee-level data structures. The alpha level for the present study was set at 0.05.

3. Results

3.1. Descriptive Analysis

Descriptive results are presented in Table 1. In general, children displayed roughly similar levels of steps per min across all testing days. Additionally, children's time spent in sedentary, Light PA and MVPA were also quite similar and relatively stable for each repeated measure. Approximately 15 to 20 min valid wearing time were captured by the accelerometers during each 30-min exergaming session. More specifically, the mean steps per min ranged from 23 to 49. Children spent around 9 to 11 min in sedentary, 3 to 6 min in light PA and only accumulated 3 to 4 min of MVPA. In particular, although the last three days had the highest scores of steps per min, students did not show a higher level of time engaged in MVPA.

Table 1. Descriptive statistics for all outcome variables.

Variable	Steps per Min		Sedentary (Min)		Light PA (Min)		MVPA (Min)	
	Mean	SD	Mean	SD	Mean	SD	Mean	SD
Day 1	23.22	15.32	9.69	3.61	3.35	1.72	2.39	2.09
Day 2	36.65	26.25	9.01	3.92	3.73	2.20	3.37	3.21
Day 3	38.40	25.21	10.39	4.3	4.26	2.45	3.31	2.90
Day 4	38.40	27.04	9.61	4.23	4.64	2.59	3.38	2.67
Day 5	42.26	25.24	8.95	3.70	4.70	2.55	3.73	2.94
Day 6	42.24	26.22	9.59	4.45	5.18	2.26	3.95	2.71
Day 7	38.64	23.13	9.61	4.53	5.23	2.36	3.70	2.67
Day 8	40.28	25.74	10.08	4.69	5.44	2.37	3.71	2.53
Day 9	37.57	24.88	9.98	4.56	5.22	2.56	3.69	2.46
Day 10	39.41	27.13	10.77	4.12	5.33	2.66	3.44	2.54
Day 11	40.85	25.28	10.56	4.46	5.46	2.45	3.25	2.49
Day 12	39.19	24.37	10.47	4.37	5.23	2.67	3.32	2.53
Day 13	38.75	23.35	10.73	4.33	5.28	2.60	3.39	2.81
Day 14	37.85	23.01	10.40	3.56	5.40	2.26	3.20	2.16
Day 15	40.29	24.17	10.89	3.95	5.46	2.50	3.19	2.41
Day 16	40.34	25.48	10.93	4.02	5.95	2.66	3.46	2.51
Day 17	36.12	20.82	11.34	4.313	5.41	2.58	3.15	2.14
Day 18	41.60	24.58	9.94	4.17	5.68	2.81	3.48	2.59
Day 19	49.06	29.94	9.64	4.42	6.10	3.04	3.87	2.78
Day 20	47.52	27.80	9.26	3.90	5.60	1.94	3.50	2.13
Day 21	47.50	30.26	9.10	3.96	5.64	2.96	3.69	2.67

SD = standard deviation; Sedentary = time spent in sedentary; Light PA = time spent in light physical activity; MVPA = time spent in moderate to vigorous physical activity.

3.2. Intraclass Correlation Coefficient and Pearson Correlation

The result of ANOVA from ICC demonstrated that there were no differences among trials for accelerometer measurements, $F (12, 185) = 0.916$, $p = 0.53$, indicating that no learning or fatigue effect was detected (Table 2). In addition, ICC for accelerometer assessments showed single measures was 0.033 with a 95% confidence interval from 0.014–0.059, which was considered a low degree of reliability. Furthermore, ANOVA analysis for pedometer assessments did detect a possible learning effect during the 21 classes, $F (26, 97) = 3.315$, $p < 0.01$, but a low degree of reliability was also found between pedometer measurements from ICC, the single measures was 0.199 with a 95% confidence interval from 0.153–0.260. The result of Pearson correlation indicated that there was no significant relationship between time spent in MVPA determined by accelerometers and steps per min determined by pedometers ($r = 0.027$, $p = 0.597$).

Table 2. Intraclass correlation coefficient (ICC) for accelerometer and pedometer assessments.

		IC	95% CI		F Test with True Value 0			
			LB	UB	Value	df1	df2	Sig.
GT3X	Single	0.033 [a]	0.014	0.059	1.450	185	2220	0.000
	Average	0.310 [c]	0.155	0.448	1.450	185	2220	0.000
NL-1000	Single	0.199 [a]	0.153	0.260	7.692	97	2522	0.000
	Average	0.870 [c]	0.830	0.904	7.692	97	2522	0.000

GT3X = ActiGraph GT3X accelerometer; NL-1000 = NL-1000 pedometer; Single = single measures; Average = average measures; IC = Intraclass correlation; 95% CI = 95% confidence interval; LB = lower bound; UB = upper bound. [a] The estimator is the same here, whether the interaction effect is present or not; [c] This estimate is computed assuming the interaction effect is absent, because it is not estimable otherwise.

3.3. Hierarchical Linear Modeling

In order to further explore the relationship between pedometer and accelerometer assessments by controlling the student background and aforementioned possible learning effect, HLM was employed. We developed the (1) null model, which did not use any predictors to gauge to what extent that a second and third level model could contribute to explain the variance of the outcome variable; (2) control model, which added background variables of students to the null model; and (3) full model, which added the major predictor to the control model. The full model is developed as following:

Level-1 Model:

$$\text{MVPAmti} = \psi 0ti + \psi 1ti*(\text{DAYmti}) + \psi 2ti*(\text{TIMEmti}) + \psi 3ti*(\text{SPMmti}) + \varepsilon mti \tag{1}$$

At level 1 (measurement level), outcome variable was the total MVPA divided by time, control variable "day" represents the "learning effect", "time" refers to "how long the measurement process took". The predictor variable, steps per min (SPM), is the pedometer steps divided by time. $\psi 0ti$ and εmti represented the initial status of student t in class i and a random effect, respectively.

Level-2 Model:

$$\psi 0ti = \pi 00i + \pi 01i*(\text{SEXti}) + \pi 02i*(\text{AGEti}) + \pi 03i*(\text{RACE1ti}) + e0ti \tag{2}$$

Level-3 Model:

$$\pi 00i = \beta 000 + r00i \tag{3}$$

Level 3 (classroom level) was added to account for the possible variability among classes, where $\beta 000$ was the grand mean score of all classes, and r00i was the random effect of classes. As a result, steps per min were found to have a significant, positive relationship with MVPA (Table 3). However, only 1.3% more variance at level 1 was explained by adding the steps per min into the full model, which means that the significant association was weak as demonstrated by small proportions of variance explained. Therefore, the results of the HLM implicitly took nesting into account and included more controls in the models, which did not contradict the ICCs results. In other words, the measurement provided by pedometer was not reliable when we assessed students' MVPA, as a low degree of reliability was also seen in pedometer outputs.

Table 3. Hierarchical linear modeling (HLM) for moderate to vigorous physical activity with three-level modeling.

Fixed Effect	Coefficient	Standard Error	*t*-Ratio	Approx. *d.f.*	*p* Value
For INTRCPT1, ψ_0	-	-	-	-	-
For INTRCPT2, π_{00}	-	-	-	-	-
INTRCPT3, β_{000} For SEX, π_{01}	0.072128	0.030573	2.359	19	0.029
INTRCPT3, β_{010} For AGE, π_{02}	−0.000908	0.011431	−0.079	343	0.937
INTRCPT3, β_{020} For RACE1, π_{03}	−0.006521	0.003386	−1.926	343	0.055
INTRCPT3, β_{030} For DAY slope, ψ_1 For INTRCPT2, π_{10}	0.032761	0.008744	3.747	343	<0.001
INTRCPT3, β_{100} For TIME slope, ψ_2 For INTRCPT2, π_{20}	−0.002019	0.000476	−4.24	5625	<0.001
INTRCPT3, β_{200} For SPM slope, ψ_3 For INTRCPT2, π_{30}	0.004824	0.001595	3.024	5625	0.003
INTRCPT3, β_{300}	0.001793	0.000145	12.38	5625	<0.001

SPM = steps per min.

4. Discussion

The manufacturer of the motion sensors now offers various instruments for analyzing movement data, but their trustworthiness in exergaming settings has not been documented in the literature. Therefore, this study was designed to provide reliability evidence for two popular motion sensors (NL-1000 pedometer and ActiGraph GT3X accelerometer) that are used as practical and objective PA measurement tools in exergaming settings. Based upon the descriptive analysis, children actually spent most time in sedentary behavior as compared to LPA and MVPA while playing exergames. Although each exergaming session had 30 min, only half to two-third PA time were captured by accelerometers. The results of ICCs showed the estimates of PA levels were inconsistent among children as the ICCs were far from ideal, indicating low reliability of two monitors in measuring elementary school children' regular PA levels during exergaming play.

While the findings are unexpected and not accordance with most previous studies indicating these motion-sensors are reliable instruments in assessing children's PA behaviors in other setting, we identified plausible reason for such discrepancies. In the present study, participants were elementary school children and they were equipped with two motion sensors simultaneously while playing exergames. That is, the inconsistency of instruments placement may lead to data loss (about one-third of PA time missed) and unreliability of motion sensors in capturing movement data in exergaming.

Unlike traditional physical education class where contents are consistently delivered by the instructors, the exergaming activities were carried out by multiple random games. Within a single game console, different games with respective difficult levels can provide varying EE. In our study, students were offered with eight different Nintendo Wii exergames and every student played different types of exergames, thus variability of EE across types of games tended to be large. For example, the "Just Dance" allowed players to perform more than 20 songs consecutively with several difficulty levels depending on how well the player was dancing. Such arrangement resulted in students being exposed to various conditions. Therefore, different types of exergames and game sequence effects might be potential confounding factors on reliability of measurements in exergaming. In addition, children rotated from stations to stations in the present study. That is, when a participant arrived at next station, he or she had to set up a different game to meet his or her interests and needs. In that case, the exergaming was not implemented in a continuous way and children were not really being physically active during these transitions. To this sense, the transition time may lead to inaccurate data because each child would have unequal PA intensities and time of game playing.

The correlation analysis suggested no significant positive relationship between accelerometers and pedometers measures. Furthermore, the HLM analysis further confirmed low reliability of two monitors, which was not contradictory with the ICCs results as very little shared variance could be explained by pedometers and accelerometers. Previous studies using similar activity monitors have shown agreement in measuring PA levels among children and youth [33,34]. These empirical studies utilized different epoch lengths (5 s and 30 s) and cut points to determine sedentary, light PA and MVPA thresholds in either school-based physical education or free-living settings. Although several validated MVPA epoch lengths have been proposed for use in children, the impact of accelerometer epoch length on PA measures remains a contentious issue, particularly with regard to application in school children. For example, researchers suggested that the 15 s epoch length for accelerometers captured more MVPA and sedentary time yet fewer steps and less light PA and total PA were tracked compared to 60 s epoch length [35]. Appukutty and colleagues [36] indicated that the MVPA time were significantly higher with 10 s epoch than 60 s epoch in children. In general, children's PA patterns tend to be varied and intermittent for differing activities and intensities. The use of shorter epochs would produce higher and more accurate estimates of MVPA time compared to longer epochs [37]. McClain and colleagues [34] further demonstrated that 5 s epoch length in ActiGraph accelerometer yielded the lowest root mean squared error in assessing MVPA, indicating shorter epochs would yield more PA amount. Because of this, children's PA may be better captured with shorter epochs. In this study, we used 1s epoch length to make sure we accurately captured children's PA as much as possible. Nevertheless, we still believe that different epoch length thresholds would explain part of the differences between our findings and previous studies.

Furthermore, it has been noted that different equation should be used when using accelerometers to children with chronic diseases such as congenital heart disease (CHD), cystic fibrosis (CF), dermatomyositis (JDM), juvenile arthritis (JA), inherited muscle disease (IMD), and hemophilia (HE) [38]. For example, Stephen et al. [38] found that agreement between predicted and measured energy expenditure (EE) varied across disease group and ranged from (ICC) 0.13–0.46. With the prediction equation specific to the disease group was presented, an improved range of results (ICC 0.62–0.88) (SE 0.45–0.78) was shown. The researchers concluded that current prediction should be replaced with disease-specific equation in children with chronic conditions as the current equation demonstrate poor agreement. In terms of testing reliability and validity of pedometers in clinical population, it has been reported that pedometers (Yamax SW digi-walker, New Lifestyles NL-2000) are useful for tracking ambulatory movement in the population [39]. For example, in their study with youth with cerebral palsy, NL-1000 pedometer demonstrated an excellent reliability (ICC 0.88–0.99) and validity (ICC 0.78–0.95) with no significant difference between the video step counts and pedometer step counts in walking and running in controlled setting. When using pedometers, however, in population with disabilities, the 3% error cutoff for accuracy may not be realistic for population with disabilities [40].

Finally, it is known that both waist-mounted accelerometers and pedometers have lower accuracy when one's PA level is at slow speeds [41,42]. For instance, McClain et al. [43] found agreement between NL-1000 and ActiGraph accelerometers estimates of free-living MVPA in 10-year old children, but large differences were also found at other settings, especially when children experienced a low PA intensity. Similarly, although Kinnunen et al. [44] found statistically significant correlations, the overall agreement between pedometer and accelerometer step counts was poor and varied with PA levels.

The strength of this study lies in that it is the first of its kind to assess the reliability of two motion sensors in measuring children's PA levels in exergaming settings. However, there are several limitations that should be noted. While multiple sessions of two objective motion sensors were used to explore their reliability, they were not compared to the gold standard measures of energy expenditure. Therefore, a rigorous design and better statistical analyses will be necessary in the future research. In fact, exergaming has several limitations when being considered a PA option. One such limitation is the limited time children spent in being moderately or even vigorously active. Exergaming oftentimes requires the players short bursts of exertion followed by considerable breaks between activities, which may lead to children not very active to the MVPA level. Although there were various difficulty levels available for children in exergames such as beginner, intermediate, and advanced levels, it is implausible to let each child play the advanced level games for every time, because games were selected randomly and varied according to how well the child performed. If children played the same games, they would lose interest in exergaming and the enjoyment of exercise would decrease over time. Therefore, the low speed and random nature of exergaming may result in accelerometers and pedometers having lower reliability in measuring children's PA levels.

5. Conclusions

In summary, the primary finding of the study was that the NL-1000 pedometers and ActiGraph GT3X accelerometers have low reliability in assessing elementary school children's PA levels during exergaming. More research is warranted in determining the reliable and accurate measurement information regarding the use of modern devices during exergaming. Although the current study does not provide promising reliability evidence for the use of NL-1000 pedometers and ActiGraph GT3X accelerometers in assessing PA in exergaming settings, the findings may render some implications for future exergaming research. First, the same exergaming activities should be employed when motion sensors are used to eliminate the variability caused by different games. Second, researchers should minimize the transition time by increasing the time of game playing to make sure children stay physically active pattern most of the time. Third, placing the monitor on ankles or using heart rate monitors may be more appropriate in assessing children's PA during exergames play. Finally, researchers should ensure the consistency of the device placement during measurement. When using these motion sensors in clinical population whom might be using exergaming as a therapeutic means, more factors need to be taken into considerations such as type of disease, presence of disabilities, and utilizing disease-specific prediction equation.

Author Contributions: During the construction of this study, N.Z. played a role in writing the manuscript. X.G., played a role in data analyses. Y.L. and J.E.L. played a role in helping write the manuscript. Z.G. played a role in developing the idea, overseeing the study, and data collection.

Acknowledgments: The authors would like to thank all the children for their participation in this study as well as the teachers for their support.

Conflicts of Interest: The authors declare no conflict of interest.

References

1. Global Strategy on Diet, Physical Activity and Health. Available online: http://www.who.int/ dietphysicalactivity/reducingsalt/en/ (accessed on 27 March 2016).
2. Gao, Z.; Chen, S.; Stodden, D.F.A. Comparison of children's physical activity levels in physical education, recess, and exergaming. *J. Phys. Act. Health* **2015**, *12*, 349–354. [CrossRef] [PubMed]
3. Sun, H. Exergaming impact on physical activity and interest in elementary school children. *Res. Q. Exerc. Sport* **2012**, *83*, 212–220. [CrossRef] [PubMed]
4. Graf, D.L.; Pratt, L.V.; Hester, C.N.; Short, K.R. Playing active video games increases energy expenditure in children. *Pediatrics* **2009**, *124*, 534–540. [CrossRef] [PubMed]
5. Lyons, E.J.; Tate, D.F.; Ward, D.S.; Bowling, J.M.; Ribisl, K.M.; Kalyararaman, S. Energy expenditure and enjoyment during video game play: Differences by game type. *Med. Sci. Sports Exerc.* **2011**, *43*, 1987–1993. [CrossRef] [PubMed]
6. Gao, Z.; Chen, S. Are field-based exergames useful in preventing childhood obesity? A systematic review. *Obes. Rev.* **2014**, *15*, 676–691. [CrossRef] [PubMed]

7. Gao, Z.; Chen, S.; Pasco, D.; Pope, Z. Effects of active video games on physiological and psychological outcomes among children and adolescents: A meta-analysis. *Obes. Rev.* **2015**, *16*, 783–794. [CrossRef] [PubMed]

8. Gao, Z.; Zhang, T.; Stodden, D. Children's physical activity levels and their psychological correlated in interactive dance versus aerobic dance. *J. Sport Health Sci.* **2013**, *2*, 146–151. [CrossRef]

9. Shayne, R.K.; Fogel, V.A.; Miltenberger, R.G.; Koehler, S. The effects of exergaming on physical activity in a third-grade physical education class. *J. Appl. Behav. Anal.* **2012**, *45*, 211–215. [CrossRef] [PubMed]

10. Fairclough, S.; Stratton, G. A review of physical activity levels during elementary school physical education. *J. Teach. Phys. Educ.* **2006**, *25*, 240–258. [CrossRef]

11. Christison, A.; Khan, H.A. Exergaming for health: A community based pediatric weight management program using active video gaming. *Clin. Pediatr.* **2012**, *51*, 382–388. [CrossRef] [PubMed]

12. Zeng, N.; Gao, Z. Exergaming and obesity in youth: Current perspectives. *Int. J. Gen. Med.* **2016**, *9*, 275. [PubMed]

13. Hilton, C.L.; Cumpata, K.; Klohr, C.; Gaetke, S.; Artner, A.; Johnson, H.; Dobbs, S. Effects of exergaming on executive function and motor skills in children with autism spectrum disorder: A pilot study. *Am. J. Occup. Ther.* **2014**, *68*, 57–65. [CrossRef] [PubMed]

14. Benzing, V.; Schmidt, M. Cognitively and physically demanding exergaming to improve executive functions of children with attention deficit hyperactivity disorder: A randomised clinical trial. *BMC Pediatr.* **2017**, *17*, 8. [CrossRef] [PubMed]

15. Sirard, J.R.; Pate, R.R. Physical activity assessment in children and adolescents. *Sports Med.* **2001**, *31*, 439–454. [CrossRef] [PubMed]

16. Liggett, L.; Gray, A.; Parnell, W.; McGee, R.; McKenzie, Y. Validation and reliability of the New Lifestyles NL-1000 accelerometer in New Zealand preschoolers. *J. Phys. Act. Health* **2012**, *9*, 295–300. [CrossRef] [PubMed]

17. Sallis, J.F. Measuring physical activity: Practical approaches for program evaluation in Native American communities. *J. Public Health Manag. Pract.* **2010**, *16*, 404–410. [CrossRef] [PubMed]

18. Gao, Z.; Hannon, J.C.; Newton, M.; Huang, C. The effects of curricular activity on students' situational motivation and physical activity levels. *Res. Q. Exerc. Sport* **2011**, *82*, 536–544. [CrossRef] [PubMed]

19. Gao, Z.; Pope, Z.; Lee, J.E.; Stodden, D.; Roncesvalles, N.; Pasco, D.; Huang, C.; Feng, D. Impact of exergaming on young children's school day energy expenditure and moderate-to-vigorous physical activity levels. *J. Sport Health Sci.* **2017**, *6*, 11–16. [CrossRef]

20. Prince, S.A.; Adamo, K.B.; Hamel, M.E.; Hardt, J.; Gorber, S.C. A comparison of direct versus self-report measures for assessing physical activity in adults: A systematic review. *Int. J. Behav. Nutr. Phys. Act.* **2008**, *5*, 56–80. [CrossRef] [PubMed]

21. Steeves, J.A.; Tyo, B.M.; Connolly, C.P.; Gregory, D.A.; Stark, N.A.; Bassett, D.R. Validity and reliability of the Omron HJ-303 tri-axial accelerometer-based pedometer. *J. Phys. Act. Health* **2011**, *8*, 1014–1020. [CrossRef] [PubMed]

22. Ozemek, C.; Kirschner, M.M.; Wilkerson, B.S.; Byun, W.; Kaminsky, L.A. Intermonitor reliability of the GT3X+ accelerometer at hip, wrist and ankle sites during activities of daily living. *Physiol. Meas.* **2014**, *35*, 129–138. [CrossRef] [PubMed]

23. Duncan, S.J.; Schofield, G.; Duncan, E.K.; Hinckson, E.A. Effects of age, walking speed, and body composition on pedometer accuracy in children. *Res. Q. Exerc. Sport* **2007**, *78*, 420–428. [CrossRef] [PubMed]

24. Schneider, P.L.; Crouter, S.E.; Lukajic, O.; Bassett, J.D. Accuracy and reliability of 10 pedometers for measuring steps over a 400-m walk. *Med. Sci. Sports Exerc.* **2003**, *35*, 1779–1784. [CrossRef] [PubMed]

25. ActiLife 6 Manual. Available online: http://actigraphcorp.com/support/manuals/actilife-6-manual/ (accessed on 30 March 2016).

26. Lee, K.Y.; Macfarlane, D.J.; Cerin, E. Do three different generations of the actigraph accelerometer provide the same output? In Proceedings of the 57th American College of Sports Medicine Annual Meeting, Baltimore, MD, USA, 2–5 June 2010.

27. Flynn, J.I.; Coe, D.P.; Larsen, C.A.; Rider, B.C.; Conger, S.A.; Bassett, J.D. Detecting indoor and outdoor environments using the ActiGraph GT3X light sensor in children. *Med. Sci. Sports Exerc.* **2014**, *46*, 201–206. [CrossRef] [PubMed]

28. Evenson, K.R.; Catellier, D.J.; Gill, K.; Ondrak, K.S.; McMurray, R.G. Calibration of two objective measures of physical activity for children. *J. Sports Sci.* **2008**, *26*, 1557–1565. [CrossRef] [PubMed]

29. Landis, J.R.; Koch, G.G. The measurement of observer agreement for categorical data. *Biometrics* **1977**, *33*, 159–174. [CrossRef] [PubMed]

30. Bryk, A.S.; Raudenbush, S.W. *Hierarchical Linear Models*; Sage: Newbury Park, CA, USA, 1992; pp. 347–396.

31. Cheval, B.; Sarrazin, P.; Pelletier, L. Impulsive approach tendencies towards physical activity and sedentary behaviors, but not reflective intentions, prospectively predict non-exercise activity thermogenesis. *PLoS ONE* **2014**, *9*, e115238. [CrossRef] [PubMed]

32. Nezlek, J.B. Multilevel random coefficient analyses of event and interval contingent data in social and personality psychology research. *Pers. Soc. Psychol. Bull.* **2001**, *27*, 771–785. [CrossRef]

33. Beets, M.W.; Morgan, C.F.; Banda, J.A.; Bornstein, D.; Byun, W.; Mitchell, J.; Munselle, L.; Rooney, L.; Beighle, A.; Erwin, H. Convergent validity of pedometer and accelerometer estimates of moderate-to-vigorous physical activity of youth. *J. Phys. Act. Health* **2011**, *8*, 295–305. [CrossRef] [PubMed]

34. McClain, J.J.; Sisson, S.B.; Washington, T.L.; Craig, C.L.; Tudor-Locke, C. Comparison of Kenz Lifecorder EX and ActiGraph accelerometers in 10-yr-old children. *Med. Sci. Sports Exerc.* **2007**, *39*, 630–638. [CrossRef] [PubMed]

35. Colley, R.C.; Harvey, A.; Grattan, K.P.; Adamo, K.B. Impact of accelerometer epoch length on physical activity and sedentary behavior outcomes for preschool-aged children. *Health Rep.* **2014**, *25*, 3–9. [PubMed]

36. Appukutty, M.; Tanaka, C.; Tanaka, S. Physical activity measurements by 10 sec and 60 sec epoch length using triaxial accelerometer among elementary school children in Japan. *Obes. Rev.* **2014**, *15*, 244–248.

37. Bailey, R.C.; Olson, J.O.D.I.; Pepper, S.L.; Porszasz, J.A.N.O.S.; Barstow, T.J.; Cooper, D.M. The level and tempo of children's physical activities: An observational study. *Med. Sci. Sports Exerc.* **1995**, *27*, 1033–1041. [CrossRef] [PubMed]

38. Stephens, S.; Takken, T.; Esliger, D.W.; Pullenayegum, E.; Beyene, J.; Tremblay, M.; Schneiderman, J.; Biggar, D.; Longmuir, P.; McCrindle, B.; et al. Validation of accelerometer prediction equations in children with chronic disease. *Pediatr. Exerc. Sci.* **2016**, *28*, 117–132. [CrossRef] [PubMed]

39. Maher, C.; Kenyon, A.; McEvoy, M.; Sprod, J. The reliability and validity of a research-grade pedometer for children and adolescents with cerebral palsy. *Dev. Med. Child Neurol.* **2013**, *55*, 827–833. [CrossRef] [PubMed]

40. Kenyon, A.; McEvoy, M.; Sprod, J.; Maher, C. Validity of pedometers in people with physical disabilities: A systematic review. *Arch. Phys. Med. Rehabil.* **2013**, *94*, 1161–1170. [CrossRef] [PubMed]

41. Mcclain, J.J.; Abraham, T.L.; Brusseau, J.T.; Tudor-Locke, C. Epoch length and accelerometer outputs in children: Comparison to direct observation. *Med. Sci. Sports Exerc.* **2008**, *40*, 2080–2087. [CrossRef] [PubMed]

42. Clemes, S.A.; O'Connell, S.; Rogan, L.M.; Griffiths, P.L. Evaluation of a commercially available pedometer used to promote physical activity as part of a national programme. *Br. J. Sports Med.* **2009**, *44*, 1178–1183. [CrossRef] [PubMed]

43. McClain, J.J.; Hart, T.L.; Getz, R.S.; Tudor-Locke, C. Convergent validity of 3 low cost motion sensors with the ActiGraph accelerometer. *J. Phys. Act. Health* **2010**, *7*, 662–670. [CrossRef] [PubMed]

44. Kinnunen, T.I.; Tennant, P.W.; McParlin, C.; Poston, L.; Robson, S.C.; Bell, R. Agreement between pedometer and accelerometer in measuring physical activity in overweight and obese pregnant women. *BMC Public Health* **2011**, *11*, 501–510. [CrossRef] [PubMed]

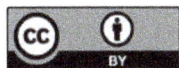

Journal of
Clinical Medicine

MDPI

Article

Cross-Sectional Associations of Environmental Perception with Leisure-Time Physical Activity and Screen Time among Older Adults

Ming-Chun Hsueh [1] , Chien-Yu Lin [2], Pin-Hsuan Huang [3], Jong-Hwan Park [4,*] and Yung Liao [3,*]

1   Department of Physical Education, National Taiwan Normal University, 162, Heping East Road Section 1, Taipei 106, Taiwan; boxeo@ntnu.edu.tw
2   Institute of Health Behaviors and Community Sciences, National Taiwan University, 17, Xuzhou Road, Taipei 100, Taiwan; chinchin019283@gmail.com
3   Department of Health Promotion and Health Education, National Taiwan Normal University, 162, Heping East Road Section 1, Taipei 106, Taiwan; victorlove1610@gmail.com
4   Institute of Convergence Bio-Health, Dong-A University, 32, Daeshingongwon-Ro, Seo-Gu, Busan 49201, Korea
*   Correspondence: jparkl@dau.ac.kr (J.-H.P.); liaoyung@ntnu.edu.tw (Y.L.); Tel.: +82-10-6228-1485 (J.-H.P.); +886-2-7734-1722 (Y.L.); Fax: +82-52-240-2971 (J.-H.P.); +886-2363-3026 (Y.L.)

Received: 14 February 2018; Accepted: 10 March 2018; Published: 13 March 2018

Abstract: This study investigated associations of perceived environmental factors with leisure-time physical activity (LTPA) and screen time (ST) among older adults. A cross-sectional study was conducted by administering computer-assisted telephone interviews to 1028 older Taiwanese adults in November 2016. Data on personal factors, perceived environmental factors, LTPA, and ST were included. Odds ratios (ORs) and 95% confidence intervals (CIs) were calculated to examine associations of environmental perception with LTPA and ST by using logistic regression analyses. The results showed that after adjusting for potential confounders, older adults who perceived their neighborhood with good access to shops (AS) and to public transportation (AT) were more likely to have sufficient LTPA (AS: OR = 1.64, 95% CI: 1.16–2.32; AT: OR = 1.43; 95% CI, 1.00–2.03) and less likely to have excessive ST (AS: OR = 0.70; 95% CI: 0.50–0.97; AT: OR = 0.64; 95% CI: 0.46–0.90). Different perceived environmental factors were also associated with LTPA and ST, respectively. This study highlights environment perception as a crucial factor for LTPA and ST. These findings suggest that policy makers and physical activity intervention designers should develop both common and individual environmental strategies to improve and increase awareness of the neighborhood environment to promote LTPA and reduce ST among older adults.

Keywords: senior citizens; perceived environmental factor; recreational physical activity; screen based sedentary behavior

---

1. Introduction

Sufficient physical activity is associated with better physical and psychological health outcomes, and reduced risks of non-communicable diseases and all-cause mortality in older adults [1]. Studies have shown that participation in leisure-time physical activity offers an opportunity to reduce the prevalence of morbidity in later life and offset a potential burden of aging on the public health sector [2]. Despite the known health benefits associated with participation in the recommended amount of leisure-time physical activity (150 min/week), nearly 40% of older Taiwanese remain inactive [3].

In terms of utilizing an ecological approach in designing effective interventions and relevant policies, it is important to understand how environmental attributes correlate with health behavior [4]. Compared with individually based interventions, environmental changes are supposed to provide a long-term impact and on behavior of the larger population. In the last decade, many studies have shown perceived neighborhood environmental factors to be associated with total physical activity in older adults [5,6]. However, leisure-time physical activity is particularly relevant as older adult tend to have significantly more leisure time available in later life [2]. Nevertheless, most existing evidence concerning associations between perceived neighborhood environment and physical activity measurement was commonly accrued across all domains, and few studies targeted leisure-time physical activity in older adults [5,6]. It is important to understand how perceived environmental facilitation or impediments associated with the neighborhood leisure-time behaviors of older adults can vary in different contexts. Moreover, few studies have examined the perceived environmental correlates of leisure-time physical activity, particularly in Asian countries, which likely have different residential densities, cultures, and infrastructure than Western countries. Thus, more evidence from Asian countries' older adults, especially in Taiwan, is beneficial for understanding how perceived neighborhood environmental factors relate to leisure-time physical activity and may provide insights for public health intervention.

In recent years, time spent in sedentary behavior has become a new risk factor for health [7]. Previous studies have shown evidence that sedentary behavior is related to an increased risk of all-cause mortality and other negative health outcomes in older adults [8]. Considering screen-based sedentary time, such as television viewing, internet and computer use are increasingly common leisure-time sedentary behaviors in older adults [9], which has the potential to negatively impact health, independent of other sedentary behaviors (e.g.,: reading, talking and transport) [10,11]. With the rapidly aging population and the high prevalence of screen time in the older age group, in Taiwan, almost 64.4% of older adult report spending excessive screen time (including television viewing time and computer use) [10].

Owen et al. [12] has emphasized that neighborhood environmental attributes may also play a role in sedentary behaviors in older adults, particularly screen-based behavior. For example, previous studies have found that older adults who reported positive perceptions of their neighborhoods in terms of local traffic safety [3,13], access to facilities, safety from crime, and walking facilities [14] had less television viewing time. However, previous studies concerning the associations between neighborhood environments and screen time were mostly conducted on adolescents [15], youth [16], and adult populations [17]. It is not clear whether the relationships of neighborhood environments and screen time are different in the older age group. Additionally, despite the fact that screen-based sedentary behavior including television time, computer or internet use may vary [12], there have been limitations in studies to date that have examined these relationships on perception of environmental factors and screen time (combined television time, computer and internet use) in older adults. Moreover, although there has been some research examining the role of neighborhood environmental factors in relation to leisure time physical activity and screen time, very few studies have concurrently considered factors associated with older adult in an Asian country, despite the fact that such investigations could potentially provide more practical and policy-related information. Consequently, to address these gaps, the purpose of this study was to adopt an ecological framework to examine the associations of perceived environmental perception with leisure-time physical activity and screen time in Taiwanese older adults. This study tested the hypothesis that good perceived neighborhood environment would be associated with high levels of leisure-time physical activity and low levels of screen time.

2. Material and Methods

2.1. Participants

This study used data collected by administering a random-digit dialing, telephone-based, cross-sectional survey in 2016 through a telephone research service company. In November 2016, Taiwan was estimated to have an older adult population of 3,089,843 (target population) and an area of 36,192.8 km^2. The required sample size for this study was calculated to be 1067 adults with a 95% confidence level and a 3% confidence interval. A stratified sampling process was used to select respondents. Trained interviewers administered a standardized questionnaire. All the interviewers had experience in administering telephone population surveys and received two days of training before the start of each survey. A total of 3546 adults were asked to participate, and 1074 of them completed the survey (response rate: 30.3%). However, after data cleaning, 1028 participants submitted valid data for analysis (eligible rate: 29.0%). The telephone research service company did not offer any rewards for participation. Verbal informed consent was obtained before the start of the telephone interviews and the study protocols were reviewed and approved by the Research Ethics Committee of National Taiwan Normal University (REC number: 201605HM006).

2.2. Outcome Variables

The outcome variables of this study were leisure-time physical activity and screen time. For leisure-time physical activity, measured from the Taiwan version of the International Physical Activity Questionnaire-long version (IPAQ-LV: https://sites.google.com/site/theipaq/questionnaire_links) [18,19]. Participants were asked to recall the frequency and average duration of vigorous intensity leisure-time activity, moderate intensity leisure-time activity, and walking during the last seven days. The questions included "During the last 7 days, on how many days did you do the activities (vigorous/moderate/walking) in your leisure time?" and "How much time did you usually spend on one of those days doing the activities in your leisure time?" The total amount of leisure-time physical activity was classified into two groups: "sufficient leisure-time physical activity" ($\geq$150 min/week) and "insufficient leisure-time physical activity" (<150 min/week). Sufficient leisure-time physical activity refers to at least 150 min per week. This criterion is in accordance with the current recommendations for the practice of physical activity in older adult's guidelines [20].

The outcome of screen time was estimated using two questions that queried participants' self-report television watching and computer/internet use. The survey items were: "During the last week, how much time in total did you spend sitting or lying down and watching television or videos/DVDs." The same question was asked with "using the computer/Internet." The items (television viewing time (intraclass correlation coefficient, ICC) = 0.76, and using the computer/Internet = 0.79) have been shown to have good test-retest reliability) in the Measure of Older Adults' Sedentary Time questionnaire (MOST) [21]. Taiwanese older adults exhibited an acceptable test-retest reliability [10]. Responses to both items were added together and dichotomized into two categories, namely, excessive screen time ($\geq$2 h/day) and low screen time (<2 h/day). This cutoff point ($\geq$2 h/day) was also reported as being associated with health risks in previous studies [22].

2.3. Perceived Environmental Variables

The perceived environmental factors were measured using the Taiwanese version of the International Physical Activity Questionnaire-environmental module (IPAQ-E). The IPAQ-E questionnaire was developed by the International Physical Activity Prevalence Study to understand the environmental factors affecting walking and bicycling in neighborhoods. The IPAQ-E was translated with the IPAQ, according to the process of translation and adaptation of instruments provided by the World Health Organization [23]. The details of IPAQ-E are described elsewhere: http://sallis.ucsd.edu/Documents/Measures_documents/PANES_survey.pdf [24]. The 17-item IPAQ-E questionnaire consisted of three categories of items, which included seven core items, four recommended items, and six optional items. In this study, 11 of the 17 items were included for measuring the perceived environmental attributes, including (1) residential density, (for this question, the five options were as follows: detached single-family housing; townhouses, row houses, apartments or condos of 2–3 stories; a mix of single-family residences and townhouses, row houses, apartments or condos; apartments or condos of 4–12 stories; and apartments or condos of more than 12 stories), (2) access to shops (Many shops are within walking distance of my home), (3) access to public transportation (It is less than a 10–15 min walk to a transit station from my home), (4) presence of sidewalks (There are sidewalks on most of the streets in my neighborhood), (5) access to recreational facilities (My neighborhood has several free or low-cost recreation facilities), (6) crime safety at night (The crime rate in my neighborhood makes it unsafe to go on walks at night), (7) traffic safety (There is so much traffic on the streets that walking is difficult or unpleasant), (8) seeing people being active (I see many people being physically active in my neighborhood), (9) aesthetics (There are many interesting things to look at while walking in my neighborhood), (10) connectivity of streets (There are many four-way intersections in my neighborhood), (11) presence of a destination (There are many places to go within easy walking distance of my home). Six optional items regarding the presence of bike lanes, traffic safety for bicyclists, maintenance of sidewalks, maintenance of bike lanes, safety from crime during the day, and number of households owning cars or motor bikes, were not included in this study.

All items were converted into binary items. For residential density, the choice of detached single-family residences formed a category indicating "low residential density," while the other possible responses were included in another category indicating "high residential density." With regard to the other questions, responses were classified into two categories of "agree" (strongly agree and somewhat agree) and "disagree" (somewhat disagree and strongly disagree). These classifications were similar to those used in previous studies from Taiwan [3] and Japan [25].

2.4. Sociodemographic Variables

Sociodemographic variables included gender, age, occupational type, educational level, marital status, living status, residential area, self-rated health status, and Body Mass Index (BMI). Age was divided into three categories: 65–74 years, 75–84 years, and 85+ years. Occupational type was categorized into "full-time job" and "not full-time job." Educational level was classified into two groups: "not tertiary degree" (less than 13 years) and "tertiary degree" (13 years and more). Marital status was classified as "married" and "unmarried" (including widowed, separated, and divorced). Living status was divided into "living with others" and "living alone." Residential area was categorized into "metropolitan" and "non-metropolitan" areas. Self-rated health status was categories into "good" and "poor." BMI was based on self-reported weight and height and was grouped into two categories: "not overweight" (<24 kg/m^2) and "overweight/obese" (≥ 24 kg/m^2). We used 24 kg/m^2 as a cut-off point of BMI is because this cut-off point for older adults is suggested by Health Promotion Administration, Ministry of Health and Welfare in Taiwan (http://health99 hpa.gov.tw/OnlinkHealth/OnlInk_BMI. aspx) [26].

2.5. Statistical Analyses

The data were analyzed from 1028 older Taiwanese adults who provided complete information for the study variables. Forced-entry adjusted logistic regression for gender, age, occupational type, educational level, marital status, living status, residential area, self-rated health status, and BMI was conducted to examine the association of 11 perceived environmental factors for leisure-time physical activity and screen time. Adjusted Odds ratios (ORs) and 95% confidence intervals (CIs) were calculated for each variable. Inferential statistics were obtained using SPSS (version 23.0, IMB, CITY, STATE, COUNTRY) and the level of significance was set at $p < 0.05$.

3. Results

3.1. Participant Characteristics

The basic information of the respondents is shown in Table 1. Of the total respondents, 49.1% were female, 33.9% were ≥75 years old, 71.2% had a non-tertiary degree, 89.8% were in a non-full-time job, 23.0% were unmarried, 13.7% were living alone, 50.7% lived in a non-metropolitan area, 19.0% had poor self-rated health status, and 41.6% were overweight or obese. The prevalence of achieving 150 min/week for leisure-time physical activity was 66.3%, and 60.2% exceeded 120 min/day of screen time.

Table 1. Basic characteristics of all respondents (*n* = 1028).

Variable	Category	Study Sample n	Study Sample %
Gender	Male	523	50.9%
	Female	505	49.1%
Age	65–74	679	66.1%
	≥75	349	33.9%
Educational	Tertiary degree	296	28.8%
	Non-tertiary degree	732	71.2%
Occupational type	Full-time job	105	10.2%
	Non-full-time job	923	89.8%
Marital status	Married	792	77.0%
	Unmarried	236	23.0%
Living status	With others	887	86.3%
	Alone	141	13.7%
Residential area	Metropolitan	507	49.3%
	Non-metropolitan	521	50.7%
Self-rated health status	Good	833	81.0%
	Poor	195	19.0%
Body Mass Index (kg/m2)	Non-overweight	600	58.4%
	Overweight/obese	428	41.6%
LTPA	Insufficient (<150 min/week)	346	33.7%
	Sufficient (≥150 min/week)	682	66.3%
ST	Low (<2 h/day)	409	39.8%
	Excessive (≥2 h/day)	619	60.2%

Abbreviations: LTPA = leisure-time physical activity; ST = screen-time.

3.2. Perceived Environmental Factors Associated with Leisure-Time Physical Activity

In Table 2, logistic regression analyses revealed that six of the 11 environmental attributes were significantly associated with 150 min/week for leisure-time physical activity. After adjusting for potential confounders, older adults who perceived that they had good access to shops (OR = 1.64; 95% CI: 1.16–2.32), good access to public transportation (OR = 1.43; 95% CI: 1.00–2.03), good access to recreational facilities (OR = 1.73; 95% CI: 1.26–2.37), seeing people being active (OR = 1.47; 95% CI: 1.10–1.93), good aesthetics (OR = 1.33; 95% CI: 1.01–1.75), and presence of a destination (OR = 1.92; 95% CI: 1.42–2.59) were more likely to achieve 150 min/week for leisure-time physical activity.

Table 2. Perceived Environmental Factors Associated with LTPA and ST.

Variable	Category	Total Sample		Sufficient LTPA	Excessive ST
		n	%	OR (95%CI)	OR (95%CI)
Residential density [a]	High	937	90.8%	0.88 (0.53–1.42)	0.67 (0.44–1.04)
	Low	95	9.2%	1.00	1.00
Access to shops	Good	838	81.2%	1.64 (1.16–2.32) *	0.70 (0.50–0.97) *
	Poor	194	18.8%	1.00	1.00
Access to public transportation	Good	836	81.0%	1.43 (1.00–2.03) *	0.64 (0.46–0.90) *
	Poor	196	19.0%	1.00	1.00
Presence of sidewalks	Yes	618	59.9%	1.30 (0.98–1.73)	0.99 (0.76–1.30)
	No	414	40.1%	1.00	1.00
Access to recreational facilities	Yes	794	76.9%	1.73 (1.26–2.37) **	0.77 (0.57–1.04)
	No	238	23.1%	1.00	1.00
Crime safety at night	Not safe	174	16.9%	1.17 (0.82–1.67)	0.87 (0.62–1.21)
	Safe	858	83.1%	1.00	1.00
Traffic safety	Not safe	345	33.4%	0.89 (0.66–1.18)	0.99 (0.75–1.29)
	Safe	687	66.6%	1.00	1.00
Seeing people being active	Yes	677	65.6%	1.47 (1.10–1.93) *	0.82 (0.63–1.07)
	No	355	34.4%	1.00	1.00
Aesthetics	Yes	562	54.5%	1.33 (1.01–1.75) *	0.79 (0.61–1.02)
	No	470	45.5%	1.00	1.00
Connectivity of streets	Good	671	65%	1.29 (0.97–1.71)	0.60 (0.46–0.78) **
	Poor	361	35%	1.00	1.00
Presence of destination	Yes	726	70.3%	1.92 (1.42–2.59) **	0.81 (0.61–1.07)
	No	306	29.7%	1.00	1.00

[a] residential density definition: single-family housing as "low residential density"; townhouses, row houses, apartments or condos of 2–3 stories; a mix of single-family residences and townhouses, row houses, apartments or condos; apartments or condos of 4–12 stories; and apartments or condos of more than 12 stories as "high residential density,". Adjusted for gender, age, occupational type, educational level, marital status, living status, residential area, self-rated health status, and Body Mass Index (BMI); * $p < 0.05$, ** $p < 0.001$. LTPA = leisure-time physical activity; ST = screen-time.

3.3. Perceived Environmental Factors Associated with Screen Time

Table 2 also shows that three of the 11 environmental attributes were significantly associated with 120 min/day for screen time behavior. Older adults who perceived that they had good access to shops (OR = 0.70; 95% CI: 0.50–0.97), good access to public transportation (OR = 0.64; 95% CI: 0.46–0.90), and good connectivity of streets (OR = 0.60; 95% CI: 0.46–0.78) were less likely to have a screen time of more than 120 min/day.

4. Discussion

The present study is the one of the few sources of evidence from an Asian country to have concurrently examined the associations of perceived environmental factors with both leisure-time physical activity and screen time among Taiwanese older adults. The main findings of the present study are that two common perceived environmental factors, good access to shops and good access to public transportation, are both related to sufficient levels of leisure-time physical activity ($\geq$150 min/week) and lower screen time (<2 h/day). Environmental and government policy initiatives aiming to improve "active aging" should promote older adults' awareness of good access to shops and public transportation in the neighborhood.

Our finding shows that good access to shops and good access to public transportation were concurrently associated with high levels of leisure-time physical activity and lower screen time in Taiwanese older adult. The present results were inconsistent with previous findings from other countries, which have reported that in older adults, perceiving good access to shops and to public transportation were not associated with leisure-time walking and moderate-to-Vigorous physical activity (MVPA) [27,28] as well as positive associations with screen time [29]. One possibility is that, as Ding et al. [30] and Rhodes et al. [31] discussed in a previous report, associations between perceived environmental attributes and both physical activity and sedentary behavior tended to differ by country. For example, Taiwanese older adults aged 65 have considerable free or low-cost public transportation services in Taiwanese neighborhoods, such as public light buses, and this policy might encourage older adults to utilize public transport to do more recreational activity. Another possible speculation for these results could be that public transport stops and shops/commercial destinations were strong correlates of activity travel in older adults [32]; thus, positive perceptions of these environmental attributes might influence older adults to partially replace their screen behaviors at home with more outdoor activity. Therefore, this suggests that accessible public transportation and neighborhood shopping are two important environmental attributes that are likely to facilitate leisure-time physical activity and less screen time, particularly in Taiwanese older adults.

Different perceived environmental factors were also associated with leisure-time physical activity. The factors concerning access to recreational facilities, seeing people being active, neighborhood aesthetics, and presence of a destination were related to higher leisure-time physical activity. This supports findings from studies conducted in older adults that differed between western and Asian countries [27,33,34]. This means that the association between these environment characteristics and leisure-time physical activity might be stronger in this population Therefore, these environment characteristics could be enabling older adult to go outside, which might be an important strategy to increase older adults' leisure-time physical activity.

There are generally consistent findings that built environment factors of street connectivity positively related to physical activity [6]. The relationships are less clear for sedentary behavior. The present study found that in older adults, reporting good connectivity of streets was significantly associated with lower screen time. The present finding is inconsistent with those of a previous study in adults from western countries [35] and older adults in Japan [29]. It is possible that street networks might enable older adults to reach destinations directly, which might indirectly reduce how much time older adults spend watching television or using the internet at home. Although the environmental factor of street connectivity was not associated with leisure-time physical activity in these results, it is important to consider that screen-based behavior and physical activity are independent behaviors that can have quite different determinants [36]. This result may strengthen the evidence for several perceived environmental factors associated with screen time, which is crucial for the literature because thus there has been a limited amount of data reported from Asian countries regarding older adults.

The major strengths of this study were its large sample of Asian older adults recruited from nationally representative settings across Taiwan, as well as its examination of a broad range of perceived environmental characteristic correlates of leisure-time physical activity and screen time. It was anticipated that the selected neighborhood design variables would be positively associated with leisure-time physical activity levels, as well as being negatively associated with screen time. Several limitations of the current analysis may have contributed to this. First, the cross-sectional design of the study does not allow us to infer causality. Second, our focus in the current analysis was personal perceptions of environmental characteristics. However, prior research suggests a discrepancy between perception-based insights and actual environmental design features and amenities and suggests that integrating objective and perceived measures may provide a more complete measure of the environment [37]. Nevertheless, it is important to understand and consider older adults' subjective perceptions of environmental features, as these may influence their levels of domain-specific physical activity and screen-based sedentary behavior. Third, the use of self-reported measures for leisure-time physical activity and screen time could be subject to recall error and social desirability bias [21,38]. Fourth, other ecological environmental factors, such as social environment and socio-economic status [39], as well as home environmental factors [3] were not measured, and could possibly have affected older adult' physical activity or screen behavior results. Finally, including segments of the population that did not have a household telephone (approximately 7.1% in 2015) was impossible, thus, the data may not to obtain representative samples [40].

5. Conclusions

The aim of this study was to examine the perceived environmental correlates of leisure-time physical activity and screen time among Taiwanese older adults. The ubiquitous presence of two common environmental features (access to shops and access to public transportation) were concurrently deemed to facilitate both recommendations for leisure-time physical activity and screen time and are likely contributors to these health behaviors. However, different sets of environmental factors were associated with high levels of leisure-time physical activity and lower screen time. This information has obvious local and culturally-specific relevance to current Taiwanese ageing populations. The present findings may provide critical evidence, alerting policy-makers simultaneously to physical activity and sedentary behavior intervention designers so that, in addition to common strategies (access to recreational facilities, seeing people being active, aesthetics, presence of a destination), different intervention strategies should also be considered when promoting leisure-time physical activity and reducing screen time among older adults.

Acknowledgments: This work was supported by a Global Research Network program through the Ministry of Education of the Republic of Korea and the National Research Foundation of Korea (NRF-Project number: NRF-2017S1A2A2038558).

Author Contributions: Conceived and designed the experiments: Ming-Chun, Hsueh, Jong-Hwan Park, Yung Liao. Analyzed the data: Yung Liao, Chien-Yu Lin, Pin-Hsuan Huang. Wrote and revised the paper: Ming-Chun, Hsueh, Chien-Yu Lin, Pin-Hsuan Huang, Jong-Hwan Park. All the authors have read and approved the final manuscript.

Conflicts of Interest: The authors declare no conflict of interest.

References

1. World Health Organization. *Global Status Report on Noncommunicable Diseases 2014*; WHO: Geneva, Switzerland, 2014; Available online: http://www.who.int/nmh/publications/ncd-status-report-2014/en/ (accessed on 1 November 2017).
2. Annear, M.J.; Cushman, G.; Gidlow, B. Leisure time physical activity differences among older adults from diverse socioeconomic neighborhoods. *Health Place* **2009**, *15*, 482–490. [CrossRef] [PubMed]
3. Hsueh, M.C.; Liao, Y.; Chang, S.H. Perceived Neighborhood and Home Environmental Factors Associated with Television Viewing among Taiwanese Older Adults. *Int. J. Environ. Res. Public Health* **2016**, *13*, 708. [CrossRef] [PubMed]
4. Sallis, J.F.; Owen, N.; Fisher, E. Ecological models of health behavior. In *Health Behavior and Health Education: Theory, Research, and Practice*, 4th ed.; John Wiley & Sons: Hoboken, NJ, USA, 2008.
5. Barnett, D.W.; Barnett, A.; Nathan, A.; van Cauwenberg, J.; Cerin, E; Council on Environment and Physical Activity (CEPA)—Older Adults Working Group. Built environmental correlates of older adults' total physical activity and walking: A systematic review and meta-analysis. *Int. J. Behav. Nutr. Phys. Act.* **2017**, *14*, 103. [CrossRef] [PubMed]
6. Van Cauwenberg, J.; de Bourdeaudhuij, I.; de Meester, F.; van Dyck, D.; Salmon, J.; Clarys, P.; Deforche, B. Relationship between the physical environment and physical activity in older adults: A systematic review. *Health Place* **2011**, *17*, 458–469. [CrossRef] [PubMed]
7. Dunstan, D.W.; Howard, B.; Healy, G.N.; Owen, N. Too much sitting—A health hazard. *Diabetes Res. Clin. Pract.* **2012**, *97*, 368–376. [CrossRef] [PubMed]
8. Rezende, L.F.M.; Sa, T.H.; Mielke, G.I.; Viscondi, J.Y.K.; Rey-Lopez, J.P.; Garcia, L.M.T. All-cause mortality attributable to sitting time: Analysis of 54 countries worldwide. *Am. J. Prev. Med.* **2016**, *51*, 253–263. [CrossRef] [PubMed]
9. Harvey, J.A.; Chastin, S.F.; Skelton, D.A. Prevalence of sedentary behavior in older adults: A systematic review. *Int. J. Environ. Res. Public Health* **2013**, *10*, 6645–6661. [CrossRef] [PubMed]

10. Hsueh, M.C.; Liao, Y.; Chang, S.H. Associations of total and domain-specific sedentary time with type 2 diabetes in taiwanese older aults. *J. Epidemiol.* **2016**, *26*, 348–354. [CrossRef] [PubMed]

11. Hu, F.B.; Li, T.Y.; Colditz, G.A.; Willett, W.C.; Manson, J.E. Television watching and other sedentary behaviors in relation to risk of obesity and type 2 diabetes mellitus in women. *JAMA* **2003**, *289*, 1785–1791. [CrossRef] [PubMed]

12. Owen, N.; Sugiyama, T.; Eakin, E.E.; Gardiner, P.A.; Tremblay, M.S.; Sallis, J.F. Adults' sedentary behavior determinants and interventions. *Am. J. Prev. Med.* **2011**, *41*, 189–196. [CrossRef] [PubMed]

13. Shibata, A.; Oka, K.; Sugiyama, T.; Ding, D.; Salmon, J.; Dunstan, D.W.; Owen, N. Perceived neighbourhood environmental attributes and prospective changes in TV viewing time among older Australian adults. *Int. J. Behav. Nutr. Phys. Act.* **2015**, *12*, 50. [CrossRef] [PubMed]

14. Van Cauwenberg, J.; de Donder, L.; Clarys, P.; de Bourdeaudhuij, I.; Owen, N.; Dury, S.; de Witte, N.; Buffel, T.; Verte, D.; Deforche, B. Relationships of individual, social, and physical environmental factors with older adults' television viewing time. *J. Aging Phys. Act.* **2014**, *22*, 508–517. [CrossRef] [PubMed]

15. Lenhart, C.M.; Wiemken, A.; Hanlon, A.; Perkett, M.; Patterson, F. Perceived neighborhood safety related to physical activity but not recreational screen-based sedentary behavior in adolescents. *BMC Public Health* **2017**, *17*, 722. [CrossRef] [PubMed]

16. Carson, V.; Janssen, I. Neighborhood disorder and screen time among 10–16 year old Canadian youth: A cross-sectional study. *Int. J. Behav. Nutr. Phys. Act.* **2012**, *9*, 66. [CrossRef] [PubMed]

17. Compernolle, S.; de Cocker, K.; Roda, C.; Oppert, J.M.; Mackenbach, J.D.; Lakerveld, J.; Glonti, K.; Bardos, H.; Rutter, H.; Cardon, G.; et al. Physical environmental correlates of domain-specific sedentary behaviours across five European regions (the SPOTLIGHT Project). *PLoS ONE* **2016**, *11*, e0164812. [CrossRef] [PubMed]

18. Liou, Y.M. *The Manual of the Short-Telephone Version of International Physical Activity Questionnaires by a Computer Assisted Telephone Interviewing (Cati) System*; The Bureau of Health Promotion, Department of Health: Taipei, Taiwan, 2006.

19. IPAQ Scoring Protocol. Available online: https://sites.google.com/site/theipaq/questionnaire_links (accessed on 1 November 2017).

20. Nelson, M.E.; Rejeski, W.J.; Blair, S.N.; Duncan, P.W.; Judge, J.O.; King, A.C.; Macera, C.A.; Castaneda-Sceppa, C. Physical activity and public health in older adults: Recommendation from the American College of Sports Medicine and the American Heart Association. *Med. Sci. Sports Exerc.* **2007**, *39*, 1435–1445. [CrossRef] [PubMed]

21. Gardiner, P.A.; Clark, B.K.; Healy, G.N.; Eakin, E.G.; Winkler, E.A.; Owen, N. Measuring older adults' sedentary time: Reliability, validity, and responsiveness. *Med. Sci. Sports Exerc.* **2011**, *43*, 2127–2133. [CrossRef] [PubMed]

22. Hamer, M.; Stamatakis, E. Screen-based sedentary behavior, physical activity, and muscle strength in the English longitudinal study of ageing. *PLoS ONE* **2013**, *8*, e66222. [CrossRef] [PubMed]

23. World Health Organization. *Process of Translation and Adaptation of Instruments*; WHO: Geneva, Switzerland, 2014; Available online: http://www.who.int/substance_abuse/research_tools/translation/en/ (accessed on 1 November 2017).

24. The International Physical Activity Prevalence Study (IPS). Environmental Module. Available online: http://sallis.ucsd.edu/Documents/Measures_documents/PANES_survey.pdf (accessed on 1 November 2017).

25. Liao, Y.; Wang, I.T.; Hsu, H.H.; Chang, S.H. Perceived environmental and personal factors associated with walking and cycling for transportation in Taiwanese adults. *Int. J. Environ. Res. Public Health* **2015**, *12*, 2105–2119. [CrossRef] [PubMed]

26. Health Promotion Administration, Ministry of Health and Welfare. Body Mass Index. 2017. Available online: http://health99.hpa.gov.tw/OnlinkHealth/Onlink_BMI.aspx (accessed on 1 November 2017).

27. Inoue, S.; Ohya, Y.; Odagiri, Y.; Takamiya, T.; Kamada, M.; Okada, S.; Oka, K.; Kitabatake, Y.; Nakaya, T.; Sallis, J.F.; et al. Perceived neighborhood environment and walking for specific purposes among elderly Japanese. *J. Epidemiol.* **2011**, *21*, 481–490. [CrossRef] [PubMed]

28. Saito, Y.; Oguma, Y.; Inoue, S.; Tanaka, A.; Kobori, Y. Environmental and individual correlates of various types of physical activity among community-dwelling middle-aged and elderly Japanese. *Int. J. Environ. Res. Public Health* **2013**, *10*, 2028–2042. [CrossRef] [PubMed]

29. Liao, Y.; Shibata, A.; Ishii, K.; Koohsari, M.J.; Oka, K. Cross-sectional and prospective associations of neighborhood environmental attributes with screen time in Japanese middle-aged and older adults. *BMJ Open* **2018**, *8*, e019608. [CrossRef] [PubMed]

30. Ding, D.; Adams, M.A.; Sallis, J.F.; Norman, G.J.; Hovell, M.F.; Chambers, C.D.; Hofstetter, C.R.; Bowles, H.R.; Hagstromer, M.; Craig, C.L.; et al. Perceived neighborhood environment and physical activity in 11 countries: Do associations differ by country? *Int. J. Behav. Nutr. Phys. Act.* **2013**, *10*, 57. [CrossRef] [PubMed]

31. Rhodes, R.E.; Mark, R.S.; Temmel, C.P. Adult sedentary behavior: A systematic review. *Am. J. Prev. Med.* **2012**, *42*, e3–e28. [CrossRef] [PubMed]

32. Cerin, E.; Nathan, A.; van Cauwenberg, J.; Barnett, D.W.; Barnett, A.; Council on Environment and Physical Activity (CEPA)—Older Adults Working Group. The neighbourhood physical environment and active travel in older adults: A systematic review and meta-analysis. *Int. J. Behav. Nutr. Phys. Act.* **2017**, *14*, 15. [CrossRef] [PubMed]

33. Salvador, E.P.; Reis, R.S.; Florindo, A.A. Practice of walking and its association with perceived environment among elderly Brazilians living in a region of low socioeconomic level. *Int. J. Behav. Nutr. Phys. Act.* **2010**, *7*, 67. [CrossRef] [PubMed]

34. Li, F.; Fisher, K.J.; Brownson, R.C.; Bosworth, M. Multilevel modelling of built environment characteristics related to neighbourhood walking activity in older adults. *J. Epidemiol. Community Health* **2005**, *59*, 558–564. [CrossRef] [PubMed]

35. Van Dyck, D.; Cerin, E.; Conway, T.L.; de Bourdeaudhuij, I.; Owen, N.; Kerr, J.; Cardon, G.; Frank, L.D.; Saelens, B.E.; Sallis, J.F. Associations between perceived neighborhood environmental attributes and adults' sedentary behavior: Findings from the USA, Australia and Belgium. *Soc. Sci. Med.* **2012**, *74*, 1375–1384. [CrossRef] [PubMed]

36. Salmon, J.; Owen, N.; Crawford, D.; Bauman, A.; Sallis, J.F. Physical activity and sedentary behavior: A population-based study of barriers, enjoyment, and preference. *Health Psychol.* **2003**, *22*, 178–188. [CrossRef] [PubMed]

37. Hinckson, E.; Cerin, E.; Mavoa, S.; Smith, M.; Badland, H.; Stewart, T.; Duncan, S.; Schofield, G. Associations of the perceived and objective neighborhood environment with physical activity and sedentary time in New Zealand adolescents. *Int. J. Behav. Nutr. Phys. Act.* **2017**, *14*, 145. [CrossRef] [PubMed]

38. Liou, Y.M.; Jwo, C.J.; Yao, K.G.; Chiang, L.C.; Huang, L.H. Selection of appropriate Chinese terms to represent intensity and types of physical activity terms for use in the Taiwan version of IPAQ. *J. Nurs. Res.* **2008**, *16*, 252–263. [CrossRef] [PubMed]

39. Yen, I.H.; Michael, Y.L.; Perdue, L. Neighborhood environment in studies of health of older adults: A systematic review. *Am. J. Prev. Med.* **2009**, *37*, 455–463. [CrossRef] [PubMed]

40. Report on the Survey of Family Income and Expendture; Directorate General of Budget, Accounting and Statistics: Taipei, Taiwan. 2015. Available online: http://win.dgbas.gov.tw/fies/doc/result/104.pdf (accessed on 1 December 2017).

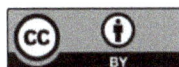

Journal of
Clinical Medicine

MDPI

Review

Exergaming for Children and Adolescents: Strengths, Weaknesses, Opportunities and Threats

Valentin Benzing * and **Mirko Schmidt**

Institute of Sport Science, University of Bern, 3012 Bern, Switzerland; mirko.schmidt@ispw.unibe.ch
* Correspondence: valentin.benzing@ispw.unibe.ch; Tel.: +41-31-631-45-48

Received: 15 October 2018; Accepted: 2 November 2018; Published: 8 November 2018

Abstract: Exergaming, or active video gaming, has become an emerging trend in fitness, education and health sectors. It is defined as digital games that require bodily movements to play, stimulating an active gaming experience to function as a form of physical activity (PA). Since exergaming is becoming more popular, claims have been made on the usefulness of exergaming. It has, for example, been entitled as being "the future of fitness" by the American College of Sports Medicine, promoting PA and health in children and adolescents. However, research also suggests that long-term engagement in exergaming is difficult to achieve, and there is a noticeable reservation towards exergaming by parents, teachers and caregivers. To provide an overview and to outline the future directions of exergaming, the aim of this review was to critically illustrate the strengths, weaknesses, opportunities and threats of exergaming to promote PA and health in children and youth. The available evidence indicates that exergaming has the potential to improve health via an increase in PA. However, it seems that this potential is frequently underexploited, and further developments such as customized exergames are needed.

Keywords: active video gaming; serious games; physical activity; physical exercise; sedentary behavior; narrative review

1. Introduction

Across the globe, the majority of adolescents are not reaching the recommended amount of physical activity [1], consequently impacting their physical and mental health [2–4]. Reasons for decreased physical activity levels may be caused by various factors, including the fact that children and adolescents spend much more time sedentary in front of the screen than in the past [5]. Because of the increased sedentary screen time, exergaming (or active video gaming) might bear potential for making children and adolescents more active, and thus positively affecting their health [6]. Therefore, the question is whether exergaming can indeed positively affect sedentary behavior and health in children and adolescents. Before discussing the effects of exergaming in children and adolescents on physical activity and health, several general issues must be addressed.

Firstly, it is important to outline what comes under the umbrella term of exergaming. To date, there is no universal definition of exergaming available. According to Bogost [7] exergaming has been labeled by the media as "the combination of exercise and videogames". Although this description has been used by both the commercial industry and in the scientific field [8,9], it does not serve as a suitable formal definition. This becomes apparent when adhering to the traditional definition of "exercise", as intentionally to improve or maintain physical fitness with a planned, repetitive, and structured format (Caspersen et al. [10]), according to which many available exergames (for example, those with alternative intentions than improving fitness) would be excluded [11]. To overcome this issue, broader definitions have been used, describing exergaming as "interactive video gaming that stimulates an active, whole-body gaming experience" [6], or according to Gao et al. [12], it "refer[s] to videogames that require bodily movement to play and function as a form of physical activity". Since some exergames do not necessarily involve whole-body movements, and considering that there is potential for the focus to be not only on the visual but on the tactile or auditory domains in the future, we propose to combine both definitions, and exchange videogames with digital games. Consequently, for the purpose of the current analysis, the term exergames will refer to digital games that require bodily movements to play, stimulating an active gaming experience to function as a form of physical activity.

Although exergames have been available since the 1980s [6], in research it has received increased attention only in the last ten years [13]. Since then, the number of articles published related to exergaming or active video gaming has substantially increased. Although exergaming is still in its infancy, several reviews and meta-analyses regarding its potential usefulness to promote physical activity and health have already been published [14,15]. The majority of these studies have been performed within the health sector, in particular public health and rehabilitation [16]. Besides medicine, however, other disciplines such as psychology, sport science, neuroscience or computer science are also involving exergames in their research, showing the interdisciplinary nature of this intervention.

Exergaming is diverse. Reflecting the manifold research disciplines, exergaming is applied in many fields of application, including prevention [17], treatment [18] and rehabilitation [19,20]. Application also reaches a vast range of individuals, including both clinical and non-clinical populations [21]. This diversity is also exhibited in the target age groups, ranging from young children [6] to the elderly [22]. Since children and adolescents seem particularly attracted to video games, these age groups have been identified as a group who will have "special interests in and benefit from exergames" [23]. Consequently, besides the elderly, exergaming research has primarily focused on younger age groups.

Moreover, similarly to traditional exercise [24,25], exergames vary in quantitative and qualitative exercise characteristics. According to Pesce [25], quantitative parameters such as duration and intensity focus on a "medical" perspective, examining dose-response relationships. Whereas, qualitative parameters, which are globally defined as type or mode of exercise, reflect non-physical aspects of exercise tasks, such as cognitive or coordinative demands [25]. In exergaming an interplay of these factors (see Figure 1) may be crucial with regard to eliciting benefits in physical, cognitive and psychosocial target variables. In summary, exergaming may be considered as multifaceted and dependent on a variety of factors.

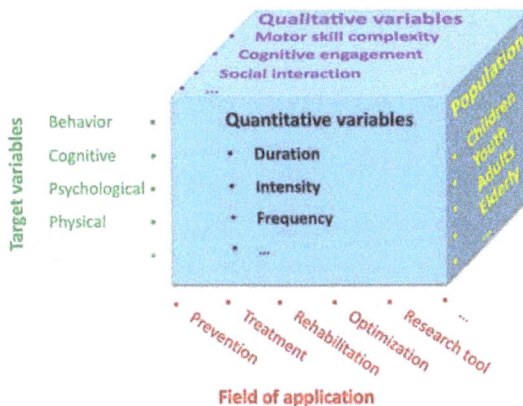

Figure 1. Overview of different dimensions associated with exergaming.

The dramatic increase in interest associated with exergaming has risen due to a variety of factors, including the technical advances which have enabled individuals to play exergames at home, and because it bears unique strengths and opportunities, such as specificity and adaptivity. In contrast to these positive factors, however, there is an uncertainty (e.g., from parents, teachers etc.) regarding the usefulness of exergaming when considering the specific weaknesses and threats associated with use in pediatric populations. Therefore, the aim of this review was to give an overview on the Strengths, Weaknesses, Opportunities and Threats (SWOT) associated with pediatric exergaming. Since exergaming is a highly diverse and a rich topic (see Figure 1), we have limited this review to include the most important dimensions for children and adolescents, basing our work on examples relevant to this population and their physical activity and health.

2. Strengths

One of the greatest strengths of exergaming (for an overview about strengths, weaknesses, opportunities and threats see Figure 2) is that it seems to increase the motivation and engagement in physical activity [26,27]. This is supported by results from previous research, demonstrating that exergaming elicits motivational gains, as well as flow, immersion and enjoyment [28,29]. The importance of enjoyment is gaining more attention in exergaming research because it seems to be an important variable in sustaining a higher physical activity level [23]. Moreover, a greater enjoyment within physical activity has been found to be important for cognitive benefits, which in turn are thought to positively influence academic achievement [30]. Although, it is currently unclear which game design characteristics maximize motivation and enjoyment, it is assumed to be important in explaining why it is easier to achieve a certain physical activity level when using the right exergame [31].

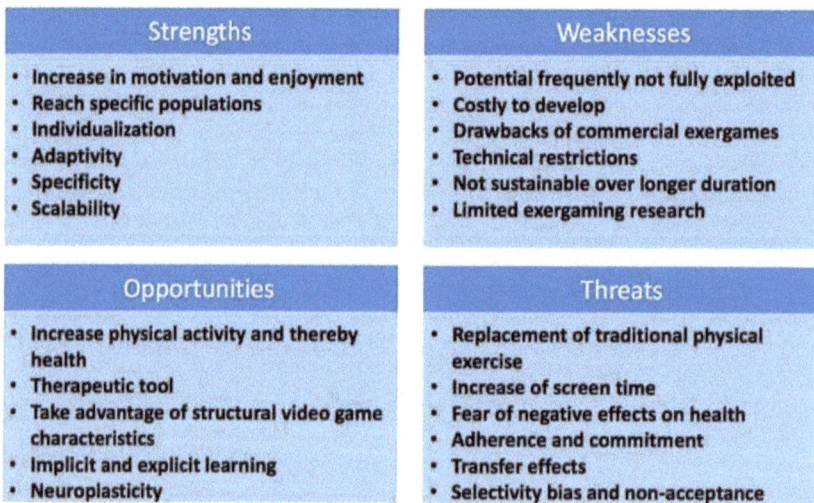

Strengths	Weaknesses
• Increase in motivation and enjoyment • Reach specific populations • Individualization • Adaptivity • Specificity • Scalability	• Potential frequently not fully exploited • Costly to develop • Drawbacks of commercial exergames • Technical restrictions • Not sustainable over longer duration • Limited exergaming research
Opportunities	**Threats**
• Increase physical activity and thereby health • Therapeutic tool • Take advantage of structural video game characteristics • Implicit and explicit learning • Neuroplasticity	• Replacement of traditional physical exercise • Increase of screen time • Fear of negative effects on health • Adherence and commitment • Transfer effects • Selectivity bias and non-acceptance

Figure 2. Strengths, weaknesses, opportunities and threats associated with exergaming in children and adolescents.

Another advantage of exergaming is that it helps to reach specific populations. This might be particularly important for children who are not meeting the recommended amount of physical activity through traditional methods, or who spend much time playing video games. In this way, it has been shown that exergaming bears the potential to reduce obesity [13,17]. Exergaming can be integrated into the school curriculum, contributing to getting children active, and consequently promoting positive effects on body mass index and fitness [26,32,33]. Moreover, children with attention deficit hyperactivity disorder, for example, who spend more time playing sedentary video games than typically developing children, might find exergames to be a viable option to replace sedentary screen time [34]. Therefore, due to the attraction of video games in specific populations, it is possible that children who are more sedentary could be reached to increase physical activity, resulting in a variety of physical and cognitive health benefits [35].

Another strength of exergaming is that it allows for individualization and adaptivity [36]. In this way, an exergaming session may be tailored to fit the needs of an individual. So, for example, important characteristics of the child such as the fitness level can be taken into account to avoid under- and overload [37]. Moreover, not only an initial assessment, but continuous measurement and adjustment can be completed with exergaming. An adjustment during the training by an algorithm combined with immediate feedback to the individual has the potential to ensure that the individual always trains at the "sweet spot". So, for example, physical and cognitive challenge may be monitored and adjusted, assuming that well-adjusted physically and cognitively engaging physical activities provide more training gains [9]. Thus, not only physical but also mental benefits may be enhanced, which in turn holds relevance for promoting academic achievement [25,38,39], creating an additional benefit of exergaming [40].

Specificity is a further advantage of exergaming. In a virtual environment, there are unlimited opportunities to create exergames for specific training purposes e.g., isolated movements may be trained and repeated in an infinite number of trials. Using such adaptations ensures that skill development in physical education [37] or in elite sports [41] can be trained. However, currently the most frequent implementation of specificity is in rehabilitation. The benefits of specificity in this field is demonstrated by studies which show that exergaming improves gross motor skills of atypically developing children [42], acting as a useful rehabilitation tool in this population (e.g., balance control) [43]. Moreover, task-specific or outcome-specific trainings seem to be a prerequisite for positive effects [44,45].

Another strength is the high scalability and economic feasibility of exergames. Most exergames use commercial game consoles and can be connected to a conventional TV screen. Therefore, exergaming can be applied almost anywhere, at any time. Since many families in developed countries have their own TV at home, and some even a game console, this results in high scalability, and the potential for distribution to reach many households.

In summary, exergaming has the potential to increase physical activity, and thus positively impact physical, cognitive and psychosocial target variables [46]. Moreover, certain populations are particularly likely to benefit from exergaming, for example, children who are inactive and not interested in traditional exercise [23]. Thus, it can be concluded that with exergaming, increased media consumption doesn't necessarily have to mean reduced physical activity. Having this in mind, exergaming could provide a useful adjunct to traditional methods of physical activity, however, there are also several potential weaknesses associated with exergaming that should be taken into consideration.

3. Weaknesses

It could be argued that one of the greatest weaknesses of exergaming is that its potential is frequently underexploited. When considering the aforementioned strengths, it becomes clear that to obtain the most beneficial effects, exergames have to be tailored to the target population, as well as the target variables [36]. However, tailoring exergames is costly and takes a long time to develop, therefore this is not often done. Although alternative factors (such as behavior change procedures) that enhance the effects of exergames and may also be applied to commercially available games have been proposed [47], more systematic collaborations between science and industry are needed.

The technical capabilities and resources of professional game publishers are substantial, consequently leading to more sophisticated, entertaining and appealing exergames. These more sophisticated exergames might be advantageous with regard to fun and enjoyment, however, there are also drawbacks specific to commercial exergames. Besides less individuality, adaptivity and specificity of these untailored exergames, generally it is difficult to access the data of the exergame, for example, to control for fidelity of implementation and energy expenditure consumption [48]. This makes it difficult to fully exploit the benefits of exergaming as a monitoring tool, for example in clinical populations or in a school setting.

Another technical consideration is that the gaming experience as well as the elicited energy expenditure of exergames is highly dependent on the virtual environment as well as on the technical capabilities, such as the sensors [47,49]. This is reflected in the finding that exergames involving lower body movements elicit more energy expenditure, thus both the virtual environment and the technical implementation is important [49]. Although there are several different sensor technologies available, including hand-held motion sensors as well as motion capture technology, there are problems attached to both. Hand-held motion sensors make it easy to cheat, whereby the computer believes that the child is engaging in the physical activity when they are in fact stationary [47]. For motion capture technology, although it seems to encourage more energy expenditure [50], it was found to be error-prone [51]. This in turn is problematic with regard to adherence and drop-out, where technical difficulties discourage the user from participation [51,52].

Besides technical issues, it seems that current exergames are not able to keep the interest of players over longer time periods [53]. This can be explained by the reasons frequently given for dropout in exergaming interventions, indicating that the played exergames became boring [51,52]. This points to a lack in variety and immersion in the currently available exergames. Although dropout rates have been found to be smaller in multiplayer modes, it seems that current exergames are not sustainable in general. Thus, although exergaming can elicit moderate to vigorous intensities [54], other factors increasing adherence have to be considered, and sustainable play is yet to be proven [55].

Considering that exergaming has only been developed in the last decades, there has already been a great amount of research done so far. Nevertheless, exergaming research is limited, and there are many issues that remain unclear. For example, it is unknown whether exergaming will replace traditional exercises or sedentary behaviors (see threats section). This is of great importance considering that a frequent goal of exergaming is to increase physical activity levels. Moreover, exergaming has rarely been compared or combined with traditional exercises in children [33,56], and it is unclear whether exergaming results in as much physical activity as traditional exercises, and also how long potential positive effects of exergaming persist [57–59]. Since exergaming is highly diverse, and most studies apply different games, more studies investigating the underlying mechanisms as well as the specific exergaming characteristics and their impact on physical activity levels are needed.

Taken together, the potential of exergaming is frequently underexploited, and in order to make the best use of exergaming in the future, more games should be customized to meet the needs of specific populations [36]. Although customizing exergames is currently costly and limited by technical considerations, exergaming technology is advancing and becoming more affordable, creating potential opportunities for future development.

4. Opportunities

Although in exergaming research, a variety of strengths have already shown its potential, a major opportunity of exergaming is to further develop these strengths. So, for example, a major opportunity of exergaming (which has been shown to some extent) is that it helps to get children and adolescents active, which would promote motor skills, cognitive performance as well as mental health. Physical inactivity is a major health factor in children and adults due to the many harmful effects on both physical [3] and mental health [4]. Considering that most children and adolescents in Europe and the US play video games [60], exergaming could become an important tool to promote physical activity, reach individuals that could not be reached by alternative methods, and promote positive effects on cognitive performance, mental and physical health [46].

The use of video games as a therapeutic tool is promising [61]. Children and adolescents in clinical as well as rehabilitative settings may benefit from exergaming. It has already been shown in rehabilitation that exergaming has the potential to improve general as well as disease specific outcomes [44]. Moreover, there is promising evidence showing that exergaming is feasible as a physiotherapeutic intervention in adults [62], and that children's motor learning may even be enhanced by practice in a virtual environment [63]. Thus, in the future, exergaming may be used by occupational or physiotherapists to reach those who cannot do traditional physical therapy due to their physical condition or location. Since exergaming is highly scalable, it could be utilizable for a variety of diseases and disorders in the future. In this way, exergaming could be used as a form of therapy/rehabilitation to help to get many children active who cannot be reached, due to their distant location for example, or their inability to leave the hospital due to their disease [64].

Additionally, the applied exergames could serve as a continuous diagnostic tool. While playing, information about the state of the user (including psychophysiological data) could be logged. The computer or a caregiver could then access the diagnostic information and automatically or manually adjust the exergame to suit the needs of the individual [36]. Furthermore, it is probable that in the future, multiple technical devices access and share their data to provide an optimized training including exergaming, augmented reality and traditional exercises.

Several factors are suggested to be important for successful interventions. These factors include both hardware and software as well as many structural characteristics, which lead to both immersion and increased motivation to play video games [65,66]. In children and adolescents, a goal would be to use comparable output hardware as well as game elements [66] and structural characteristics of video games [65] in exergaming. In further detail, these characteristics could include multiple levels, such as social, manipulation and control, narrative and identity, reward and punishment and presentation features [65]. A systematic inclusion of these characteristics could help to enhance exergaming, facilitate initiation and maintenance and finally replace sedentary behavior with physical activity.

As another opportunity, learning (of motor skills for example) can occur both implicitly and explicitly in exergaming, since it is possible to learn movements embedded in a story without formal instruction [45]. This combination of playful non-instructive learning with informative instructive learning bears great potential for children and adolescents, but must be investigated further in the future.

Moreover, exergaming has the potential to stimulate neuroplasticity through environmental enrichment and task complexity. Neuroplasticity refers to "the capacity of the nervous system to modify its organization" [67]. These adaptations for example can occur as a consequence of skill training, resulting in learning and skill acquisition [68]. Since research has shown that environmental enrichment seems to stimulate cognitive functions [69] as well as neural and synaptic growth [70], exergaming consequently has the potential to promote neuroplasticity. However, not only novel or enriched environments, but also physical exercise [68] and task complexity [71] seems to facilitate neuroplasticity. Since as mentioned before, a strength of exergaming is adaptivity, task complexity can be kept on a (optimal) challenging level in a changing virtual environment, altogether contributing to facilitated neuroplasticity.

Considering the mentioned opportunities, it is suggested to specifically implement existing strengths of exergames such as adaptivity, specificity and individuality in a more systematic fashion. Furthermore, to enhance potential benefits and increase adherence, one could include structural video game characteristics as well as sound exergaming procedures, such as involving parents in game play [47,65,72]. However, these advances might also be associated with a variety of new and unexpected threats which should be considered.

5. Threats

The most likely risk of exergaming, whilst also being responsible for some of the greatest strengths, is that exergaming takes place in a virtual environment. Because of this circumstance, there are concerns that exergaming replaces traditional physical exercises and increases screen time.

One of the greatest threats of exergaming revolves around the question of whether traditional physical activity is replaced by exergaming. Given that in exergaming research a major aim is to increase physical activity levels and impact physical health (e.g., in obesity), a replacement of traditional exercises would have an adverse effect. There is first evidence in overweight and obese adolescent girls, indicating that an exergaming intervention may result in increased self-reported physical activity and less TV watching. However, the results are somewhat inconclusive since there was no increase in physical activity provided by accelerometry [73]. Nevertheless, in the scientific community, it is well established that exergaming should not, and cannot replace traditional physical exercise [46]. On the contrary, the underlying idea is that it should replace sedentary behavior such as video gaming. Since there is currently not enough scientific evidence on this issue, this risk must be researched in future studies and monitored carefully.

Whether exergaming increases screen time substantially is also unclear from a scientific standpoint. On the one hand, it is possible that applied exergaming interventions, in physical education (PE) for example, increase screen time to a smaller extent. On the other hand, research has shown that PE combined with exergaming revealed greater improvements with regard to fitness and BMI than PE alone [33]. Therefore, exergaming might be a gateway to sedentary people. Consequently, to fully evaluate the effects caused by the added active screen time, further research is needed to investigate both the positive effects of more physical activity and the negative effects evolving from more screen time.

Related to this issue, the underlying assumption of people who fear increases in screen time is that exergaming has negative effects on the mental health of children and adolescents. Here it is thought that exergames will cause social isolation due to excessive video gaming, or increase aggression [74]. This fear, however, is likely based on previous research about sedentary violent video games [75] and problematic gaming behavior [76]. In contrast to these findings, research also revealed positive effects of sedentary video games on cognition, motivation, emotion and social benefits [77,78], meaning that the hypothesized negative effects of sedentary video gaming are currently subject to controversial debate [79]. Most importantly, it is questionable whether the negative effects of specific types of sedentary video games can be easily transferred to active video games, since these games can only be played limitedly due to the level of physical exertion and reaching fatigue. Nevertheless, this fear leads to a reservation towards exergaming, which consequently threatens adherence and commitment.

The transferability from exergaming to the real world is uncertain. Another risk refers to the controversial debate in the cognitive training literature regarding the transferability of skills from a (virtual) training to the real world [80,81]. Since near transfer effects are easier obtained, the virtual environment can be systematically designed to come as close to real world settings as possible [41,82]. Although exergaming offers this unique potential to increase transfer effects compared with previous video games, it is also likely that transfer effects are limited by the choice of exergames. Thus, theory driven approaches [72] for example using the identical elements theory [83] in order to increase transfer effects are needed.

Finally, exergaming might attract certain individuals, which potentially introduces selectivity bias. Research has shown a non-acceptance of potential users because of the digital nature of the games [51]. Thus, due to the technical implementation of exergaming utilizing game consoles and the virtual environment, exergaming itself might lead to an attraction of certain individuals [34]. Since, for example, more boys are playing video games than girls [76], a risk might be that boys in particular are attracted by exergaming. This in turn could lead to a selectivity bias in research and practice [34]. Notably, as with every novel technology, exergaming must first prove its value to convince different potential users, parents, teachers and caregivers. Nevertheless, researchers and game developers should pay attention to the inclusion of different target groups.

Taken together, these potential threats indicate that exergaming should not be a substitute for traditional sports or exercises [46], and that an increase in screen time has to be monitored carefully in order to prevent potential negative effects. Among others, the most important future challenges include the increase of transfer effects by using theory driven approaches, such as the identical elements theory, which might help to specifically target intended outcome variables during exergaming [83].

6. Summary

The current SWOT analysis reveals that exergaming has a variety of strengths, most notably identifying the potential for individualization, adaptivity and specificity. Additionally, the increased motivation and engagement, and the potential to reach specific populations lay the foundations for exergaming to promote physical activity and health in children and adolescents successfully.

However, there are also weaknesses associated with exergaming, which mostly involve its implementation. In further detail, it seems that the potential of exergaming is frequently underexploited, and that in previous exergaming studies, there is limited systematic inclusion of theories and underlying mechanisms.

Since exergaming is a relatively new technological achievement, promising opportunities such as getting people active as well as promoting motor skills, cognitive performance and mental health warrant further investigation. However, substantial modifications must be monitored continuously and carefully regarding potential threats, most importantly considering the risk of replacement of traditional physical exercise, and the risk of increased screen time.

Taken together, since most children and adolescents in Europe and the US play video games [60], we are already past the point of no return. Thus, the question is no longer whether children and adolescents are playing video games and how can we prevent them from doing so, but how we can positively impact what type of digital games they use, and for what purpose they are playing. Considering this, exergaming could be a viable tool to positively influence the screen time experience of children and adolescents.

7. Limitations

This SWOT analysis suffers from weaknesses which are worth noting. First, it might be that strengths and positive effects are more likely to become published than null or even negative effects. Having this publication bias in mind, the current analysis might also lean towards the strengths of exergaming. Thus, more empirical research, not only investigating whether there is a positive effect or no effect of exergaming on specific variables, but specifically focusing on the potential negative effects is needed. Second, it is impossible to make a truly objective SWOT analysis [84]. One could even say that a SWOT analysis is subjective by definition, since a weighting on the importance of aspects must be done. Therefore, this analysis also contains subjective opinions. Third, the current SWOT analysis has no claim to be complete. The aim was to collect and identify the most important aspects, however, this review is not exhaustive.

Author Contributions: All listed authors made substantial contributions to this manuscript. V.B. wrote a first draft of the manuscript. M.S. reviewed and commented on the manuscript. All authors approved the final version of the manuscript.

Funding: This research received no external funding.

Acknowledgments: Many thanks to Amie Wallman-Jones for her helpful comments on the manuscript.

Conflicts of Interest: The authors declare no conflict of interest.

References

1. Kalman, M.; Inchley, J.; Sigmundova, D.; Iannotti, R.J.; Tynjälä, J.A.; Hamrik, Z.; Haug, E.; Bucksch, J. Secular trends in moderate-to-vigorous physical activity in 32 countries from 2002 to 2010: A cross-national perspective. *Eur. J. Public Health* **2015**, *25*, 37–40. [CrossRef] [PubMed]
2. Swinburn, B.A.; Sacks, G.; Hall, K.D.; McPherson, K.; Finegood, D.T.; Moodie, M.L.; Gortmaker, S.L. The global obesity pandemic: Shaped by global drivers and local environments. *Lancet* **2011**, *378*, 804–814. [CrossRef]
3. Poitras, V.J.; Gray, C.F.; Borghese, M.M.; Carson, V.; Chaput, J.; Janssen, I.; Katzmarzyk, P.T.; Pate, R.R.; Connor Gorber, S.; Kho, M.E.; et al. Systematic review of the relationships between objectively measured physical activity and health indicators in school-aged children and youth. *Appl. Physiol. Nutr. Metab.* **2016**, *41*, S197–S239. [CrossRef] [PubMed]
4. Lubans, D.; Richards, J.; Hillman, C.; Faulkner, G.; Beauchamp, M.; Nilsson, M.; Kelly, P.; Smith, J.; Raine, L.; Biddle, S. Physical activity for cognitive and mental health in youth: A systematic review of mechanisms. *Pediatrics* **2016**, *138*, e20161642. [CrossRef] [PubMed]

5.   Owen, N.; Sparling, P.B.; Healy, G.N.; Dunstan, D.W.; Matthews, C.E. Sedentary behavior: Emerging evidence for a new health risk. *Mayo Clin. Proc.* **2010**, *85*, 1138–1141. [CrossRef] [PubMed]
6.   Best, J.R. Exergaming in youth. *Zeitschrift für Psychol.* **2013**, *221*, 72–78. [CrossRef] [PubMed]
7.   Bogost, I. *Persuasive Games: The Expressive Power of Videogames*; The MIT Press: Cambridge, MA, USA; London, UK, 2007; ISBN 9780262026147.
8.   Best, J.R. Exergaming immediately enhances children's executive function. *Dev. Psychol.* **2012**, *48*, 1501–1510. [CrossRef] [PubMed]
9.   Benzing, V.; Heinks, T.; Eggenberger, N.; Schmidt, M. Acute cognitively engaging exergame-based physical activity enhances executive functions in adolescents. *PLoS ONE* **2016**, *11*, e0167501. [CrossRef] [PubMed]
10. Caspersen, C.J.; Powell, K.E.; Christenson, G.M. Physical activity, exercise, and physical fitness: Definitions and distinctions for health-related research. *Public Health Rep.* **1985**, *100*, 126–131. [PubMed]
11. Yang, S. Defining Exergames & Exergaming. *Proc. Meaningful Play* **2010**, 1 17.
12. Gao, Z.; Lee, J.E.; Pope, Z.; Zhang, D. Effect of active videogames on underserved children's classroom behaviors, effort, and fitness. *Games Health J.* **2016**, *5*, 318–324. [CrossRef] [PubMed]
13. Gao, Z.; Chen, S.; Pasco, D.; Pope, Z. A meta-analysis of active video games on health outcomes among children and adolescents. *Obes. Rev.* **2015**, *16*, 783–794. [CrossRef] [PubMed]
14. Donath, L.; Rössler, R.; Faude, O. Effects of virtual reality training (exergaming) compared to alternative exercise training and passive control on standing balance and functional mobility in healthy community-dwelling seniors: A meta-analytical review. *Sport. Med.* **2016**, *46*, 1293–1309. [CrossRef] [PubMed]
15. Ennis, C.D. Implications of exergaming for the physical education curriculum in the 21st century. *J. Sport Health Sci.* **2013**, *2*, 152–157. [CrossRef]
16. Taylor, M.J.D.; Griffin, M. The use of gaming technology for rehabilitation in people with multiple sclerosis. *Mult. Scler.* **2015**, *21*, 355–371. [CrossRef] [PubMed]
17. Gao, Z.; Chen, S. Are field-based exergames useful in preventing childhood obesity? A systematic review. *Obes. Rev.* **2014**, *15*, 676–691. [CrossRef] [PubMed]
18. Barry, G.; Galna, B.; Rochester, L. The role of exergaming in Parkinson's disease rehabilitation: A systematic review of the evidence. *J. Neuroeng. Rehabil.* **2014**, *11*, 33. [CrossRef] [PubMed]
19. Benzing, V.; Eggenberger, N.; Spitzhüttl, J.; Siegwart, V.; Pastore-Wapp, M.; Kiefer, C.; Slavova, N.; Grotzer, M.; Heinks, T.; Schmidt, M.; et al. The Brainfit study: Efficacy of cognitive training and exergaming in pediatric cancer survivors—A randomized controlled trial. *BMC Cancer* **2018**, *18*, 18. [CrossRef] [PubMed]
20. Benzing, V.; Schmidt, M. Cognitively and physically demanding exergaming to improve executive functions of children with attention deficit hyperactivity disorder. *BMC Pediatr.* **2017**, *17*, 8. [CrossRef] [PubMed]
21. Stanmore, E.; Stubbs, B.; Vancampfort, D.; de Bruin, E.D.; Firth, J. The effect of active video games on cognitive functioning in clinical and non-clinical populations: A meta-analysis of randomized controlled trials. *Neurosci. Biobehav. Rev.* **2017**, *78*, 34–43. [CrossRef] [PubMed]
22. Zeng, N.; Pope, Z.; Lee, J.E.; Gao, Z. A systematic review of active video games on rehabilitative outcomes among older patients. *J. Sport Health Sci.* **2017**, *6*, 33–43. [CrossRef] [PubMed]
23. Baranowski, T. Exergaming: Hope for future physical activity? or blight on mankind? *J. Sport Health Sci.* **2017**, *6*, 44–46. [CrossRef] [PubMed]
24. Garber, C.E.; Blissmer, B.; Deschenes, M.R.; Franklin, B.A.; Lamonte, M.J.; Lee, I.-M.; Nieman, D.C.; Swain, D.P. Quantity and quality of exercise for developing and maintaining cardiorespiratory, musculoskeletal, and neuromotor fitness in apparently healthy adults. *Med. Sci. Sport. Exerc.* **2011**, *43*, 1334–1359. [CrossRef] [PubMed]
25. Pesce, C. Shifting the focus from quantitative to qualitative exercise characteristics in exercise and cognition research. *J. Sport Exerc. Psychol.* **2012**, *34*, 766–786. [CrossRef] [PubMed]
26. Vaghetti, C.A.O.; Monteiro-Junior, R.S.; Finco, M.D.; Reategui, E.; Silva da Costa Botelho, S. Exergames experience in physical education: A review. *Phys. Cult. Sport. Stud. Res.* **2018**, *78*, 23–32. [CrossRef]
27. Kato, P.M. Video games in health care: Closing the gap. *Rev. Gen. Psychol.* **2010**, *14*, 113–121. [CrossRef]
28. Lee, S.; Kim, W.; Park, T.; Peng, W. The psychological effects of playing exergames: A systematic review. *Cyberpsychol. Behav. Soc. Netw.* **2017**, *20*, cyber.2017.0183. [CrossRef] [PubMed]
29. Feltz, D.L.; Forlenza, S.T.; Winn, B.; Kerr, N.L. Cyber buddy is better than no buddy: A test of the Köhler Motivation Effect in exergames. *Games Health J.* **2014**, *3*, 98–105. [CrossRef] [PubMed]

30. Schmidt, M.; Benzing, V.; Kamer, M. Classroom-based physical activity breaks and children's attention: Cognitive engagement works! *Front. Psychol.* **2016**, *7*, 1474. [CrossRef] [PubMed]
31. Mellecker, R.; Lyons, E.J.; Baranowski, T. Disentangling fun and enjoyment in exergames using an expanded design, play, experience framework: A narrative review. *Games Health J.* **2013**, *2*, 142–149. [CrossRef] [PubMed]
32. Gao, Z.; Pope, Z.; Lee, J.E.; Stodden, D.; Roncesvalles, N.; Pasco, D.; Huang, C.C.; Feng, D. Impact of exergaming on young children's school day energy expenditure and moderate-to-vigorous physical activity levels. *J. Sport Health Sci.* **2017**, *6*, 11–16. [CrossRef] [PubMed]
33. Ye, S.; Lee, J.; Stodden, D.; Gao, Z. Impact of exergaming on children's motor skill competence and health-related fitness: A quasi-experimental study. *J. Clin. Med.* **2018**, *7*, 261. [CrossRef] [PubMed]
34. Benzing, V.; Chang, Y.-K.; Schmidt, M. Acute physical activity enhances executive functions in children with ADHD. *Sci. Rep.* **2018**, *8*, 12382. [CrossRef] [PubMed]
35. Finco, M.D.; Reategui, E.; Zaro, M.A.; Sheehan, D.D.; Katz, L. Exergaming as an alternative for students unmotivated to participate in regular physical education classes. *Int. J. Game-Based Learn.* **2015**, *5*, 1–10. [CrossRef]
36. Mishra, J.; Anguera, J.A.; Gazzaley, A. Video games for neuro-cognitive optimization. *Neuron* **2016**, *90*, 214–218. [CrossRef] [PubMed]
37. Staiano, A.E.; Calvert, S.L. Exergames for physical education courses: Physical, social, and cognitive benefits. *Child Dev. Perspect.* **2011**, *5*, 93–98. [CrossRef] [PubMed]
38. Budde, H.; Voelcker-Rehage, C.; Pietraßyk-Kendziorra, S.; Ribeiro, P.; Tidow, G. Acute coordinative exercise improves attentional performance in adolescents. *Neurosci. Lett.* **2008**, *441*, 219–223. [CrossRef] [PubMed]
39. Vazou, S.; Pesce, C.; Lakes, K.; Smiley-Oyen, A. More than one road leads to Rome: A narrative review and meta-analysis of physical activity intervention effects on cognition in youth. *Int. J. Sport Exerc. Psychol.* **2016**, 1–26. [CrossRef]
40. Moreau, D.; Conway, A.R.A. The case for an ecological approach to cognitive training. *Trends Cogn. Sci.* **2014**, *18*, 334–336. [CrossRef] [PubMed]
41. Neumann, D.L.; Moffitt, R.L.; Thomas, P.R.; Loveday, K.; Watling, D.P.; Lombard, C.L.; Antonova, S.; Tremeer, M.A. A systematic review of the application of interactive virtual reality to sport. *Virtual Real.* **2018**, *22*, 183–198. [CrossRef]
42. Page, Z.E.; Barrington, S.; Edwards, J.; Barnett, L.M. Do active video games benefit the motor skill development of non-typically developing children and adolescents: A systematic review. *J. Sci. Med. Sport* **2017**, *20*, 1087–1100. [CrossRef] [PubMed]
43. Pope, Z.; Zeng, N.; Gao, Z. The effects of active video games on patients' rehabilitative outcomes: A meta-analysis. *Prev. Med.* **2017**, *95*, 38–46. [CrossRef] [PubMed]
44. Hickman, R.; Popescu, L.; Manzanares, R.; Morris, B.; Lee, S.P.; Dufek, J.S. Use of active video gaming in children with neuromotor dysfunction: A systematic review. *Dev. Med. Child Neurol.* **2017**, *59*, 903–911. [CrossRef] [PubMed]
45. Smits-Engelsman, B.; Vinçon, S.; Blank, R.; Quadrado, V.H.; Polatajko, H.; Wilson, P.H. Evaluating the evidence for motor-based interventions in developmental coordination disorder: A systematic review and meta-analysis. *Res. Dev. Disabil.* **2018**, *74*, 72–102. [CrossRef] [PubMed]
46. Gao, Z. Fight fire with fire? Promoting physical activity and health through active video games. *J. Sport Health Sci.* **2017**, *6*, 1–3. [CrossRef] [PubMed]
47. Baranowski, T.; Maddison, R.; Maloney, A.; Medina, E.; Simons, M. Building a better mousetrap (exergame) to increase youth physical activity. *Games Health J.* **2014**, *3*, 72–78. [CrossRef] [PubMed]
48. Tanaka, K.; Parker, J.; Baradoy, G.; Sheehan, D.; Holash, J.R.; Katz, L. A comparison of exergaming interfaces for use in rehabilitation programs and research. *Loading* **2012**, *6*, 69–81.
49. Biddiss, E.; Irwin, J. Active video games to promote physical activity in children and youth. *Arch. Pediatr. Adolesc. Med.* **2010**, *164*, 664–672. [CrossRef] [PubMed]
50. O'Donovan, C.; Hirsch, E.; Holohan, E.; McBride, I.; McManus, R.; Hussey, J. Energy expended playing Xbox Kinect™ and Wii™ games: A preliminary study comparing single and multiplayer modes. *Physiotherapy* **2012**, *98*, 224–229. [CrossRef] [PubMed]
51. Radhakrishnan, K.; Baranowski, T.; Julien, C.; Thomaz, E.; Kim, M. Role of digital games in self-management of cardiovascular diseases: A scoping review. *Games Health J.* **2018**, *8*, g4h.2018.0011. [CrossRef] [PubMed]

52. Chin A Paw, M.J.M.; Jacobs, W.M.; Vaessen, E.P.G.; Titze, S.; van Mechelen, W. The motivation of children to play an active video game. *J. Sci. Med. Sport* **2008**, *11*, 163–166. [CrossRef] [PubMed]

53. Liang, Y.; Lau, P.W.C. Effects of active videogames on physical activity and related outcomes among healthy children: A systematic review. *Games Health J.* **2014**, *3*, 122–144. [CrossRef] [PubMed]

54. Howe, C.A.; Barr, M.W.; Winner, B.C.; Kimble, J.R.; White, J.B. The physical activity energy cost of the latest active video games in young adults. *J. Phys. Act. Health* **2015**, *12*, 171–177. [CrossRef] [PubMed]

55. Barnett, A.; Cerin, E.; Baranowski, T. Active video games for youth: A systematic review. *J. Phys. Act. Health* **2011**, *8*, 724–737. [CrossRef] [PubMed]

56. Hasselmann, V.; Oesch, P.; Fernandez-Luque, L.; Bachmann, S. Are exergames promoting mobility an attractive alternative to conventional self-regulated exercises for elderly people in a rehabilitation setting? Study protocol of a randomized controlled trial. *BMC Geriatr.* **2015**, *15*, 108. [CrossRef] [PubMed]

57. Gao, Z.; Hannon, J.C.; Newton, M.; Huang, C. Effects of curricular activity on students' situational motivation and physical activity levels. *Res. Q. Exerc. Sport* **2011**, *82*, 536–544. [CrossRef] [PubMed]

58. Gao, Z.; Zhang, T.; Stodden, D. Children's physical activity levels and psychological correlates in interactive dance versus aerobic dance. *J. Sport Health Sci.* **2013**, *2*, 146–151. [CrossRef]

59. Foley, L.; Maddison, R. Use of active video games to increase physical activity in children: A (virtual) reality? *Pediatr. Exerc. Sci.* **2010**, *22*, 7–20. [CrossRef] [PubMed]

60. Müller, K.W.; Janikian, M.; Dreier, M.; Wölfling, K.; Beutel, M.E.; Tzavara, C.; Richardson, C.; Tsitsika, A. Regular gaming behavior and internet gaming disorder in European adolescents: Results from a cross-national representative survey of prevalence, predictors, and psychopathological correlates. *Eur. Child Adolesc. Psychiatry* **2015**, *24*, 565–574. [CrossRef] [PubMed]

61. Shah, A.; Kraemer, K.R.; Won, C.R.; Black, S.; Hasenbein, W. Developing digital intervention games for mental disorders: A review. *Games Health J.* **2018**, *7*, 213–224. [CrossRef] [PubMed]

62. Schumacher, H.; Stüwe, S.; Kropp, P.; Diedrich, D.; Freitag, S.; Greger, N.; Junghanss, C.; Freund, M.; Hilgendorf, I. A prospective, randomized evaluation of the feasibility of exergaming on patients undergoing hematopoietic stem cell transplantation. *Bone Marrow Transplant.* **2018**, *53*, 584–590. [CrossRef] [PubMed]

63. Levac, D.E.; Jovanovic, B.B. Is children's motor learning of a postural reaching task enhanced by practice in a virtual environment? In Proceedings of the 2017 International Conference on Virtual Rehabilitation (ICVR), Montreal, QC, Canada, 19–22 June 2017; pp. 1–7.

64. Knols, R.H.; Vanderhenst, T.; Verra, M.L.; de Bruin, E.D. Exergames for patients in acute care settings: Systematic review of the reporting of methodological quality, FITT Components, and program intervention details. *Games Health J.* **2016**, *5*, 224–235. [CrossRef] [PubMed]

65. King, D.; Delfabbro, P.; Griffiths, M. Video game structural characteristics: A new psychological taxonomy. *Int. J. Ment. Health Addict.* **2010**, *8*, 90–106. [CrossRef]

66. Howard, M.C. Virtual reality interventions for personal development: A meta-analysis of hardware and software. *Hum. Comput. Interact.* **2018**, 1–35. [CrossRef]

67. Bavelier, D.; Neville, H.J. Cross-modal plasticity: Where and how? *Nat. Rev. Neurosci.* **2002**, *3*, 443–452. [CrossRef] [PubMed]

68. Hötting, K.; Röder, B. Beneficial effects of physical exercise on neuroplasticity and cognition. *Neurosci. Biobehav. Rev.* **2013**, *37*, 2243–2257. [CrossRef] [PubMed]

69. Van Praag, H.; Kempermann, G.; Gage, F.H. Neural consequences of environmental enrichment. *Nat. Rev. Neurosci.* **2000**, *1*, 191–198. [CrossRef] [PubMed]

70. Brown, J.; Cooper-Kuhn, C.M.; Kempermann, G.; van Praag, H.; Winkler, J.; Gage, F.H.; Kuhn, H.G. Enriched environment and physical activity stimulate hippocampal but not olfactory bulb neurogenesis. *Eur. J. Neurosci.* **2003**, *17*, 2042–2046. [CrossRef] [PubMed]

71. Carey, J.R.; Bhatt, E.; Nagpal, A. Neuroplasticity promoted by task complexity. *Exerc. Sport Sci. Rev.* **2005**, *33*, 24–31.

72. Holtz, B.E.; Murray, K.; Park, T. Serious games for children with chronic diseases: A systematic review. *Games Health J.* **2018**, *7*, g4h.2018.0024. [CrossRef] [PubMed]

73. Staiano, A.E.; Beyl, R.A.; Hsia, D.S.; Katzmarzyk, P.T.; Newton, R.L. Twelve weeks of dance exergaming in overweight and obese adolescent girls: Transfer effects on physical activity, screen-time, and self-efficacy. *J. Sport Health Sci.* **2017**, *6*, 4–10. [CrossRef] [PubMed]

74. Spiegel, J.S. The ethics of virtual reality technology: Social hazards and public policy recommendations. *Sci. Eng. Ethics* **2017**, *24*, 1537–1550. [CrossRef] [PubMed]

75. Calvert, S.L.; Dodge, K.A.; Nagayama Hall, G.C.; Fasig-Caldwell, L.G.; Galloway, D.P.; Appelbaum, M.; Graham, S.; Hamby, S.; Citkowicz, M.; Hedges, L.V. The American Psychological Association Task Force assessment of violent video games: Science in the service of public interest. *Am. Psychol.* **2017**, *72*, 126–143. [CrossRef] [PubMed]

76. Desai, R.A.; Krishnan-Sarin, S.; Cavallo, D.; Potenza, M.N. Video-gaming among high school students: Health correlates, gender differences, and problematic gaming. *Pediatrics* **2010**, *126*, e1414–e1424. [CrossRef] [PubMed]

77. Bavelier, D.; Bediou, B.; Green, C.S. Expertise and generalization: Lessons from action video games. *Curr. Opin. Behav. Sci.* **2018**, *20*, 169–173. [CrossRef]

78. Granic, I.; Lobel, A.; Engels, R.C.M.E. The benefits of playing video games. *Am. Psychol.* **2014**, *69*, 66–78. [CrossRef] [PubMed]

79. Ferguson, C.J. Do angry birds make for angry children? A meta-analysis of video game influences on children's and adolescents' aggression, mental health, prosocial behavior, and academic performance. *Perspect. Psychol. Sci.* **2015**, *10*, 646–666. [CrossRef] [PubMed]

80. Au, J.; Buschkuehl, M.; Duncan, G.J.; Jaeggi, S.M. There is no convincing evidence that working memory training is NOT effective: A reply to Melby-Lervåg and Hulme (2015). *Psychon. Bull. Rev.* **2016**, *23*, 331–337. [CrossRef] [PubMed]

81. Melby-Lervåg, M.; Hulme, C. There is no convincing evidence that working memory training is effective: A reply to Au et al. (2014) and Karbach and Verhaeghen (2014). *Psychon. Bull. Rev.* **2016**, *23*, 324–330. [CrossRef] [PubMed]

82. Noack, H.; Lövdén, M.; Schmiedek, F. On the validity and generality of transfer effects in cognitive training research. *Psychol. Res.* **2014**, *78*, 773–789. [CrossRef] [PubMed]

83. Woodworth, R.S.; Thorndike, E.L. The influence of improvement in one mental function upon the efficiency of other functions. (I). *Psychol. Rev.* **1901**, *8*, 247–261. [CrossRef]

84. Pickton, D.W.; Wright, S. What's swot in strategic analysis? *Strateg. Chang.* **1998**, *7*, 101–109. [CrossRef]

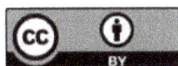

Journal of
Clinical Medicine

MDPI

Review

Virtual Reality Exercise for Anxiety and Depression: A Preliminary Review of Current Research in an Emerging Field

Nan Zeng [1] , Zachary Pope [1], Jung Eun Lee [2] and Zan Gao [1,*]

[1]   School of Kinesiology, University of Minnesota Twin Cities, Minneapolis, MN 55455, USA;
      zengx185@umn.edu (N.Z.), popex157@umn.edu (Z.P.)
[2]   Department of Applied Human Sciences, University of Minnesota Duluth, Duluth, MN 55812, USA;
      junelee@d.umn.edu
*   Correspondence: gaoz@umn.edu; Tel.: +1-612-626-4639

Received: 20 December 2017; Accepted: 28 February 2018; Published: 4 March 2018

Abstract: Objective: Although current evidence supports the use of virtual reality (VR) in the treatment of mental disorders, it is unknown whether VR exercise would be beneficial to mental health. This review synthesized literature concerning the effect of VR exercise on anxiety and depression among various populations. Methods: Ten electronic databases were searched for studies on this topic from January 2000 through October 2017. Studies were eligible if the article: (1) was peer-reviewed; (2) was published in English; and (3) used quantitative measures in assessing anxiety- and depression-related outcomes. Results: A total of five empirical studies met the eligibility criteria. These studies included two randomized clinical trials, one control trial, and two cross-sectional studies. Four studies reported significant improvements in anxiety- and depression-related measures following VR exercise, including reduced tiredness and tension, in addition to increased energy and enjoyment. Nonetheless, one study failed to support the effectiveness of VR exercise over traditional exercise alone on depressive symptoms. Conclusions: Findings favor VR exercise in alleviating anxiety and depression symptomology. However, existing evidence is insufficient to support the advantages of VR exercise as a standalone treatment over traditional therapy in the alleviation of anxiety and depression given the paucity of studies, small sample sizes, and lack of high-quality research designs. Future studies may build upon these limitations to discern the optimal manner by which to employ VR exercise in clinical settings.

Keywords: anxiety; depression; exercise; mental health; virtual reality

---

1. Introduction

Anxiety is a psychological disorder characterized by worried thoughts, feelings of tension, and physical changes such as increased blood pressure [1]. Individuals with anxiety disorders tend to have recurring intrusive thoughts or concerns, as well as specific physical symptoms such as trembling, sweating, a rapid heartbeat, or dizziness [1]. Today, anxiety disorders are the most common mental illness in the U.S., affecting approximately 40 million adults (18.1% of the U.S. population) annually. However, only 36.9% of those suffering from any anxiety disorder receive treatment [2]. Depression is another major psychological disorder. Depressed individuals present not only with poor mood, but also with disturbed sleep or appetite, significant weight loss or gain, loss of interest or pleasure in daily activities, lack of energy, inability to concentrate, feelings of worthlessness, and recurrent thoughts of death or suicide [1]. In 2015, 16.1 million U.S. adults had experienced at least one major depressive episode within the past year (6.7% of all U.S. adults) [2]. Remarkably, while anxiety and depression disorders are different, individuals who develop depression may have experienced an anxiety disorder earlier in life. Indeed, individuals with depression often experience symptomology similar to that characteristic of anxiety disorders, including nervousness, irritability, disturbed sleep or appetite, and poor concentration, among other symptoms [2]. Fortunately, anxiety and depression disorders are treatable, with most individuals able to be helped with the appropriate professional care. Concerted and novel efforts, therefore, must continue to be made to promote mental health among individuals with anxiety and depression through innovative treatment approaches.

Many treatments are available to treat anxiety and depression disorders, including medication, exercise, meditation, and cognitive behavioral therapy. In many cases, these treatments can be tailored to a client to help reduce symptomology of anxiety and/or depression. To date, the application of emerging technology in health promotion has generated substantial public interest. Among the emerging technologies that may potentially aid in the treatment of anxiety and depression, virtual reality (VR) is arguably the most exciting and technologically-advanced. VR is a digital technology that artificially creates sensory experiences—including visual, auditory, touch, and scent stimuli—while allowing the user to manipulate objects within the virtual environment created [3]. Two types of VR exist: (1) immersive VR, which frequently uses head-mounted displays, body-motion sensors, real-time graphics, and advanced interface devices (e.g., specialized helmets) in the simulation of a completely virtual environment for the user; and (2) non-immersive VR, which uses interfaces such as flat-screen televisions/computer screens with associated keyboards, gamepads, and joysticks. Simply stated, immersive VR seeks to envelop the players in a virtual world, making the players feel as though they are "actually there", whereas the non-immersive VR does not simulate a virtual world to as deep a degree.

Over the past decade, VR applications were widely used for rehabilitation medicine (e.g., stroke, Parkinson's disease, and developmental disabilities) and behavioral medicine (e.g., phobias, post-traumatic stress disorder, and autism) [4–6]. Notably, VR-based treatments for different mental health conditions have observed positive findings. Specifically, VR has been investigated in the treatment of phobias, obesity, chronic pain, and eating disorders [7–10]. Recently, VR exposure therapy (VRET) has become popular in the treatment of anxiety and depression, with a growing body of literature suggesting that VRET is a successful tool for the treatment of anxiety- and depression-related symptomology [11–15]. Yet, the current literature concerning the effects of VR-based treatments on anxiety and depression primarily focuses on VRET, with VR exercise in the treatment of these conditions being seldom reviewed. VR exercise refers to equipping traditional exercise equipment like bikes and treadmills with VR capabilities. Specifically, some new exercise apparatus has been equipped with integrated sensors that sync with a computer or gaming console and allow the player to engage in strenuous physical exertion on the apparatus while simultaneously engaging in VR gameplay. Researchers and health professionals have documented that combining VR with exercise equipment (a.k.a., VR exercise) may serve to enhance the psychological benefits of exercise and increase the chances of long-term adherence to exercise [16,17]. For example, the latest commercially-available VR exercise apparatus—the VirZoom, a VR exercise bike compatible with most VR headsets (e.g., the Oculus Rift, PlayStation VR, Samsung Gear VR, HTC Vive, etc.)—is presenting researchers and health professionals with the opportunity to implement VR exercise to promote improved health. Thus, given the enjoyable nature of currently-available VR exercise games and the demonstrated positive effects exercise has on anxiety and depression [16,18,19], VR exercise might be viewed as a potentially effective approach to alleviate anxiety- and depression-related symptomology.

As VR exercise is increasing in popularity given the compatibility of VR systems with traditional exercise apparatus such as bikes and treadmills, the potential of VR exercise to be used in the treatment of anxiety and depression is great. Unfortunately, there have been no known comprehensive reviews that have specifically examined the effectiveness of VR exercise on anxiety- and depression-related outcomes. The purpose of this review, therefore, is to systematically evaluate the available evidence concerning the effects of VR exercise on anxiety and depression. In detail, this preliminary review aims to identify, synthesize, and interpret the best available evidence for the use of VR exercise in promoting anxiety- and depression-related outcomes. Findings of this review will help inform scholars and health professionals of the potential benefits VR exercise has in the treatment of anxiety- and depression-related symptomology and where improvements can be made to VR exercise interventions that seek to reduce these symptoms among patients.

2. Methods

The Preferred Reporting Items for Systematic Review and Meta-Analysis Protocols (PRISMA-P) 2015 statement was consulted and provided the framework for this review [20].

2.1. Information Sources and Search Strategies

The following electronic databases were employed for the literature search: Academic Search Complete, Communication and Mass Media Complete, Education Resources Information Center (ERIC), Google Scholar, Medline, PsycINFO, PubMed, Scopus, SPORTDiscus, and Web of Science. The literature search was conducted independently by the co-authors, with all studies queried placed within a shared research folder. Search terms were discussed among the research team and used in combination: ("virtual reality" OR "head-mounted display") AND ("exercise" OR "physical activity" OR "sports" OR "bike" OR "treadmill") AND ("mental illness" OR "mental disorders" OR "mental health" OR "anxiety" OR "depression").

2.2. Eligibility Criteria

The eligibility criteria used to evaluate each study included: (1) published in English between January 2000 through October 2017 as peer-reviewed study; (2) employed the use of immersive VR only (e.g., head-mounted display(s)), with studies of non-immersive VR (e.g., Xbox 360 Kinect and Nintendo Wii) excluded; (3) involved human participants; (4) used quantitative measures in assessing anxiety- and depression-related outcomes; and (5) employed an established study design that allowed for examination of the effect of VR exercise on anxiety- and depression-related outcomes (e.g., randomized controlled trials (RCTs), cohort, and observational studies), meaning case studies were excluded.

2.3. Data Extraction

Three reviewers (NZ, ZP, and JL) separately screened the titles of potentially relevant articles. If the reviewers were unable to determine the relevance of an article to the topic, then the abstract was reviewed. Data extraction was completed by one reviewer (NZ) and checked by another (ZP) for accuracy. All potential articles were downloaded as full text and stored in a shared folder, after which three authors (NZ, ZP, and JL) reviewed each article independently to ensure that only relevant entries were included. A list of published articles on the topic was then created in a Microsoft Excel spreadsheet (Microsoft Corporation, Redmond, WA, USA). The following information was extracted: (1) year of publication and country of origin, (2) methodological details (e.g., study design, sample characteristics, study duration, VR exposure, anxiety- and depression-related outcomes, and instruments), and (3) key findings concerning the effectiveness of VR exercise on anxiety- and depression-related outcomes. Finally, relevant studies were further identified through cross-referencing the bibliographies of selected articles. Notably, reviewers were not blinded to the authors or journals, and no attempts were made to contact investigators or correspondents of the original studies to acquire any information missing from the included articles.

2.4. Risk of Bias in Individual Studies

To assess the risk of bias in each study, two reviewers (NZ, ZP) independently rated each study using an 8-item quality assessment tool (see Table 1) employed in previous literature [21–23]. Each item within each study was rated as "positive" (when the item was explicitly described and present) or "negative" (when the item was inadequately described or absent). Two reviewers (NZ, ZP) separately scored each article to ensure reliable scoring of the quality assessment. When disagreements occurred between the two reviewers, unresolved differences were evaluated by a third reviewer (JL). In particular, Items 1, 3, 4, and 6 in Table 1 were deemed the most important, as these items had greater potential to significantly affect the research findings. Of note, the final score for each study was calculated by summing up the all "positive" ratings. A study was considered "high-quality and at low risk of bias" when scored above the median score of 4.5 following the scoring of all studies. Studies below the median score were considered "low-quality and at high risk of bias".

Table 1. Design Quality Analysis.

Articles	Randomization	Control	Pre-Post	Retention	Missing Data	Power Analysis	Validity Measure	Follow-Up	Score	Effectiveness
Lee et al. [24]	+	+	+	+	−	−	+	+	6	Yes
Monteiro-Junior et al. [25]	+	+	+	+	−	+	+	+	7	No
Chen et al. [26]	−	+	+	+	−	−	+	−	4	Yes
Plante et al. [27]	+	−	+	+	−	−	+	−	4	Yes
Plante et al. [28]	+	−	+	+	−	−	+	−	4	Yes

Note: "+" Refers to Positive (Explicitly Described and Present in Details); "−" Refers to Negative (Inadequately Described and Absent); "Yes" Indicates Significant Positive Effect; "No" Indicates No Significant Effect; Median Score = 4.5.

3. Results

3.1. Study Selection

A total of 407 potentially relevant articles were identified. After removing duplicates, titles and abstracts of the remaining articles were screened and further identified as potentially meeting the eligibility criteria. An additional study was located through the search of reference lists. Following a thorough securitization of the full-text articles, five studies fully met the eligibility criteria and were included in this review (see Figure 1). Reasons for excluding articles included: non-English language articles, ineligible VR type (i.e., non-immersive VR), and no measures of anxiety and depression, among others. Notably, a high inter-rater agreement (97%) of the articles included was obtained between the authors.

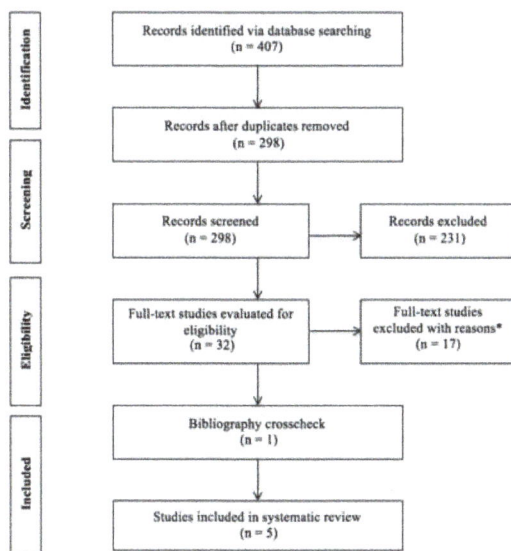

Figure 1. PRISMA flow diagram of studies through the review process; * reasons for study exclusion included non-English language articles, ineligible VR type (i.e., non-immersive VR), and no measures of anxiety and depression. Many studies were excluded for multiple reasons.

3.2. Study Characteristics

The characteristics of included studies are shown in Table 2. Among the five studies, two were RCTs [24,25], one was a controlled trial (CTs; quasi-experimental pre posttest design without randomization) [26], and two were pre-experimental designs with pre-post-test design among same participants) [27,28]. The studies were conducted in different countries: two in the U.S. [27,28], one in Brazil [25], one in Korea [24], and one in Taiwan [26], reflecting the global nature of the phenomenon under study. Among these studies, one was conducted in a clinical setting [26], but the other four were completed in a laboratory setting [24,25,27,28]. Participants' ages ranged from 22 years to 84 years. Populations were diverse, including patients suffering from spinal-cord injuries [26], college students and faculty/staff [27,28], and older adults [24,25]. Notably, a relatively large variability in sample size and VR exposure was observed across studies, with samples varying from 30 to 154 participants (median number of participants being 70) and VR exposure length ranging from 30 min to 8 weeks (median period of exposure being 90 min). All studies examined the effects of VR exercise on health-related outcomes including physical fitness, cognitive functioning, mental health, and anxiety and depression. Measures employed to assess anxiety- and depression- related outcomes were most often the Activation-Deactivation Adjective Check List (AD-ACL) [26–28], Geriatric Depression Scale (GDS) [25], and Short-Form Health Survey (SF-36) [24].

3.3. Quality and Risk of Bias Assessment

Following the rating of each study using the 8-item quality and risk of bias assessment tool, scores ranged from 4 to 7 (see Table 1). In detail, two studies received an overall rating of high-quality/low risk of bias (scored above the median score of 4.5), while three studies received an overall rating of low-quality/high risk of bias. Notably, all studies succeeded in retaining at least 70% of the participants. The most common issues with the study quality and risk of bias were related to lack of follow-up measurements, no power calculations to determine appropriate sample sizes, and omission of discussion regarding missing data interpretation. Additionally, relevant discussions concerning potential bias and methodological efforts to minimize confounding effects were rarely mentioned within the low-quality studies. Given the poorer quality of research designs among the literature on this topic, a meta-analysis was prohibited.

3.4. Key Findings

Of the five studies examining the effects of VR exercise on participants' anxiety- and depression-related outcomes, four reported significant improvements in outcomes associated with these conditions, such as reduced tiredness and tension, and increased energy and enjoyment [24,26–28]. Notably, one study failed to support the effectiveness of VR exercise over traditionally active exercise (without virtual reality stimulation) on depressive symptoms [25]. Specifically, Chen and colleagues [26] investigated the psychological benefits of VR exercise in patients suffering from spinal-cord injuries. An experimental group ($n = 15$, $M_{age} = 51.3$, $SD = 15.8$) underwent treatment using a VR exercise bike, while a comparison group ($n = 15$, $M_{age} = 45.4$, $SD = 14.24$) received an identical exercise treatment but without VR equipment. Significant differences for AD-ACL-measured calmness and tension were observed between groups, with experimental group participants experiencing the greatest reductions in tension and improvements in feelings of calmness. Additionally, Lee et al. [24] examined the effect of individualized feedback-based VR exercise on health-related quality of life in older women. Participants were randomized to either a VR exercise (motions based on Tai Chi) group ($n = 26$, $M_{age} = 68.7$, $SD = 4.6$) or group-based exercise group ($n = 28$, $M_{age} = 67.7$, $SD = 4.3$). Both groups received a 60-min intervention three times a week for eight weeks. The SF-36 was administered. The findings indicated that the VR exercise group not only achieved greater decreases depression compared to the group-based exercise group, but also larger improvements in quality of life, social functioning, and physical fitness.

Moreover, Plante et al. [27] conducted a cross-sectional study to assess the psychological benefits of VR-based treadmill exercise among college students ($n = 154$, 102 females). Participants were randomly assigned to one of three 20-min conditions: (1) walking on a laboratory treadmill while using VR, (2) walking on the treadmill without VR, (3) experiencing a virtual walk using VR without any exercise performed (i.e., sedentary condition), and (4) walking outside around campus. The AD-ACL was used to assess mood states, including energy, calmness, tension, and tiredness. Findings indicated that VR-based treadmill walking enhanced energy and reduced tiredness and tension to the greatest degree versus the other three groups. Similarly, Plante and colleagues [28] conducted another cross-sectional study of VR biking exercise study among University faculty and staff ($n = 88$, 44 females). Participants were randomly assigned to one of three 30-min conditions including: (1) playing a VR computer bicycle game, (2) an interactive VR bicycle experience on a computer while exercising on a stationary bike at moderate intensity, and (3) bicycling at a moderate intensity (60–70% maximum heart rate) on a stationary bicycle. The AD-ACL was administered to assess mood states before and after each exercise session, and findings favored VR-based biking exercise for the enhancement of enjoyment and energy, as well as the reduction of tiredness compared to the other two conditions.

Table 2. Descriptive Characteristics of Included Studies.

Study Description	Design/Sample	Type	Outcomes/Instrument	Exposure	Duration	Findings
Chen et al. [26] 2009, Taiwan	Quasi-experiment; $N = 30$ Patients suffering from spinal-cord injury; Intervention ($n = 15$, $M_{age} = 51.3$, $SD = 15.8$); Control ($n = 15$, $M_{age} = 45.4$, $SD = 14.24$)	VR-based exercise bike	Mood states were assessed via Activation–Deactivation Adjective Check List (AD-ACL)	Rehabilitation therapy with a VR-based exercise bike Vs. same therapy without VR	Not applicable	A virtual-reality-based rehabilitation program can ease patients' tension and induce calm
Lee et al. [24] 2015, Korea	Randomized controlled trial (RCT); $N = 54$; Intervention ($n = 26$, $M_{age} = 68.7$, $SD = 4.6$); Control ($n = 28$, $M_{age} = 67.7$, $SD = 4.3$)	Individualized feedback-based VR exercise	Psychological outcomes were measured via Short-Form Health Survey (SF-36)	Individualized feedback-based VR exercise Vs. group-based exercise	a 60-min intervention three times a week for eight weeks.	Individualized feedback-based virtual reality group (IFVRG) showed greater improvement in mental health (increased social functioning and decreased depression)
Monteiro-Junior et al. [25] 2017, Brazil	RCT; $N = 70$ older adults; Intervention ($n = 29$, $M_{age} = 85$, $SD = 8$); Control ($n = 41$, $M_{age} = 86$, $SD = 5$)	VR-based physical exercise	Depressive symptoms were assessed via Geriatric Depression Scale (GDS)	Exercises with VR stimulation Vs. same exercises without VR stimulation	30–45 min/session, 12–16 sessions twice a week	There was no significant difference between groups in depressive symptoms
Plante et al. [27] 2003, USA	Cross-sectional; $N = 154$ (102 females) students were assigned to 4 different conditions	VR with walking on treadmill	Mood states were assessed via AD-ACL, including energy, calmness, tension, and tiredness	Brisk outdoor walk Vs. VR with walking on treadmill Vs. Walking on the treadmill without VR Vs. VR without exercise	4×20-min experiments	VR may enhance energy and reduce tiredness and tension when paired with actual exercise
Plante et al. [28] 2003, USA	Cross-sectional; $N = 88$ (44 females, $M_{age} = 38.1$, $SD = 12.31$) university faculty and staffs were assigned to 3 different conditions	VR in combination with stationary bike	Mood states were assessed via AD-ACL, including energy, calmness, tension, and tiredness	Stationary bicycling at a moderate intensity (60–70% maximum heart rate) Vs. VR-based bicycle game without actual exercise Vs. (3) VR-based stationary bike at moderate intensity	3×30-min experiments	VR when paired with exercise enhances enjoyment, energy, and reduces tiredness. Notably, VR without exercise was found to increase tension, tiredness, and lower energy level

Although a majority of the included studies (*n* = 4) supported the claim that VR exercise can improve anxiety- and depression-related outcomes, it is worth noting that one study failed to back these findings. Monteiro-Junior et al. [25] evaluated the effects of VR exercise on cognitive functions, physical performance, fear of falling, and depressive symptoms among older adults. Participants were randomly allocated to either VR-based physical exercise with exergames (*n* = 29, M_{age} = 85, *SD* = 8) or active control group (*n* = 41, M_{age} = 86, *SD* = 5), with the latter group performing same exercises without VR stimulation. Both groups received a one-week intervention lasting 30–45 min per session for 12–16 sessions. Depressive symptoms were assessed via the GDS. No significant differences between groups for depressive symptoms were observed. Notably, depressive symptoms in this study were assessed as a secondary outcome.

4. Discussion

The primary focus of this article was to comprehensively review the available literature regarding the effectiveness of VR exercise on anxiety and depression while attempting to provide practitioners and health professionals future directions for the use of VR exercise in treating these and other mental disorders. Five studies were included in the final analysis. Findings revealed that VR exercise had significant beneficial effects on anxiety- and depression-related outcomes in 4 of included studies. Notably, no detrimental effects were observed within any study. Overall, the present review provides initial evidence of the potential of using VR exercise to treat individuals with anxiety and depression.

The majority of the five articles included in this review indicated VR exercise to have positive effects on anxiety- and depression-related outcomes [24,26–28]. Although the results are encouraging, several limitations should be noted. First, relatively small sample sizes and short or unclear VR exercise exposure periods may limit the ability to generalize the findings and confirm an optimal dose (i.e., type, duration, intensity, and frequency) of VR exercise needed to treat anxiety and depression. Second, as most of the included studies were conducted in a laboratory setting (*n* = 4), integrating VR exercise into clinical practice must be viewed cautiously. Third, as technology advances, some types of VR may have been phased out by newer systems. For example, three included studies were conducted before 2010 [26–28]. Thus, while the VR technology used in these studies was research-grade, this technology might be antiquated compared to currently-available VR systems. These outdated VR systems may have affected the participant experience within these studies and thereby had an impact on the treatment effects. Nonetheless, the largely positive findings of this body of VR exercise literature on anxiety and depression are encouraging, as VR systems continue to improve in quality.

VR is a technology-based interface that allows users to experience computer-generated virtual environments [29]. Over the past decade, VR technology has experienced increasing application in the treatment of individuals with mental disorders [5]. As previously stated, most available VR literature focused on effects of VRET on mental disorders. VRET is based upon emotion-processing theory, which postulates that fear memories are structures and contain information regarding fear stimuli, responses, and meaning [29]. As such, VRET has been widely used in clinical research to trigger and adjust those fear structures by presenting novel incompatible information and advancing emotional processing (e.g., creating a virtual environment containing the trigger(s) of an individual's anxiety and/or depression) [29]. Within these clinical research studies, a growing body of literature has demonstrated that VRET is related to large declines in symptoms of both anxiety and depression, and is similar in efficacy to traditional exposure therapy [13,30–32]. Yet, the effects of commercially-available VR exercise on mental health are rarely investigated. More research needs to be done in this area of inquiry.

Currently, only 41% of U.S. adults with a mental disorder received mental health services in the past year. This fact is concerning and suggests the need for new and enjoyable treatments for mental disorders to be included exclusively or as an adjunct to traditional treatments [33]. Fortunately, VR exercise continues to become more mainstream for health promotion and, given the demonstrated effects of exercise on anxiety and depression in addition to the enjoyable nature of VR [16,18,19],

VR exercise may be a potential treatment option for these two mental disorders and others. Indeed, the latest commercially-available immersive VR headsets, such as the PlayStation VR, Samsung Gear VR, and Oculus Rift are increasingly becoming popular worldwide, presenting scholars and health professionals with opportunities to implement VR exercise interventions with the objective of promoting mental health among various populations. For instance, Zeng and colleagues (2017) [34] conducted a pilot study using a state-of-the-art VR exercise apparatus (VirZoom) and demonstrated the feasibility of using VR exercise for enhancing psychological outcomes including enjoyment and self-efficacy, indicating the potential of VR exercise technology for use in the promotion of mental health to be great. Yet, VR exercise studies akin to those of Zeng and colleagues that employ the newest VR systems among individuals with anxiety or depression, with the objective to improve the symptomology associated with these two disorders, remain to be observed.

It is noteworthy that employing the newest VR exercise systems in the promotion of psychological health among individuals with anxiety or depression offers several advantages. Specifically, the newest VR exercise systems allow for the precise presentation and control of stimuli within a dynamic multi-sensory three-dimensional computer-generated environment [35] while creating a safe and motivating exercise condition that may avoid the injury and burnout sometimes associated with exercise in a real-world setting. Given these advantages and the fact that regular exercise can have a profoundly positive impact on depression, anxiety, and other mental disorders [36,37], clinicians and health professionals should take into account the 2008 Physical Activity Guidelines for Americans [38] when considering a VR exercise prescription as an adjunctive or alternative approach to mental health treatments. As such, more research is warranted in order to determine the optimal dose of VR exercise (i.e., intensity, duration, and frequency) needed to promote the most positive psychological outcomes, which would assist in the advancement of VR exercise toward personalized medicine. Yet, if empirical research continues to demonstrate effectiveness, the use of VR exercise could offer adjunctive or alternative options for the treatment of mental disorders such as anxiety or depression.

As with any other groundbreaking innovation, VR is not devoid of potentially negative aspects. To begin, emerging evidence has suggested that the use of contemporary, consumer-oriented head-mounted display devices (e.g., Oculus Rift, Samsung Gear VR, HTC Vive, etc.) may cause motion sickness, with females at greater risk [39]. The common symptoms of motion sickness include eye strain, headache, stomach awareness, sweating, fatigue, drowsiness, disorientation, and, in some cases, nausea and vomiting [40]. Thus, VR exercise may not be a good option for those who suffer from or are at higher risk of motion sickness and live with symptoms of epilepsy such as severe dizziness, blackouts, and seizures. Further, while VR games make exercise more appealing, the equipment used for VR exercise is relatively expensive compared to traditional exercise. For example, the VirZOOM exercise bike—a virtual reality fitness game platform, which integrates a traditional stationary bike with a VR headset (e.g., PlayStation VR), costs approximately $1000 prior to purchasing compatible games. As such, the high price of VR exercise may result in potential stakeholders within the medical field adopting a "wait-and-see" approach toward the implementation of this novel technology. Additionally, as with other forms of technology, there may be some risk for VR obsession/dependence—factors that need to be considered when treating individuals with other mental disorders. Finally, while exercise has been proven to be effective in the treatment of anxiety and depression [41,42], it is worth noting that most VR exercise apparatuses are still in the exploratory phase of development and have yet to advance beyond feasibility and small case studies [43]. Therefore, VR exercise still remains widely unexplored, suggesting more research is warranted.

Although the current study's strength lies in the provision of the first known synthesis of the effects of VR exercise on anxiety and depression in a systematic manner, the study is not without limitations. To begin, the current review only included peer-reviewed full-text and English language publications, despite the fact that other unpublished and non-English research may be available on the topic. Second, qualitative perspectives such as user experience were excluded, because they fell outside the review's primary aim. These viewpoints, however, would have significant relevance for the treatment of mental disorders. Third, it is possible that other VR exercises exist and, as such, it is possible the search terms used in the current study limited our ability to locate all relevant studies. Finally, given a small number of empirical studies and the relatively low quality of the study designs and methodology, a conclusive statement regarding the effectiveness of VR exercise on anxiety and depression should be interpreted with caution—providing further indication of the need for greater study on this topic.

5. Conclusions

This preliminary review synthesizes the available experimental evidence regarding the effects of VR exercise on anxiety- and depression-related outcomes. Findings favor VR exercise, as this small group of studies indicates improvements in mental health for those who had these two mental disorders. Yet, the paucity of literature on this topic and the need for higher-quality study designs among large samples necessitates further research prior to large-scale implementation of VR exercise treatments for anxiety and depression within clinical settings.

Author Contributions: The author would like to thank the co-authors for their help to complete this study. During the construction of this study, Nan Zeng played a role in data collection, sorting, analysis, and writing the article. Zachary Pope played a role in data collection and helped to write the article. Jung Eun Lee played a role in data collection and helped to write the article. Zan Gao played a role in developing the research ideas, designing the research design, overseeing data collection and analysis, and revising the article.

Conflicts of Interest: The authors declare no conflicts of interest.

References

1. Kazdin, A.E. *Encyclopedia of Psychology*; Oxford University Press: Washington, DC, USA, 2000.
2. Anxiety and Depression Association of America. Facts & Statistics. 2017. Available online: https://adaa. org/about-adaa/press-room/facts-statistics (accessed on 23 November 2017).
3. Pasco, D. The potential of using virtual reality technology in physical activity settings. *Quest* **2013**, *65*, 429–441. [CrossRef]
4. McEwen, D.; Taillon-Hobson, A.; Bilodeau, M.; Sveistrup, H.; Finestone, H. Virtual reality exercise improves mobility after stroke: An inpatient randomized controlled trial. *Stroke* **2014**, *45*, 1853–1855. [CrossRef] [PubMed]
5. Morina, N.; Ijntema, H.; Meyerbröker, K.; Emmelkamp, P.M. Can virtual reality exposure therapy gains be generalized to real-life? A meta-analysis of studies applying behavioral assessments. *Behav. Res. Ther.* **2015**, *74*, 18–24. [CrossRef] [PubMed]
6. Didehbani, N.; Allen, T.; Kandalaft, M.; Krawczyk, D.; Chapman, S. Virtual reality social cognition training for children with high functioning autism. *Comput. Hum. Behav.* **2016**, *62*, 703–711. [CrossRef]
7. Rothbaum, B.O.; Hodges, L.; Smith, S.; Lee, J.H.; Price, L. A controlled study of virtual reality exposure therapy for the fear of flying. *J. Consult. Clin. Psychol.* **2000**, *68*, 1020–1026. [CrossRef] [PubMed]
8. Llobera, J.; González-Franco, M.; Perez-Marcos, D.; Valls-Solé, J.; Slater, M.; Sanchez-Vives, M.V. Virtual reality for assessment of patients suffering chronic pain: A case study. *Exp. Brain Res.* **2013**, *225*, 105–117. [CrossRef] [PubMed]
9. Riva, G.; Bacchetta, M.; Baruffi, M.; Molinari, E. Virtual reality–based multidimensional therapy for the treatment of body image disturbances in obesity: A controlled study. *Cyberpsychol. Behav.* **2001**, *4*, 511–526. [CrossRef] [PubMed]
10. Gutiérrez-Maldonado, J.; Wiederhold, B.K.; Riva, G. Future directions: How virtual reality can further improve the assessment and treatment of eating disorders and obesity. *Cyberpsychol. Behav. Soc. Netw.* **2016**, *19*, 148–153. [CrossRef] [PubMed]
11. McCann, R.A.; Armstrong, C.M.; Skopp, N.A.; Edwards-Stewart, A.; Smolenski, D.J.; June, J.D.; Metzger-Abamukong, M.; Reger, G.M. Virtual reality exposure therapy for the treatment of anxiety disorders: An evaluation of research quality. *J. Anxiety Disord.* **2014**, *28*, 625–631. [CrossRef] [PubMed]
12. Krijn, M.; Emmelkamp, P.M.; Olafsson, R.; Biemond, R. Virtual reality exposure therapy of anxiety disorders: A review. *Clin. Psychol. Rev.* **2004**, *24*, 259–281. [CrossRef] [PubMed]

13. Powers, M.B.; Emmelkamp, P.M.G. Virtual reality exposure therapy for anxiety disorders: A meta-analysis. *J. Anxiety Disord.* **2008**, *22*, 561–569. [CrossRef] [PubMed]
14. Valmaggia, L.R.; Latif, L.; Kempton, M.J.; Rus-Calafell, M. Virtual reality in the psychological treatment for mental health problems: A systematic review of recent evidence. *Psychiatry Res.* **2016**, *236*, 189–195. [CrossRef] [PubMed]
15. Falconer, C.J.; Rovira, A.; King, J.A.; Gilbert, P.; Antley, A.; Fearon, P.; Ralph, N.; Slater, M.; Brewin, C.R. Embodying self-compassion within virtual reality and its effects on patients with depression. *Br. J. Psychiatry Open* **2016**, *2*, 74–80. [CrossRef] [PubMed]
16. Mestre, D.R.; Dagonneau, V.; Mercier, C.S. Does virtual reality enhance exercise performance, enjoyment, and dissociation? An exploratory study on a stationary bike apparatus. *Presence Teleoper. Virtual Environ.* **2011**, *20*, 1–14. [CrossRef]
17. Plante, T.G.; Aldridge, A.; Bogden, R.; Hanelin, C. Might virtual reality promote the mood benefits of exercise. *Comput. Hum. Behav.* **2003**, *19*, 495–509. [CrossRef]
18. Plante, T.G.; Cage, C.; Clements, S.; Stover, A. Psychological benefits of exercise paired with virtual reality: Outdoor exercise energizes whereas indoor virtual exercise relaxes. *Int. J. Stress Manag.* **2006**, *13*, 108–117. [CrossRef]
19. Mestre, D.R.; Ewald, M.; Maiano, C. Virtual reality and exercise: Behavioral and psychological effects of visual feedback. *Stud. Health Technol. Inf.* **2011**, *167*, 122–127.
20. Moher, D.; Shamseer, L.; Clarke, M.; Ghersi, D.; Liberati, A.; Petticrew, M.; Shekelle, P.; Stewart, L.A. Preferred reporting items for systematic review and meta-analysis protocols (PRISMA-P) 2015 statement. *Syst. Rev.* **2015**, *4*, 1. [CrossRef] [PubMed]
21. Zeng, N.; Pope, Z.; Lee, J.E.; Gao, Z. A systematic review of active video games on rehabilitative outcomes among older patients. *J. Sport Health Sci.* **2017**, *6*, 33–43. [CrossRef]
22. Pope, Z.; Zeng, N.; Gao, Z. The effects of active video games on patients' rehabilitative outcomes: A meta-analysis. *Prev. Med.* **2017**, *95*, 38–46. [CrossRef] [PubMed]
23. Gao, Z.; Chen, S. Are field-based exergames useful in preventing childhood obesity? A systematic review. *Obes. Rev.* **2014**, *15*, 676–691. [CrossRef] [PubMed]
24. Lee, M.; Son, J.; Kim, J.; Yoon, B. Individualized feedback-based virtual reality exercise improves older women's self-perceived health: A randomized controlled trial. *Arch. Gerontol. Geriatr.* **2015**, *61*, 154–160. [CrossRef] [PubMed]
25. Monteiro-Junior, R.S.; Figueiredo, L.F.; Maciel-Pinheiro, P.D.; Abud, E.L.; Engedal, K.; Barca, M.L.; Nascimento, O.J.; Laks, J.; Deslandes, A.C. Virtual reality-based physical exercise with exergames (PhysEx) improves mental and physical health of institutionalized older adults. *J. Am. Med. Dir. Assoc.* **2017**, *18*, 454.e1–454.e9. [CrossRef] [PubMed]
26. Chen, C.; Jeng, M.; Fung, C.; Doong, J.; Chuang, T. Psychological benefits of virtual reality for patients in rehabilitation therapy. *J. Sport Rehabil.* **2009**, *18*, 258–268. [CrossRef]
27. Plante, T.G.; Aldridge, A.; Su, D.; Bogdan, R.; Belo, M.; Kahn, K. Does virtual reality enhance the management of stress when paired with exercise? An exploratory study. *Int. J. Stress Manag.* **2003**, *10*, 203–216. [CrossRef]
28. Russell, W.D.; Newton, M. Short-term psychological effects of interactive video game technology exercise on mood and attention. *J. Educ. Technol. Soc.* **2008**, *11*, 294–308.
29. Maples-Keller, J.L.; Bunnell, B.E.; Kim, S.J.; Rothbaum, B.O. The use of virtual reality technology in the treatment of anxiety and other psychiatric disorders. *Harv. Rev. Psychiatry* **2017**, *25*, 103–113. [CrossRef] [PubMed]
30. Parsons, T.D.; Rizzo, A.A. Affective outcomes of virtual reality exposure therapy for anxiety and specific phobias: A meta-analysis. *J. Behav. Ther. Exp. Psychiatry* **2008**, *39*, 250–261. [CrossRef] [PubMed]
31. Opriş, D.; Pintea, S.; García-Palacios, A.; Botella, C.; Szamosközi, S.; David, D. Virtual reality exposure therapy in anxiety disorders: A quantitative meta analysis. *Depress. Anxiety* **2012**, *29*, 85–93. [CrossRef] [PubMed]
32. Anderson, P.L.; Price, M.; Edwards, S.M.; Obasaju, M.A.; Schmertz, S.K.; Zimand, E.; Calamaras, M.R. Virtual reality exposure therapy for social anxiety disorder: A randomized controlled trial. *J. Consult. Clin. Psychol.* **2013**, *81*, 751–760. [CrossRef] [PubMed]

33. Hedden, S.L.; Joel, K.; Lipari, R.; Medley, G.; Tice, P. Substance Abuse and Mental Health Services Administration, Results from the 2014 National Survey on Drug Use and Health: Mental Health Findings (NSDUH) 2015. Available online: http://www.samhsa.gov/data/sites/default/files/NSDUH-FRR1-2014/NSDUH-FRR1-2014.pdf (accessed on 20 October 2017).

34. Zeng, N.; Pope, Z.; Gao, Z. Acute effect of virtual reality exercise bike games on college students' physiological and psychological outcomes. *Cyberpsychol. Behav. Soc. Netw.* **2017**, *20*, 453–457. [CrossRef] [PubMed]

35. Rizzo, A.; Difede, J.; Rothbaum, B.O.; Daughtry, J.M.; Reger, G. Virtual reality as a tool for delivering PTSD exposure therapy. In *Post-Traumatic Stress Disorder: Future Directions in Prevention, Diagnosis, and Treatment*; Springer: New York, NY, USA, 2013.

36. Taylor, C.B.; Sallis, J.F.; Needle, R. The relation of physical activity and exercise to mental health. *Public Health Rep.* **1985**, *100*, 195–202. [PubMed]

37. Penedo, F.J.; Dahn, J.R. Exercise and well-being: A review of mental and physical health benefits associated with physical activity. *Curr. Opin. Psychiatry* **2005**, *18*, 189–193. [CrossRef] [PubMed]

38. U.S. Department of Health and Human Services. *2008 Physical Activity Guidelines for Americans*; U.S. Department of Health and Human Services: Washington, DC, USA, 2008.

39. Munafo, J.; Diedrick, M.; Stoffregen, T.A. The virtual reality head-mounted display Oculus Rift induces motion sickness and is sexist in its effects. *Exp. Brain Res.* **2017**, *235*, 889–901. [CrossRef] [PubMed]

40. D'Amour, S.; Bos, J.E.; Keshavarz, B. The efficacy of airflow and seat vibration on reducing visually induced motion sickness. *Exp. Brain Res.* **2017**, *235*, 2811–2820. [CrossRef] [PubMed]

41. Craft, L.L.; Perna, F.M. The benefits of exercise for the clinically depressed. *Prim. Care Companion J. Clin. Psychiatry* **2004**, *6*, 104–111. [CrossRef] [PubMed]

42. Wegner, M.; Helmich, I.; Machado, S.E.; Nardi, A.; Arias-Carrión, O.; Budde, H. Effects of exercise on anxiety and depression disorders: Review of meta-analyses and neurobiological mechanisms. *CNS Neurol. Disord. Drug Targets* **2014**, *13*, 1002–1014. [CrossRef] [PubMed]

43. Proffitt, R.; Lange, B. Considerations in the efficacy and effectiveness of virtual reality interventions for stroke rehabilitation: Moving the field forward. *Phys. Ther.* **2015**, *95*, 441–448. [CrossRef] [PubMed]

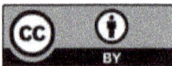

MDPI

St. Alban-Anlage 66

4052 Basel

Switzerland

Tel. +41 61 683 77 34

Fax +41 61 302 89 18

www.mdpi.com

Journal of Clinical Medicine Editorial Office

E-mail: jcm@mdpi.com

www.mdpi.com/journal/jcm

www.ingramcontent.com/pod-product-compliance
Lightning Source LLC
Chambersburg PA
CBHW051858210326
41597CB00033B/5949